Sustainable Development Goals Series

The **Sustainable Development Goals Series** is Springer Nature's inaugural cross-imprint book series that addresses and supports the United Nations' seventeen Sustainable Development Goals. The series fosters comprehensive research focused on these global targets and endeavours to address some of society's greatest grand challenges. The SDGs are inherently multidisciplinary, and they bring people working across different fields together and working towards a common goal. In this spirit, the Sustainable Development Goals series is the first at Springer Nature to publish books under both the Springer and Palgrave Macmillan imprints, bringing the strengths of our imprints together.

The Sustainable Development Goals Series is organized into eighteen subseries: one subseries based around each of the seventeen respective Sustainable Development Goals, and an eighteenth subseries, "Connecting the Goals," which serves as a home for volumes addressing multiple goals or studying the SDGs as a whole. Each subseries is guided by an expert Subseries Advisor with years or decades of experience studying and addressing core components of their respective Goal.

The SDG Series has a remit as broad as the SDGs themselves, and contributions are welcome from scientists, academics, policymakers, and researchers working in fields related to any of the seventeen goals. If you are interested in contributing a monograph or curated volume to the series, please contact the Publishers: Zachary Romano [Springer; zachary.romano@springer.com] and Rachael Ballard [Palgrave Macmillan; rachael.ballard@palgrave.com].

Daniela Kietzmann

Anaesthesia in Remote Hospitals

A Guide for Anaesthesia Providers

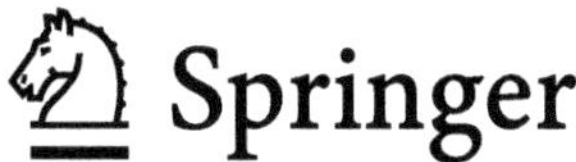

Daniela Kietzmann
Anaesthesia and Intensive Care Department
Uppsala University
Uppsala, Sweden
e-mail: danielakietzmann@yahoo.com

Sustainable Development Goals Series

ISSN 2523-3084 ISSN 2523-3092 (electronic)

ISBN 978-3-031-46612-0 ISBN 978-3-031-46610-6 (eBook)
https://doi.org/10.1007/978-3-031-46610-6

This Springer imprint is published by the registered company Springer Nature Switzerland AG
The registered company address is: Gewerbestrasse 11, 6330 Cham, Switzerland

Paper in this product is recyclable.

This handbook was written for non-specialist anaesthesia providers in remote hospitals with limited resources, especially for nurses, nurse anaesthetists, clinical officers, and general practitioners who are just trained on the job and working without supervision by an anaesthesiologist. They are doing a heroic work in their struggle to provide safe anaesthesia under difficult conditions.

Notices

Anaesthesia like any other speciality in medicine is changing and developing rather quickly due to new research and clinical experience. The author of this book has carefully checked with sources believed to be reliable to provide information that is generally in accord with the standards and guidelines accepted at the time of publication.

Practitioners must rely on their own knowledge, experience, and assessment in evaluating and applying any information, method, or drug described in this book. In view of the possibility of human error or changes in medical sciences, neither the author nor the publisher of this book warrants that the information contained herein is in every respect accurate or complete. To the fullest extent of the law, no responsibility is assumed by the author, the editors, or the publisher for any injury or damage to persons or equipment from any use or operation of any methods, instructions, drug dosage, or ideas contained in the material herein.

Preface

Several million people die each year due to a lack of access to affordable and safe anaesthesia and surgery. Most of the anaesthesia-related deaths are occurring in low- and middle-income countries (LMIC). Many of these deaths could be prevented if some conditions would improve.

Lack of reliable infrastructure: Accessibility to the hospital by all-year roads with public transportation, a continuous supply of clean running water, and reliable electricity. Electrical power cuts mean there is no light for the operation lamp, the suction machine cannot work, and the oxygen concentrator is failing. During anaesthesia induction and surgery, a power cut can quickly lead to a life-threatening complication.

Lack of functioning equipment: Oxygen source, suction machine, anaesthesia machine, vital signs monitor or pulse oximeter, laryngoscope with different sizes of blades, face masks and airways in all sizes, self-inflating bags, and defibrillator, only to mention some of the most important ones.

Lack of uninterrupted supply: Oxygen, essential drugs, and consumables may be out of stock or unavailable.

Lack of professionally trained staff: The urgent need to scale up trained nurse anaesthetists/clinical officers and specialist physicians for anaesthesia and intensive care is recognised by the WHO, but it will take a couple of years to solve that problem. In the meantime, many AP will have to continue working entirely on their own, starting at the preoperative visit, planning, and performing the anaesthesia until the postoperative recovery phase. Since it is possible to provide high quality of safe anaesthesia with affordable drugs and basic equipment, the author would like to encourage all of you who are striving for that aim.

However, this handbook does not replace any anaesthesia textbook. It does not contain regional anaesthesia other than spinal anaesthesia, and it does not refer to anaesthesia for highly specialised surgery. It is a guide for the everyday work of anaesthesia providers in many remote hospitals, whether they are small and offer only surgery for a few different, mostly emergency, indications or whether they are larger hospitals with multiple operation rooms for elective and emergency surgery but lack a continuously present anaesthesiologist.

The head of any anaesthesia department and the medical officer in charge of a hospital may refer to the "International standards for a safe practice of anaesthesia", 2018, by the World Federation of Societies of Anesthesiology and the WHO, free download available.

Remember that team-based work is key for providing safe anaesthesia. Always form a team with your anaesthesia colleague if you have one or with a person who is trained on the job to be your assistant, and with the nurses in the operation room and the doctor who is performing the surgery.

Anaesthesia like any other speciality in medicine is changing and developing rather quickly due to new research and clinical experience. The author of this book has carefully checked with sources believed to be reliable to provide information that is generally in accord with the standards accepted at the time of publication. International guidelines, chapters in appropriate textbooks as well as current reviews are cited in the "Further reading" sections at the end of the chapters. However, in view of the possibility of human error or changes in medical sciences, neither the author nor the publisher of this book warrants that the information contained herein is in every respect accurate or complete, and they disclaim all responsibility for any errors or omissions or for the results obtained from use of the information contained in this work. Readers are encouraged to confirm the information contained herein with other sources. In particular, anaesthesia practitioners are advised to check the product information of each drug they plan to administer to be certain that the information contained in this work is accurate and that changes have not been made in the recommended dose or in the contraindications for administration. This recommendation is of particular importance in connection with new or infrequently used drugs.

The author would like to encourage readers to provide feedback, especially regarding any drugs or anaesthesia methods that they find missing in this book.

Uppsala, Sweden Daniela Kietzmann

2023

Acknowledgements

I am extremely grateful for all colleagues who gave advice, proofread chapters, and sent me their remarks, shared ideas, or provided me with valuable literature. Their commitment was very encouraging for me: Michael Dobson, University of Oxford, UK (anaesthesia equipment); Andrea Maria Kollman Camaiora, University Hospital of Uppsala, Sweden (obstetric anaesthesia); Caroline Larkin, Beaumont Hospital, Ireland (spinal anaesthesia), Judith Pfänder, Matyaso Health Centre, Kigoma, Tanzania (anaesthesia equipment, difficult airway, basic physiology); Oskar Sandqvist, University Hospital of Uppsala and Nurse anaesthetist in the Swedish Army (difficult airway, trauma, and emergencies); Ulrich Spandau, St. Erik's Ophthalmologic Hospital, Stockholm, Sweden (physiology); and Bengt Sporre, University Hospital of Uppsala, Sweden (paediatric anaesthesia); thank you so much.

I would like to express special thanks to Sarah Winter, a graphic and book designer from Hamburg, Germany, for her creative and professional illustrations that perfectly match my ideas. It was a pleasure to work with you, Sarah.

I would like to thank Elizabeth Pope and Anand Shanmugam at Springer Nature who made this handbook *Anaesthesia in Remote Hospitals* possible. Without their initiative and excellent support, this project would not have become reality.

Daniela Kietzmann, Uppsala 2023

Contents

1 Introduction 1
Further Reading 2

2 Basic Physiology for Anaesthesia Providers 3
2.1 Respiratory Physiology and Ventilation During Anaesthesia 3
2.2 Oxygen and Carbon Dioxide Transport 7
2.2.1 Oxygen Transport in the Blood 7
2.2.2 Carbon Dioxide Transport in the Blood 9
2.3 The Heart and Circulation 9
2.3.1 The Heart 9
2.3.2 Systemic Circulation 11
2.3.3 The Arterial Part of the Circulation 11
2.3.4 The Venous Part of the Circulation 12
2.4 Body Water, Fluid Compartments, and the Role of the Kidneys 13
2.5 Body Temperature Regulation 15
Further Reading 16

3 Anaesthesia Equipment and Infrastructure 17
3.1 Electricity 18
3.2 Oxygen Supply 19
3.2.1 How to Assure Continuous Availability of Oxygen . . . 19
3.2.2 Piped Gas Supply 21
3.2.3 Oxygen Cylinders 21
3.2.4 Oxygen Concentrators 22
3.2.5 How to Assure an Adequate, Uninterrupted Supply of Oxygen During Anaesthesia 23
3.3 Anaesthetic Machine 24
3.3.1 Draw-Over System 25
3.3.2 Draw-Over Vaporiser 26
3.3.3 Compressed Gas Machines 27
3.3.4 Breathing Circuit and CO_2 Absorption with Soda Lime 28
3.3.5 Plenum Vaporisers 29
3.3.6 Catheter Mounts, Angle Pieces, Tube Connectors, T-piece System 30

3.4 Patient Monitoring Devices . . . 31
3.4.1 Pulse Oximetry. . . . 31
3.4.2 Non-invasive Blood Pressure Measurement 32
3.4.3 Electrocardiogram (ECG) 32
3.4.4 Capnography (CO_2 Monitoring) 33
3.4.5 Body Temperature Monitoring. . . . 34
3.4.6 Oxygen Concentration Analysers 34
3.5 Airway Equipment 35
3.5.1 Face Masks. . . . 35
3.5.2 Endotracheal Tubes 36
3.5.3 Laryngeal Mask Airways 36
3.5.4 Laryngoscopes 36
3.5.5 Filters and Heat and Moisture Exchangers 37
3.6 Other Equipment 37
3.6.1 TOF Monitors and Other Nerve Stimulators 37
3.6.2 Suction Machine 38
3.6.3 Soda Lime 38
3.6.4 Defibrillator 39
3.7 List of Minimal Equipment for Safe Anaesthesia 39
Further Reading 40

4 Preparing for Anaesthesia 41
4.1 Preoperative Evaluation 41
4.1.1 Anaesthesia Assessment by Preoperative Visit 41
4.1.2 ASA Risk Classification 42
4.1.3 Fasting Before Anaesthesia 43
4.1.4 Patients with Chronic Disease Like Hypertension, Diabetes Mellitus, or COPD 43
4.2 Anaesthesia Working Place, Trolley, Drugs, and Equipment 44
4.2.1 Anaesthesia Machine, Oxygen Source 44
4.2.2 Essential Equipment Per Operating Room 44
4.2.3 Essential Drugs for Anaesthesia Management. . . . 45
4.3 Preparing the Patient in the Operation Room 46
4.3.1 The Anaesthesia Record. . . . 46
4.3.2 Patient Preparation, Venous Access, Monitoring, Preloading with Fluid. . . . 46
4.3.3 Prevention of Wound Infection During and After Surgery. . . . 47
4.4 Positioning on the Operation Table 48
4.4.1 Supine Position Flat, with Head Up or Head Down 48
4.4.2 Lateral Position 48
4.4.3 Prone Position 48
4.4.4 Lithotomy Position 49
4.5 Patient Safety and Checklists 49
Further Reading 50

5 Post-anaesthesia Care 51
5.1 Recovery Area, Equipment 51
5.2 Admission to Recovery Area, ABCDE Assessment, Managing Complications, Discharge 52
5.2.1 Complications in the Early Post-Anaesthesia Phase . . 53
5.3 Postoperative Analgesia 54
5.4 Intermediate or High-Dependency Care Unit 55
5.4.1 Criteria for and Management of Delayed Extubation 56
Further Reading 56

6 Airway Management 57
6.1 General Considerations 57
6.2 Guedel Oropharyngeal Airway (OPA) 58
6.3 Nasopharyngeal Airway (NPA) 59
6.4 Face Mask 59
6.5 Endotracheal Intubation 60
6.5.1 Assessment Before Planned Endotracheal Intubation with Direct Laryngoscopy 60
6.5.2 Preoxygenation 61
6.5.3 The Technique for Endotracheal Intubation 62
6.5.4 Complications of Laryngoscopy/Intubation 64
6.6 Laryngeal Mask Airway (LMA) 65
6.6.1 Size of the LMA 66
6.6.2 Indications 66
6.6.3 Contraindications 66
6.6.4 Practical Considerations and Complications 66
6.7 Difficult Airway Management 67
6.7.1 Intubation with a Gum Elastic Bougie (Eschmann Stylet) 68
6.7.2 Emergency Surgical Airway with Front of Neck Access (FONA) 69
6.8 Rapid Sequence Induction 70
6.8.1 Indications for RSI 70
6.8.2 Procedure 70
Further Reading 71

7 Basic Pharmacology for Anaesthesia Providers 73
7.1 General Considerations 74
7.1.1 Storage of Drugs 74
7.1.2 Drugs for Injection Must Be Kept Sterile 74
7.1.3 Anaesthesia and Hospital Pharmacy 75
7.1.4 Variability of Drug Response and Titrating a Drug to Effect 75
7.1.5 Labelling Syringes 75
7.2 Anaesthetic Drugs 76
7.2.1 Ketamine 76
7.2.2 Thiopentone 76

7.2.3 Propofol 77
7.2.4 Etomidate 78
7.3 Opioid Analgesics 78
7.3.1 Morphine 78
7.3.2 Fentanyl 79
7.3.3 Pethidine 79
7.3.4 Tramadol 80
7.3.5 Codeine 80
7.3.6 Naloxone 80
7.3.7 Pentazocine 81
7.3.8 Buprenorphine 81
7.4 NSAIDs and Other Non-opioid Analgesics 81
7.4.1 Diclofenac 81
7.4.2 Ketorolac 82
7.4.3 Ibuprofen 82
7.4.4 Paracetamol 82
7.4.5 Metamizole 82
7.5 Sedatives 82
7.5.1 Diazepam 83
7.5.2 Midazolam 83
7.5.3 Lorazepam 83
7.5.4 Chlorpromazine 84
7.5.5 Promethazine 84
7.5.6 Clonidine 84
7.6 Muscle Relaxants and Reversal Agents 84
7.6.1 Suxamethonium 85
7.6.2 Pancuronium 86
7.6.3 Vecuronium 86
7.6.4 Atracurium 86
7.6.5 Rocuronium 86
7.6.6 Reversal Agents for MR (NMBA) 87
7.7 Local Anaesthetics 88
7.7.1 Lidocaine 88
7.7.2 Bupivacaine 88
7.8 Cardiovascular Drugs for Increasing Heart Rate and Treating Hypotension During Anaesthesia and Critical Care 89
7.8.1 Adrenaline (Epinephrine) 89
7.8.2 Atropine 89
7.8.3 Ephedrine 90
7.8.4 Noradrenaline (Norepinephrine) 90
7.8.5 Dopamine 90
7.8.6 Phenylephrine 90
7.9 Diuretics and Antihypertensive Drugs During Anaesthesia and Critical Care 91
7.9.1 Furosemide 91
7.9.2 Glyceryl Trinitrate 91
7.9.3 Hydralazine 91
7.9.4 Labetalol 92

7.9.5 Nifedipine 92
7.9.6 Mannitol 92
7.10 Antiemetic Drugs 92
7.10.1 Ondansetrone 93
7.10.2 Metoclopramide 93
7.10.3 Droperidol 93
7.10.4 Promethazine 93
7.11 Antibiotic Prophylaxis 93
7.11.1 Cloxacillin/Flucloxacillin 94
7.11.2 Ampicillin/Amoxicillin 94
7.11.3 Clindamycin 94
7.11.4 Gentamicin 94
7.11.5 Ceftriaxone 95
7.11.6 Cefuroxime 95
7.11.7 Metronidazole 95
7.12 Hormones: Corticoids, Insulin, Oxytocin 95
7.12.1 Hydrocortisone 95
7.12.2 Dexamethasone 96
7.12.3 Insulin 96
7.12.4 Oxytocin 96
7.13 Bronchorelaxation 96
7.13.1 Salbutamol 96
7.13.2 Aminophylline 97
7.14 Pharmacological Treatment of Severe Bleeding 97
7.14.1 Tranexamic Acid (TXA) 97
7.14.2 Aminocaproic Acid 97
7.14.3 FFP 98
Further Reading 98

8 General Anaesthesia for Major Operations 99
8.1 General Principles of Inhalation Anaesthesia 100
8.2 Inhalational Anaesthetic Drugs 101
8.2.1 Halothane 102
8.2.2 Isoflurane 103
8.2.3 Sevoflurane 104
8.2.4 Other Inhalational Agents 104
8.3 Total Intravenous Anaesthesia TIVA 106
8.4 Balanced Anaesthesia 106
Further Reading 107

9 Short General Anaesthesia for Minor Procedures 109
9.1 Indications 110
9.2 Relative Contraindications 110
9.3 Drugs for Short GA 110
9.3.1 Effects 110
9.3.2 Side Effects 111
9.3.3 Doses 111
9.3.4 Short GA Without Available Anaesthesia Staff for Emergency Procedures 111

9.3.5 Duration of Effect 111
9.3.6 Short GA for Patients with Hypertension 112
9.3.7 Short GA for Patients with Respiratory Disease 112
9.3.8 Short GA for Patients with Kidney Disease. 112
9.3.9 Short GA for Patients with Diabetes 112
9.3.10 Table of Doses for Short General Anaesthesia "Short GA". 112

10 Spinal Anaesthesia 115
10.1 General Considerations and Anatomy 115
10.1.1 Indications 116
10.1.2 Contraindications. 116
10.2 Technique. 116
10.3 Local Anaesthetic Drugs for Spinal Anaesthesia. 118
10.3.1 Doses of LA for Spinal Anaesthesia 119
10.3.2 Duration of Effect 119
10.3.3 Pethidine for Spinal Anaesthesia. 119
10.4 Side Effects and Complications of Spinal Anaesthesia 120
10.4.1 Post Dural Puncture Headache. 120
10.4.2 High Spinal 121
10.4.3 Total Spinal Anaesthesia 121
10.4.4 Hypotension and Bradycardia 121
10.4.5 Infection. 122
10.4.6 Spinal or Epidural Haematoma 122
Further Reading 122

11 Obstetric Anaesthesia. 123
11.1 Physiologic Changes During Pregnancy 123
11.2 Anaesthesia for Caesarean Section 124
11.2.1 Spinal Anaesthesia. 125
11.2.2 General Anaesthesia. 125
11.3 Complications of Anaesthesia for Caesarean Section 126
11.4 Anaesthesia in Preeclampsia and Eclampsia 127
11.5 Dilatation and Curettage 129
11.6 Pre- or Postpartum Bleeding, Major Bleeding During Caesarean Section, and Ruptured Ectopic Pregnancy 129
11.7 Neonatal Resuscitation. 131
11.7.1 Equipment 131
11.7.2 Procedure: Temperature, Airway, and Breathing. 131
11.7.3 Chest Compressions and Drugs. 132
Further Reading 133

12 Anaesthesia for Major Abdominal Surgery 135
12.1 General Considerations 135
12.1.1 Body Temperature 137
12.1.2 Spinal Anaesthesia. 137
12.1.3 Balanced Anaesthesia. 137
12.1.4 How to Perform Anaesthesia for Abdominal Surgery if Muscle Relaxants Are Out of Stock 138

12.1.5 Intravenous Induction and Intubation Without Neuromuscular Blocking Agent. 138
12.1.6 Inhalational Induction and Intubation Without Neuromuscular Blocking Agent. 138
12.1.7 Intubation Without Succinylcholine but with a Non-depolarising Muscle Relaxant 139
12.1.8 Postoperative Care 139
12.2 Elective Laparotomy 139
12.3 Emergency Laparotomy 140
12.3.1 Patients with Acute Abdomen: Presentation and Pathophysiology. 140
12.3.2 Common Causes for Acute Abdomen Requiring Urgent Operation 141
12.3.3 Management. 141
12.4 Laparoscopy 142
12.4.1 Anaesthesia Specific Considerations for Laparoscopic Surgery 142
12.4.2 Potential Complications During Laparoscopy 143
12.4.3 Postoperative Considerations. 144
Further Reading 144

13 Anaesthesia for Trauma Surgery 145
13.1 Initial Management 145
13.1.1 Handover 146
13.1.2 Primary Survey (c)ABCDE 146
13.2 Abdominal and Thoracic Trauma. 147
13.2.1 Anaesthesia for Abdominal Trauma. 148
13.2.2 Postoperative Care 148
13.3 Fractures, ORIF, and Amputation 149
13.4 Head Injury with Traumatic Brain Injury (TBI) 149
13.4.1 Prevention of Secondary Brain Injury 150
13.4.2 Anaesthesia for Burr Hole Evacuation of Epidural or Subdural Haematoma 150
13.4.3 Anaesthesia for Craniotomy 151
13.5 Burns 152
Further Reading 154

14 Paediatric Anaesthesia 155
14.1 General Considerations 155
14.2 Physiological Characteristics and Their Implications for Anaesthesia 156
14.2.1 Respiratory System 157
14.2.2 Circulatory System. 158
14.2.3 Kidneys and Liver 158
14.3 Preoperative Assessment and Preparation 158
14.4 Airway Management and Ventilation. 160
14.4.1 General Considerations 160
14.4.2 Sizes of Artificial Airways 162

14.4.3 Appropriate Size of the Laryngeal Mask Airway (LMA) . . . 163
14.4.4 Artificial Ventilation in Children . . . 163
14.4.5 Rapid Sequence Induction . . . 164
14.4.6 Laryngospasm, Bronchospasm, and Post-Extubation Stridor . . . 165
14.5 Perioperative IV Fluid Management and Blood Transfusion . . . 166
14.5.1 Venous Access . . . 166
14.5.2 Fluid Management and Blood Transfusion . . . 168
14.5.3 Blood Transfusion . . . 170
14.6 The Conduct of General Anaesthesia . . . 170
14.6.1 Induction of Anaesthesia for Major Surgery . . . 170
14.6.2 Maintenance of Anaesthesia . . . 173
14.6.3 Inhalational Anaesthesia . . . 173
14.6.4 Recovery from Anaesthesia . . . 175
14.7 Postanaesthesia Care . . . 176
14.7.1 Postoperative Observation . . . 176
14.7.2 Postoperative Analgesia . . . 176
14.8 Pharmacological Characteristics and Their Implications for Anaesthesia in Paediatric Patients . . . 178
14.8.1 General Considerations . . . 178
14.8.2 Dilutions and Doses of Drugs Used During Anaesthesia and Resuscitation . . . 179
14.9 Anaesthesia for Some Typical Procedures . . . 181
14.9.1 Hernia Repair . . . 181
14.9.2 Appendectomy, Intussusception, Ileus . . . 181
14.9.3 Colostomy in Neonates with Imperforate Anus . . . 181
14.9.4 Pyloromyotomy . . . 182
14.9.5 Trauma and Fractures . . . 182
14.9.6 Burns . . . 184
14.9.7 Adenotomy and Tonsillectomy . . . 185
14.9.8 Removal of Foreign Body from the Oesophagus or Airways . . . 187
Further Reading . . . 189

15 Emergencies and Critical Incidents . . . 191
15.1 Assessment, ABCDE Approach . . . 192
15.1.1 Working Systematically by ABCDE Approach . . . 193
15.1.2 The AVPU Method to Assess Level of Consciousness . . . 193
15.1.3 The Glasgow Coma Scale (GCS) . . . 193
15.2 Circulatory Shock . . . 194
15.2.1 Definition, Pathophysiology, and Compensation Mechanisms . . . 194
15.2.2 Hypovolaemic Shock . . . 195
15.2.3 Management . . . 195
15.2.4 Anaphylactic Shock . . . 197

15.3 Circulatory Arrest and Advanced Life Support (ALS). 198
15.3.1 Basic and Advanced Life Support 198
15.3.2 Resuscitating in the Operation Room 199
15.4 Laryngospasm, Bronchospasm, and Pneumothorax 200
15.4.1 Laryngospasm 200
15.4.2 Bronchospasm 201
15.4.3 Pneumothorax 201
15.5 Pulmonary Aspiration of Gastric Contents 201
15.6 Transfusion Reactions 202
15.7 Malignant Hyperthermia 203
15.8 Local Anaesthetic Toxicity. 204
15.8.1 Maximum Doses of LA 204
15.8.2 Early Signs and Management of LA Toxicity 204
15.9 Prolonged and Severe Adverse Effects of Muscle Relaxants 205
15.10 Tetanus. 207
Further Reading 207

16 Case Scenarios. 209
16.1 Case Scenarios for Discussion in Groups 209
16.1.1 Case 1. 209
16.1.2 Case 2. 209
16.1.3 Case 3. 209
16.1.4 Case 4. 210
16.1.5 Case 5. 210
16.1.6 Case 6. 210
16.1.7 Case 7. 210
16.1.8 Case 8. 210
16.2 Points for Discussion and Results of the Case Scenarios 210
16.2.1 Case 1. 210
16.2.2 Case 2. 211
16.2.3 Case 3. 211
16.2.4 Case 4. 212
16.2.5 Case 5. 212
16.2.6 Case 6. 212
16.2.7 Case 7. 213
16.2.8 Case 8. 213

Appendices. 215

Epilogue 219

Index. 221

List of Abbreviations

AC	Air condition
ACLS	Advanced Cardiac Life Support
ALS	Advanced Life Support
AP	Anaesthesia provider
APL valve	Adjustable pressure limiting valve
ASA	American Society of Anesthesiologists
ATLS	Advanced Trauma Life Support
AVS	Automatic voltage stabiliser
BD	Twice daily
BW	Bodyweight
C/S	caesarean section
CNS	Central nervous system
CO	Cardiac output
CO_2	Carbon dioxide
COPD	Chronic obstructive lung (pulmonary) disease
CPAP	Constant positive airway pressure
CPP	Cerebral perfusion pressure
CPR	Cardiopulmonary resuscitation
CRT	Capillary refill time
CSF	Cerebrospinal fluid
CT scan	Computed tomography scan
CTZ	Chemoreceptor trigger zone
CVP	Central venous pressure
D&C	Dilatation and curettage
D5%	Dextrose 5% = glucose 5%
DAP	Diastolic arterial blood pressure
DCR	Damage control resuscitation
DIC	Disseminated intravascular coagulation
DNS	Dextrose 5% in normal saline 0.9%
EACA	Epsilon-amino-caproic acid
ECF	Extracellular fluid
ECG	Electrocardiogram
ENT	Ear, nose and throat surgery
$ETCO_2$	End-tidal carbon dioxide
ETT	Endotracheal tube
FFP	Fresh frozen plasma
FGF	Fresh gas flow

FONA	Front of neck airway
FRC	Functional residual capacity
GA	General anaesthesia
H_2O	Water
Hb	Haemoglobin
HDU	High dependency unit
HES	Hydroxyethyl starch plasma expander
HIC	High-income countries
HME	Heat and moisture exchanger
I/C	In charge
IAP	Intraabdominal pressure
ICF	Intracellular fluid
ICP	Intracranial pressure
ICS	Intercostal space
ICU	Intensive care unit
IM	Intramuscular
IO	Intraosseous
IPPV	Intermittent positive pressure ventilation
ITA	Intubation anaesthesia
IV	Intravenous
kPa	Kilopascal
LA	Local anaesthetic, local anaesthesia
LMA	Laryngeal mask airway
LMIC	Low- and middle-income countries
LV	Left ventricle of the heart
MABL	Maximum allowable blood loss
MAC	Minimum alveolar (or anaesthetic) concentration
MAP	Mean arterial blood pressure
MD	Medical doctor
MH	Malignant hyperthermia
MIS	Minimally invasive surgery (laparoscopy)
MR	Muscle relaxant
MRI	Magnetic resonance imaging
MV	Minute ventilation
N_2O	Nitrous oxide
NA	Not applicable
NGT	Nasogastric tube
NIBP	Non-invasive blood pressure
NICU	Neonatal intensive care unit
NMBA	Neuromuscular blocking agents (muscle relaxants)
No.	Number
NPA	Nasopharyngeal airway
NPO	Non-profit organisation
NS	Normal saline
NSAID	Non-steroidal anti-inflammatory drugs
O/S	Out of stock
O_2	Oxygen
OD	Once daily

OMV	Oxford miniature vaporiser
OPA	Oropharyngeal airway (Guedel airway)
OR	Operation room
ORIF	Open reduction and internal fixation (of fractures)
OSA	Obstructive sleep apnoea
PACU	Post-anaesthesia care unit
PEEP	Positive end-expiratory pressure
PICU	Paediatric intensive care unit
PONV	Postoperative nausea and vomiting
PRBC	Packed red blood cells
RA	Regional anaesthesia
RBC	Red blood cells (erythrocytes)
RL	Ringer's lactate (Hartmann solution)
RR	Respiratory rate
RV	Right ventricle of the heart
SAD	Supraglottic airway device
SAP	Systolic arterial blood pressure
SC	Subcutaneous
SIB	Self-inflating bellows
SPA	Spinal anaesthesia
SPO_2	Saturation of oxygen with pulse oximetry
SVR	Systemic vascular resistance
TBI	Traumatic brain injury
TBV	Total blood volume
TDS	Three times daily
TIVA	Total intravenous anaesthesia
TOF	Train of four—test for residual muscle paralysis
TV	Tidal volume
TXA	Tranexamic acid
UPS	uninterruptible power supply
VS	Vital signs
WBC	White blood cells (leucocytes)
WFSA	World Federation of Societies of Anesthesiologists

1 Introduction

Abstract

This book is a short, comprehensive handbook for non-specialist anaesthesia providers who are working with limited resources and without a specialist anaesthesiologist.

Different methods of general anaesthesia for the most frequently performed types of surgery and for patients of all ages are described with the components of amnesia (no memory), analgesia (no pain), hypnosis (unconsciousness), muscle relaxation (immobile patient), and decreased response to stressful stimuli. For regional anaesthesia, this book only describes intrathecal block with spinal anaesthesia for surgery below the umbilicus.

Drugs for anaesthesia are very strong and may impair vital functions like breathing and circulation markedly. A high level of expertise and basic knowledge of physiology and pharmacology is needed, which is provided in special chapters of this book.

The book is suitable for training at a school of anaesthesia as well as for on-the-job training of anaesthetists. It may also help experienced anaesthetists to update their knowledge, or to learn more about how to solve problems with unavailable equipment or drugs. Since many anaesthesia-related complications are avoidable, update of knowledge can lead to improved outcomes and safer anaesthesia. The book is a contribution to the United Nations 2030 Sustainable Development Goal number 3 of "Good Health and Well-being".

Keywords

Anaesthesia training in LMICs · Anaesthesia in resource-limited settings

Anaesthesia is a state of amnesia (no memory from the onset of anaesthetic effect until some time after recovery), analgesia, hypnosis (sleep, unconsciousness), immobilisation or muscle relaxation, and decreased response to stressful stimuli. These effects can either be achieved with a single anaesthetic drug that is a volatile inhalational agent or with a combination of drugs to produce balanced anaesthesia or total intravenous anaesthesia (TIVA). Alternatively, regional anaesthesia may be suitable where a local anaesthetic drug is applied to block sensory and motor fibres of the nerves which are innervating the part of the body where surgery is to be performed.

Drugs which produce anaesthesia are very strong and can produce severe side effects, especially on circulation and breathing. Basic knowledge of physiology and pharmacology is therefore needed. Additionally, at least some sophisticated technical equipment is essential for safe anaesthesia but not always available in LMIC.

The WHO together with the WFSA (World Federation of Societies of Anaesthesiologists) has defined international standards for a safe practise of Anaesthesia, published in 2018.

Anaesthesia belongs to basic health care but is complex and potentially hazardous. The safe

D. Kietzmann, *Anaesthesia in Remote Hospitals*, Sustainable Development Goals Series,
https://doi.org/10.1007/978-3-031-46610-6_1

provision of anaesthesia requires a high level of expertise and carefulness. Even for smaller hospitals where major operations (especially caesarean section) are performed the WHO highly recommends the presence of an anaesthesiologist at least as regular supervisor. As it will take many years to achieve this goal in most of LMIC, efforts must be made on supporting all anaesthesia providers to perform safe anaesthesia despite all restraints. Each hospital where surgery is performed should aim for reducing avoidable complications by organising CME sessions (continuous medical education), establishing check lists before starting anaesthesia and surgery and by promoting further education of operation theatre staff. This short, comprehensive, and up-to-date handbook for anaesthesia can be used for teaching at the schools of anaesthesia in many countries, and also for informal on-job training of anaesthesia staff in remote hospitals. Learning during supervised patient care and performing anaesthesia, individual reading of basic textbooks and discussions in groups are some of the corner stones for professional anaesthesia training. This book may help experienced anaesthetists to update their knowledge and offers much practical advice for anaesthesia and perioperative care of the most common types of surgery, always making suggestions how to solve problems with unavailable equipment or drugs. It is also useful for anaesthetists from HICs who are going for a mission to a remote place with limited resources. It was written in the spirit of the WFSA (World Federation of Societies of Anaesthesiologists) which aims for uniting anaesthetists around the world to improve patient care and access to safe anaesthesia and perioperative medicine. The book is a little contribution to the United Nations 2030 Sustainable Development Goal of "Good Health and Well-being" by "building sustainable resilient surgical systems".

Further Reading

Check "Update in Anesthesia" and choose from the list. Or choose from "Tutorial of the week". The WFSA is also offering a YouTube channel with very useful short training videos. They can also be found either via the above mentioned website or via https://www.youtube.com/channel/UC4B28Tt4K6hc4tJ239CLS_Q

Gelb AW, Morriss WW et al (2018) World Health Organization – World Federation of Societies of Anaesthesiologists (WHO – WFSA) international standards for a safe practice of anesthesia. Anesth Analg 126:2047–2055

The WFSA is providing regular training material and updates which are freely downloadable via their website: www.wfsahq.org

2 Basic Physiology for Anaesthesia Providers

Abstract

Key concepts of basic physiology for anaesthesia providers: The respiratory tract consists of the upper and lower airways which form together the anatomical dead space, 2 ml/kg BW. The trachea and the bronchi form the bronchial tree with the branches of the bronchi and respiratory bronchioles from where the 300 million alveoli originate. Each breath consists of around one third dead space ventilation and two thirds of alveolar ventilation with gas exchange (CO_2 is removed and oxygen taken up into the lung capillaries).

During general anaesthesia, respiratory drive may be depressed and muscles may be weak so that the patient loses a free airway and stops breathing.

Oxygen is transported in the blood which contains up to 20 ml/100 ml O_2 in the arteries, bound to haemoglobin. The oxygen-haemoglobin dissociation curve, its normal shape, and changes during ventilation and disease are described in this section.

The function of the heart, the systemic, and the pulmonary circulation are described with changes during anaesthesia. Monitoring of circulation during anaesthesia with BP, pulse oximeter, ECG, and CRT is explained.

The role of the kidney in maintaining volume and composition of the body fluids, extracellular fluid space ECF, and intracellular fluid space ICF, is explained including differences between infants and adults.

Body temperature regulation is affected by general and regional anaesthesia. Patients are at risk to drop temperature, and measures must be taken to keep them warm, because hypothermia impairs platelet function and the immune system; and shivering increases oxygen consumption markedly.

Keywords

Basic physiology for anaesthesia providers · Body temperature during anaesthesia · Circulation during anaesthesia · Oxygen transport in the blood · Respiratory physiology during anaesthesia

2.1 Respiratory Physiology and Ventilation During Anaesthesia

The **respiratory tract** consists of the upper and the lower airways.

Upper Airways Nose and paranasal sinuses, nasopharynx, mouth and oropharynx, hypopharynx and larynx. The pharynx can easily collapse during anaesthesia when the muscles are relaxed and the tongue is falling behind, so that breathing

D. Kietzmann, *Anaesthesia in Remote Hospitals*, Sustainable Development Goals Series,
https://doi.org/10.1007/978-3-031-46610-6_2

is insufficient or impossible unless an intervention is performed to keep the airway open (jaw thrust, oropharyngeal airway). The entrance of the larynx, formed by the epiglottis, the arytenoid cartilage and the vocal cords, must be kept open during breathing. Even small amounts of secretions which enter the vocal cords may cause laryngospasm (spastic closure of the vocal cords by reflex) if anaesthesia is not deep. In deep anaesthesia or after muscle relaxation, the vocal cords are open.

Lower Airways Trachea which branches at the carina into the left and right main bronchus and bronchial tree (so called because the bronchi with all their branches are looking like a tree), see Fig. 2.1. In children below 3 years, the right and left bronchus are leaving the trachea at the same angle, while in older children and adults the right bronchus is leaving at a steeper angle. Therefore, if inserted too deep, the ETT will more often reach the right bronchus than the left one. The trachea is about 4 cm short in neonates and 12 cm long in adults. In adults, the carina can move nearly 4 cm with flexion and extension of the neck. This is important in intubated patients where the tube can dislocate after changing patient position (listen with your stethoscope every time after patient position on the operation table has been changed).

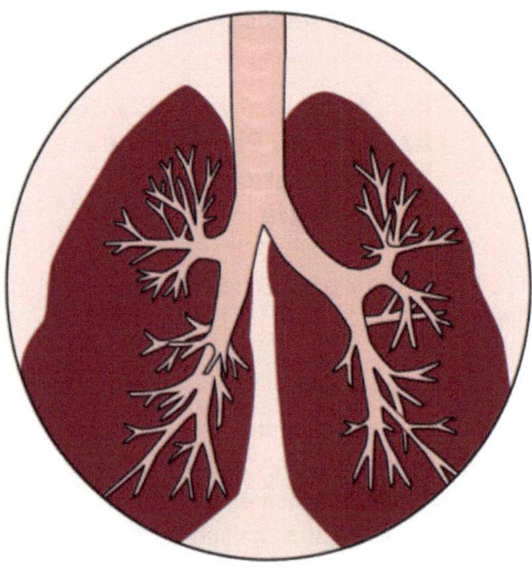

Fig. 2.1 The lungs and the bronchial tree

The upper and lower airways together form the anatomical **dead space**. Dead space is the part of each breath which is just moving in and out of the airways without being involved in gas exchange. *Dead space ventilation* is normally around one-third of the volume of each breath or 2 ml/kg BW. The remaining two-thirds make the *alveolar ventilation*. The function of the dead space ventilation is to humidify the inhaled air which takes place in the airways and reaches 100% humidity in the smallest bronchi. If the trachea is intubated, the upper airways are without function, and the gas mixture which reaches the alveoli might not be completely humid, especially if the patient is not breathing room air but medical oxygen and compressed air which are completely dry. If available, a HME (heat and moisture exchanger filter) should be attached to the endotracheal tube (ETT) or the laryngeal mask (LM) which would help humidifying the inspiratory gas mixture. During longer operations with general anaesthesia, the lower airways may accumulate mucus. If the patient is not coughing effectively during recovery, risk for postoperative pneumonia is significant. Highest incidence of pneumonia is after upper abdominal surgery. Alveolar ventilation means the air which is reaching perfused alveoli where O_2 is exchanged with CO_2.

The **lungs** are consisting of 300 million of **alveoli**, very tiny bubbles at the end of the respiratory bronchioles with a membrane and a net of capillaries surrounding them. All alveoli together are creating a surface area of 70 m^2 in adults for exchange of oxygen and carbon dioxide. Oxygen and carbon dioxide can easily cross the alveolar membrane. A red blood cell needs less than 1 second to move from the venous side to the arterial side through the pulmonary capillary, leaving CO_2 and loading with O_2. The volume in the alveoli is forming the ***total lung capacity*** and is approximately 4–7 L in adults depending on body size and weight.

Please note that with each single breath only about 10% of the lung volume is exchanged. This means, it takes some time to fill the whole lungs with oxygen when a patient is breathing pure oxygen, and it takes several minutes until the onset of effect of an inhalational anaesthetic agent. During exercise, the TV is increasing to a maximum which is called the ***vital capacity*** of the lung which is around 3.5–4.5 L. It is not possible to exhale all air inside the lung. Around 1.2–1.5 L are always remaining and forming the ***residual volume***. Together with the expiratory reserve volume, the residual volume is forming the ***functional residual capacity FRC***. The FRC is the volume which is remaining in the lungs at the end of a normal expiration. It is approximately half of the total lung capacity. The FRC is decreasing in supine position when the lungs are compressed by the weight of the thorax, and it is decreasing further after anaesthesia induction. Abdominal surgery, pregnancy, and all conditions of acute abdominal pathology are further decreasing FRC. The FRC is like a reservoir of oxygen during expiration and even short periods of apnoea. A decrease of FRC means hypoxia will occur more quickly when the patient is not breathing. Before anaesthesia induction, ***pre-oxygenation*** with 80% or with pure oxygen for approximately 3 min is necessary to get the whole lung capacity filled with oxygen and thereby the maximum time of preventing hypoxia during apnoea which may then last as long as 3–5 min without causing dangerous hypoxia. Remember that an oxygen concentrator needs to be switched on at least 5 min before giving oxygen because the machine needs that time for concentrating of oxygen. Immediately after switching it on, only air will leave the outlet of the concentrator, then oxygen concentration will increase gradually. Oxygen from a cylinder or wall outlet is immediately delivered with its concentration of 93–100%.

Ventilation means air movement in and out of the lungs. Spontaneous ventilation means the patient is breathing him/herself using the diaphragm as the major muscle for ventilation and, as some contribution, the intercostal muscles and muscles of the abdominal wall. The diaphragm is innervated by the phrenic nerve which originates from the 4th cervical interspace. Therefore, even during high spinal anaesthesia, usually the patient is still able to breathe with the diaphragm. Manual ventilation means the patient is ventilated via a bag, e.g. a SIB (self-inflating bag) with intermittent positive pressure (IPPV) by the hands of an anaesthesia provider or other health caretaker. Patients who are not breathing sufficiently due to critical illness or the effects of anaesthesia can also be ventilated mechanically with the ventilator of an anaesthesia machine or an intensive care ventilator if ventilation needs to be performed longer and provided that a functioning ventilator is available as well as staff who is trained to use that device. Avoid unnecessary extensions between ETT/LM/facemask and the breathing circuit since these items are increasing dead space. Inspiratory and expiratory tubes of the breathing circuit do not add to the dead space, because a valve is separating inspiratory air from expiratory air so that no rebreathing of inhaled air can happen. For the dead space it does not matter if the breathing tubes of the circuit are very long or rather short. Especially infants are at risk for rebreathing exhaled air if dead space volumes are too large, e.g. too big face mask, big HME filter, extensions to the circuit. Always use the smallest fitting face mask.

Dead space can also increase due to lung pathology, when some of the alveoli are ventilated but not perfused, e.g. after lung embolism (see Fig. 2.2), and even more common, if cardiac output decreases and thereby lung perfusion does not reach to all capillaries of the alveoli. Lung disease, e.g. pneumonia, is often leading to atelectasis formation that is part of the lungs where the alveoli are collapsed and are not ventilated. That means the blood from the venous side is shunted to the arterial side without gas exchange of carbon dioxide with oxygen, see Fig. 2.2.

Tidal Volume (TV) When a patient is ventilated manually or mechanically, it is important to use a tidal volume (the volume of each breath) that is physiological, neither too small (would increase the percentage of dead space ventilation) nor too

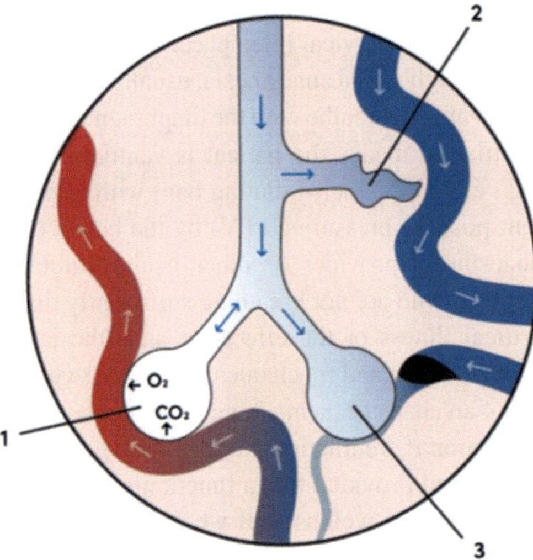

Fig. 2.2 lung alveoli and capillaries; 1 = normal ventilation and perfusion, 2 = no ventilation (atelectasis) with arteriovenous shunt perfusion 3 = dead space ventilation without perfusion (in this example caused by a clot obstructing the capillary)

big (would increase the peak inspiratory pressure in the lung alveoli and may cause lung damage). A thumb rule is not to increase the peak inspiratory pressure > 20 cmH_2O.

Minute ventilation (MV) = respiratory rate (RR) × tidal volume (TV). TV = 7 ml/kg or 6–8 ml/kg. While the TV per kg at rest is the same during all ages the respiratory rate is changing, see Table 2.1 for age-related breathing parameters. It is important to use a proper respiratory rate when ventilating patients. A simple thumb rule for **manual ventilation** is to ventilate an adult as often as you self are breathing and to ventilate a child twice as frequently as you are breathing yourself. It is much more exact, however, to use a clock with second hand or the stopwatch of your mobile phone. One breath each 5 s means a RR of 12/min. The student who is to be trained performing manual ventilation should use a clock to assure the respiratory rate, and he/she should learn how much to squeeze the ventilation bag. Be careful not to overinflate the lungs, especially in children! If anaesthesia machines are used with monitoring of the inspired pressure, this should never exceed 20 cmH_2O, while often

Table 2.1 Normal ventilation parameters related to age

Age	RR per min	TV ml / kg	TV ml
Neonate	40–60	6–8	20–30
<1 year	30–40	6–8	35–70
1–2 year	25–35	6–8	70–100
2–6 year	20–30	6–8	100–200
7–10 year	16–25	6–8	200–300
11–14 year	12–20	6–8	300–400
Adult	10–16	6–8	400–600

RR respiratory rate, *TV* tidal volume that is the volume of each breath

10–15 cm H_2O will be sufficient. If you have capnography, a normal $ETCO_2$ (end-tidal carbon dioxide) should be achieved, that is 35–45 mmHg or 4.5–6.5 kPa.

Mechanical Ventilation with a Ventilator If you are using the ventilator of an anaesthesia machine, you can choose RR and TV according to the following table. If your machine is pressure-controlled instead of volume-controlled then you can only choose the RR and the peak inspiratory pressure and the positive end-expiratory pressure (PEEP). PEEP should normally be 0–5 cm H_2O, while 5 is recommended for all adults and larger children, small children 0–3 cm H_2O. PEEP can be used to keep the lung alveoli a little open at the end of expiration. The higher the peak pressure, the higher will be the tidal volume. Many, but not all, anaesthesia machines have a respirometer or an electronic monitor which would show the expired TV. If that monitor is not available, you will have to rely on observing chest movement (adequate, too little, or too much) and on the peak inspiratory pressure instead.

Anaesthesia Is Affecting Respiration Significantly Lying supine and being anaesthetised is causing a decrease of the functional capacity of the lung, especially in obese patients. Atelectasis of the lungs may occur, which means part of the alveoli remain closed and do not participate in gas exchange. The risk for hypoxia is increased by this problem; patients need often extra oxygen during and after anaesthesia. The respiratory drive is controlled by the respiratory centre in the brain stem. Most anaesthesia drugs are causing respiratory depression. Respiratory drive is depressed, and patients are at risk of hypoventilation with increasing carbon dioxide and decreasing oxygen saturation. Therefore, it is highly recommended to have a reliable source of oxygen available during general anaesthesia and in the recovery period until the patient is fully awake and breathing sufficiently. Means to ventilate the patient must also be available, e.g. a self-inflating ventilation bag and well-fitting face masks.

While most hypnotic drugs (ketamine less than all others) depress the respiratory drive, muscle relaxants weaken the respiratory muscles. Long-acting muscle relaxants like pancuronium may cause insufficient breathing and difficulties to keep the airway patent even after the end of surgery. Narcotic drugs like fentanyl, pethidine, morphine cause respiratory depression if given in higher dose or combined with sedating drugs like diazepam. Therefore, patients should be monitored carefully even for some time after surgery.

2.2 Oxygen and Carbon Dioxide Transport

2.2.1 Oxygen Transport in the Blood

Air is containing 20.9% oxygen. Oxygen enters the lungs via inspiration and crosses the alveolar membrane thereby entering the capillaries and then the arterioles. At the same time, CO_2 is leaving the blood by crossing the alveolar membrane and then being exhaled.

Only 2% of the oxygen in arterial blood is simply dissolved gas, 98% are immediately after diffusion from alveoli into the capillary taken up into the red blood cell by diffusion and bound to haemoglobin. Haemoglobin increases the capacity of the blood to transport oxygen by nearly 50 times compared to simply dissolve oxygen. Anaemia is decreasing the amount of O_2 in the blood significantly and below 7 g/dl critically. People with anaemia can hardly exercise as the consumption of O_2 is increasing with exercise but not enough O_2 can be delivered at low levels of Hb.

Each molecule of Hb can bind 4 molecules of oxygen. Each gram of Hb can bind 1.34 ml of oxygen. With Hb of 15 g/dl, arterial blood can carry 20 ml of oxygen per 100 ml if Hb is fully saturated with O_2 that is if SaO_2, the oxygen saturation in the arterial blood, is almost 100%, while venous blood is containing about 15 ml of oxygen, with an oxygen saturation of 75% in venous blood at average.

Note that the oxygen-haemoglobin dissociation curve is not linear, see Fig. 2.3. That is very important for the body: The oxygen tension (partial pressure), that is the amount of dissolved oxygen in the blood, decreases while the blood is moving from the lung capillaries to the tissues, but the saturation of oxygen, that is the oxygen bound to Hb is changing differently: at first there is only little change in oxygen saturation, meaning that the total amount of oxygen in the blood is

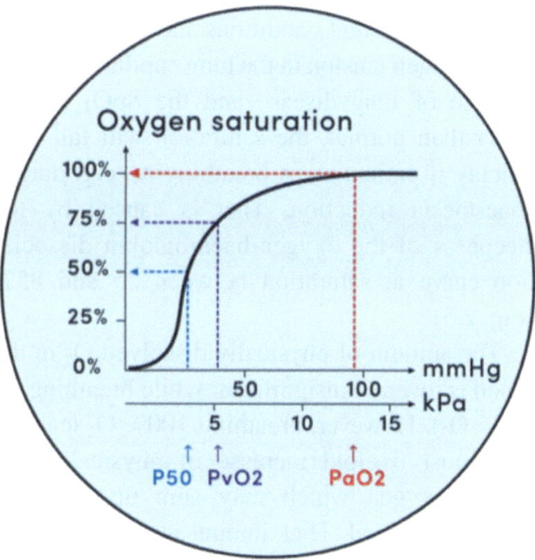

Fig. 2.3 Oxygen-haemoglobin dissociation curve. It describes the relationship between oxygen saturation of the haemoglobin and the amount of dissolved oxygen in the blood, measured as the partial pressure of oxygen (PO_2 in mmHg or kPa, where 1 kPa is equal to 7.5 mmHg). P_{50} = 27 mmHg = 3.6 kPa and means the partial pressure at which the saturation is 50%. P_vO_2 means the partial pressure in venous blood; P_aO_2 means the partial pressure in arterial blood which is around 100 mmHg or 12.5-13.5 kPa

roughly the same (changing only between 90 and 100% SaO_2) whether the oxygen tension is very different with 60 mmHg (8 kPa), 100 or 500 mmHg (13 resp. 66 kPa), 100 mmHg (13 kPa) being the O_2 tension in the lung capillaries while breathing ambient air, 500 mmHg (66 kPa) being the maximum while breathing 100% oxygen. During mild to moderate lung disease when less oxygen can cross the alveolar membranes and enter the arterial blood, it is lifesaving that a relatively low oxygen tension (partial pressure) in the blood is still combined with a relatively high saturation of >85%. That allows patient not to die from hypoxia unless the severity of the disease leads to respiratory failure with markedly too low oxygen amount in the arterial blood. In the capillaries of the tissues, on the other hand, a lot of oxygen is to be delivered; and there the oxygen saturation falls more rapidly so that the required amount of O_2 can be delivered since the affinity of haemoglobin to oxygen is decreasing and releasing oxygen from the binding sites in the red blood cells. In the venous blood the remaining saturation is around 75% but may differ from 60 to 80% in different conditions and disease states. If the oxygen tension in the lung capillaries is low because of lung disease and the SpO_2 is also lower than normal, the saturation will fall very quickly if patient stops breathing as, e.g. during anaesthesia induction. That is caused by the steepness of the oxygen-haemoglobin dissociation curve at saturation between 25 and 85% (Fig. 2.3).

The amount of physically dissolved O_2 in the blood is low and insignificant while breathing air (21% O_2). However, breathing 100% O_2 leads to an almost fivefold increase of physically dissolved oxygen which may sum up to 1.5–2 ml/100 ml blood. That amount is approximately equivalent to the oxygen which can be bound to Hb in the red blood cells of one unite transfused blood! Therefore, in severe haemorrhage, it is very important and effective to administer pure oxygen until the bleeding is stopped, the circulation is stabilised, and the Hb is acceptable. The oxygen stores in the body (in haemoglobin, in myoglobin in the skeletal muscles, and in the lungs) are only equal to the oxygen consumption during few minutes (5–6 min at rest provided patient is not suffering from fever). Thereafter, tissues would develop hypoxia. *During anaesthesia and recovery, it is highly recommended to provide at least 30–40% oxygen (or 1–2 l/min added to room air) to the patients to have a safety margin.*

It is highly recommended to use a pulse oximeter during every anaesthesia, even short GA, sedation, and spinal anaesthesia, since it is very difficult and unreliable to assess the oxygenation of patients clinically. Cyanosis (bluish colour of the skin) may be a sign of low oxygen saturation. Cyanosis may be visible at saturation <85%, that is too late. Oxygen saturation below 94% is already regarded as a limit of intervention. However, cyanosis is only visible if skin colour is not very dark and provided the patient is not suffering from severe anaemia. Cyanosis is not correlating well with SpO_2. Fingers which are cold may look bluish although saturation is good. The pulse oximeter estimates the oxygen saturation and the pulse rate independent of the level of Hb and skin colour. The saturation, SpO_2, means the percentage of binding sites of the haemoglobin molecules which are occupied by oxygen. Normally, over 96% of Hb is saturated with O_2 at sea level. When arterial blood reaches the capillaries, each Hb molecule is delivering one O_2 molecule (in conditions of increased oxygen demand and in the capillaries of the coronary circulation of the heart even 2 or 3 molecules) to the tissues. In the venous blood, oxygen saturation S_vO_2 is around 75% and can be measured with a blood gas analysis if such a machine is available in the laboratory and if such information is important (mainly in intensive care).

While the normal oxygen saturation of arterial blood can increase only slightly, from 96% while breathing air to 100% when breathing pure oxygen, the amount of physically dissolved oxygen in the blood can rise markedly, nearly five times and may sum up to 1.5 or 2 ml O_2 per 100 ml of arterial blood. The total amount of oxygen (bound to Hb and physically dissolved) which can be carried in 100 ml arterial blood is around 20 ml.

The oxygen saturation depends even on geographic location since the barometer pressure and thereby the amount of oxygen in the air is highest at sea level and several times lower at high altitude. Around 100 million people worldwide are living at altitudes above 2500 m where the air is "thin", and SPO_2 <95%. In the cities of Cusco (Peru), La Paz (Bolivia), or Quito (capital of Ecuador), people hardly have more than 90% SPO_2, and that means little margin in case of hypoxia. But even in the highlands of Ethiopia or in Addis Ababa, the oxygen saturation of normal people is only around 94%. The same applies for Darjeeling, India, and countries like Bhutan, Nepal, or Tibet where altitude is high above sea level. Tourists who are climbing high mountains in South America, the Himalaya, or East Africa can suffer from dangerous altitude sickness due to the extreme exercise and unavoidable hypoxia. On top of Mt. Kilimanjaro, Tanzania, SPO_2 is only 75–85%. People who are living permanently at high altitude get adapted, but they are at higher risk of hypoxia during anaesthesia and critical illness, and they are dependent on higher Hb concentrations than lowlanders. A functioning oxygen source is very important in all hospitals, even the smallest and especially the most remote ones.

2.2.2 Carbon Dioxide Transport in the Blood

While normally only 2% of O_2 in the blood are transported as dissolved gas, the remaining 98% needing to be bound to haemoglobin, a much greater portion of CO_2 can be dissolved in the blood. The remaining is transformed in the red blood cells: In the erythrocytes, CO_2 is metabolised to bicarbonate by the enzyme carboanhydrase according to the reaction $CO_2 + H_2O = H_2CO_3^- = H^+ + HCO_3^-$. In the lungs, this reaction is the other way round and CO_2 is exhaled after crossing the alveolar capillary membrane. Venous blood is slightly acidic compared to arterial blood because it contains more CO_2. Hypoventilation (e.g. due to respiratory depression during or after anaesthesia) would let the CO_2 level rise. As CO_2 increases the amount of acid, respiratory acidosis would develop with decreased blood pH. Clinically, such a rise in CO_2 could cause cardiac dysrhythmia, pulmonary vasoconstriction, peripheral vasodilatation, and elevated intracranial pressure.

The kidneys are playing a major role in keeping the balance of H^+ and HCO_3^- since they can excrete H^+ and reabsorb HCO_3^- thereby keeping the blood pH normal and preventing from acidosis or alkalosis. This renal adaptation takes some time and would not help in acute situations but is important in patients with chronic lung disease and hypercapnia (elevated $PaCO_2$, e.g. in COPD patients).

2.3 The Heart and Circulation

2.3.1 The Heart

The heart is a muscle pump which consists of four chambers: RA (right atrium), RV (right ventricle), LA (left atrium), and LV (left ventricle).

RV and LV are pumping the same amount of blood, the cardiac output, through the lungs (right heart) and the body (left heart), see Fig. 2.4.

The lungs are the only organs in the body besides the heart itself which are perfused by the whole cardiac output of around 5 L/min at rest for the average adult.

The heart as a muscle gets its blood supply from the left and the right coronary artery which originate from the ascending aorta. The venous blood from the coronary circulation enters the RA at the coronary sinus. Coronary artery disease is a pathologic condition where the oxygen demand of the heart is higher than the oxygen delivery so that parts of the heart muscle are prone to suffer from ischaemia. This can be caused by stenotic areas in one or more coronary arteries or branches of the arteries preventing blood flow to be sufficient especially during exercise. Or it can be caused by a situation with too low blood pressure when the blood flow in the coronary arteries can be insufficient and leading to myocardial ischaemia.

With each single heartbeat, a so-called stroke volume (SV) is ejected by the right and left ventricle. In adults, it is approximately 70 ml at rest

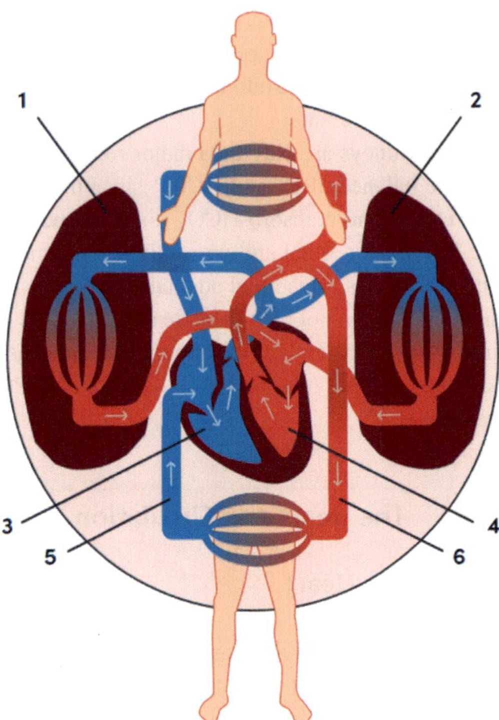

Fig. 2.4 Pulmonary and systemic blood circulation. 1 = right lung, 2 = left lung, 3 = right ventricle of the heart, 4 = left ventricle of the heart, 5 = vena cava, 6 = aorta

and can increase by 40–50% in the untrained healthy person. SV times HR (heart rate) equals cardiac output (CO) . If SV = 70 ml and HR 72/min, CO = 5 l/min (more precisely 5.040 L/min).

During exercise, the HR can be increased more than twice, and stroke volume with 50% to make a CO of about 25 L/min in the very well-trained athlete and 15 L/min in normal adults. The CO cannot be measured directly and monitored during anaesthesia (unless with advanced monitoring which may be available in large teaching hospitals and at centres for cardiac surgery). However, it is very important to assess the function of the heart during anaesthesia because anaesthetic drugs can affect the heart negatively. Blood loss or dehydration can more likely lead to circulatory failure in the anaesthetised patient. Fluid losses in the circulation would lead to smaller SV which would be compensated by higher HR and vasoconstriction. The SV is dependent on filling of the venous circulation and the strength of the heart as a muscle that is so-called contractility of the heart. If blood volume in the veins is lower, stroke volume will also decrease. Blood pressure might still be normal due to vasoconstriction while the CO is decreased. The combination of fluid losses and effects of anaesthesia drugs (vasodilatation and decreased contractility of the heart caused by propofol, thiopentone, halothane, isoflurane, or sevoflurane) can quickly lead to decompensation while ketamine is safer. Patients with risk factors for congestive heart failure or any other heart disease as well as patients older than 65 years are particularly at risk. Very small infants, especially neonates, are also prone to negative effects of anaesthetics to the heart.

The performance of the heart can be assessed by heart and pulse frequency that is listening to the heart sounds with the stethoscope and feeling the peripheral pulse, measuring the blood pressure, and checking the capillary refill time. The heart rate is normally the same as the pulse rate but in case of arrhythmia or atrial fibrillation the pulse is irregular, and pulse rate will be lower than heart rate because the left ventricle will not be filled properly when the irregular heart rate is fast and filling time for the chambers of the heart is too short. Thereby no pulse wave will occur after heart beats which are too weak.

It is recommended to monitor not only the pulse rate with a pulse oximeter or by feeling the pulse but simultaneously the heart rate with ECG monitor or precordial stethoscope.

The blood pressure needs to be measured frequently, at least every 5 min since it can change markedly and very quickly during anaesthesia and surgery.

The capillary refill time, CRT, is a useful and simple additional tool to assess circulation and cardiac output. It is performed by pressing the tip of the thumb so that it is blanching. Sudden release will lead to capillary refill as indicated by returning normal colour. Use the stop-watch function of your mobile phone to measure the CRT exactly. It is normally <2 s. In old patients, it is longer, around 3 seconds. Limitations of the method: If fingers are cold, CRT can falsely be prolonged although cardiac output might be normal. Instead of a thumb, other parts of the skin, e.g. on the chest or the forehead may be chosen to press until blanching, and then be released to stop the time until normal skin colour is back.

A heart rate below 60/min is called bradycardia while a heart rate above 100/min is tachycardia. Irregular heart rate is called arrhythmia. Heart rate may vary between 40 and 180/min in otherwise healthy young people. In the elderly, tachycardia, especially above 150/min may be associated with cardiac ischaemia since oxygen consumption of the heart muscle increases with increased HR and might become greater than the amount of oxygen which can be delivered to the heart by the coronary arteries. In young children, the stroke volume of the left ventricle can hardly increase. Therefore, infants are dependent on a sufficient heart rate to maintain cardiac output. A HR below 60–80 can be critical in small babies and needs action to be taken. Atropine is first choice drug to increase heart rate, and in severe cases, small doses of adrenaline are needed. During pregnancy, the CO is increased, and the pregnant mother needs a heart rate of >60. Atropine is first choice to increase heart rate during caesarean section.

2.3.2 Systemic Circulation

The heart pumps the blood through all tissues of the body. Thereby it is delivering oxygen, glucose, and all other nutrients to the tissues which were absorbed from the guts and metabolised in the liver. At the same time, it is removing carbon dioxide which is then exhaled from the lungs and other waste products which are metabolised by the liver or excreted by the kidneys or the faeces.

Only 15% of the circulating blood volume is within the arteries, 85% in the venous system.

The veins act as a reservoir for blood. Increased venous tone by contraction of veins is increasing the venous return that is the amount of blood per time which is filling the right heart. From the right ventricle, the blood flows through the pulmonary artery through the low-pressure vessels of the pulmonary circulation of the lungs. The pulmonary veins then collect the oxygen-enriched blood from the lung alveoli which is flowing to the left heart. Only in the left ventricle high pressure is generated which equals systolic blood pressure during contraction. During relaxation of the left ventricle (diastole) the pressure is decreasing markedly to <15 mmHg while in the aorta and all arteries the diastolic blood pressure is much higher than in the heart due to the systemic peripheral resistance. This pressure is necessary to let the blood quickly reach all peripheral parts of the body. The velocity of the pulse wave is about 20 cm/s.

It takes about 30–45 s for the blood in a forearm vein to move via the right heart, the lungs, and the left heart to the brain. Therefore, it takes at least 30 s until a patient falls asleep during IV induction of anaesthesia. For patients with low cardiac output, it takes longer to become unconscious.

Side effects on circulation as seen by drop of blood pressure or lengthening of CRT may occur already before the patient is sleeping since the anaesthetic reaches the heart and arterial blood vessels before achieving an effective concentration in the brain.

2.3.3 The Arterial Part of the Circulation

The smallest vessels of the arterial side of circulation are the arterioles just before the capillaries. The arterioles are mainly responsible for creating an adequate systemic vascular resistance which can suddenly be increased when needed, for example as compensation for acute blood loss. By contracting or dilating, the arterioles are controlling the amount of blood flow to the organs like liver, kidney, guts, muscles, skin, and so on depending on the metabolic demands of the tissues. During acute blood loss, the blood flow is mainly directed to the vital organs like brain and heart while the rest of the body is receiving less blood flow and in situation of severe blood loss might suffer from ischaemia and acidosis. The reduced renal blood flow in situation of circulatory shock can cause acute kidney failure. A shock cannot only be caused by bleeding but also by fluid losses, e.g. acute abdominal disease with bowel obstruction. Those patients are also prone to acute renal failure.

The peak blood pressure is the systolic arterial blood pressure, SAP, normally between 100 and 140 mmHg. It is caused by the contraction of the left ventricle. The lowest blood pressure in arteries is the diastolic arterial blood pressure, DAP, normally between 60 and 85 mmHg and mainly caused by systemic peripheral resistance of the arterial blood vessels. MAP, or mean arterial blood pressure, is in between SAP and DAP. It is approximately 1/3 higher than DAP plus the difference between SAP and DAP. A BP of 140/80 mmHg would result in a MAP = 80 + (140–80)/3 = 80 + 60/3 = 80 + 20 = 100 mmHg. A BP of 90/60 mmHg would result in a MAP of 60 + (90–60)/3 = 70 mmHg, still sufficient to maintain blood flow to the body. BP 80/50 mmHg is borderline with a MAP of 60 mm Hg. With a MAP of <60 mmHg, sufficient blood flow to all organs is often not possible. 70/40 in adults would mean a MAP of only 50 mmHg and needs urgent action to be taken by the health care provider.

The MAP is the most important of the BP measurements since it gives the best information about organ blood flow (together with CRT). Automatic BP machines are displaying the results of SAP, DAP, and MAP. If you have automatic BP monitor during anaesthesia, then you should also record the MAP by small lines on the anaesthesia record together with SAP and DAP.

A MAP of >60 mmHg is regarded as sufficient during anaesthesia while a MAP of 50 mmHg is the minimally required BP to maintain sufficient blood flow through heart, brain, or kidneys in otherwise healthy young people. In older or hypertensive people, MAP needs to be higher, at least 70 mmHg, and systolic BP should be at least 90–100 mmHg to keep adequate blood flow to vital organs.

2.3.4 The Venous Part of the Circulation

In the veins, the blood flow is directed towards the heart while arteries are carrying blood away from the heart. The venous pressure is much lower than arterial blood pressure, normally between 0–10 mmHg while the central venous pressure in the vena cava superior and inferior and in the right atrium is 2–12 mmHg. Deoxygenated, CO_2 enriched blood is transported from the tissues to the right heart and from the right ventricle through the pulmonary arteries into the lungs. In the lungs, the situation is opposite compared to the systemic circulation. The pulmonary arteries are carrying deoxygenated blood away from the heart. The pressure in the pulmonary arteries is only around 25/15 mmHg, much lower than in the systemic circulation. Pulmonary hypertension is a pathology which may lead to right heart failure. It is often caused by chronic lung disease as COPD. The pulmonary veins are carrying oxygenated blood to the left heart from where it is pumped to the aorta and the body. In the liver, the situation is also special since there are two capillary beds. One is from the portal vein carrying deoxygenated, but nutrient-rich blood from the guts towards the liver for metabolism. From the second capillary bed in the liver, the blood is collected in the inferior vena cava and flowing towards the right heart.

The foetus is receiving venous blood from the mother's placenta with oxygen saturation around 75%. The foetus is adapted to that situation with a special kind of foetal haemoglobin which does bind oxygen easier than the maternal blood so that the oxygen saturation in the foetal arterial blood is nearly 90%.

The veins have one-way valves every few centimetres which are necessary because of the low pressure in the venous system. Otherwise, the blood would flow back again instead of moving into one direction only and may cause varices to develop.

Venous return is the amount of blood flowing in the venous system to the right heart. During anaesthesia, high speed of intravenous infusion is increasing venous return. Mechanical or manual ventilation with high pressure is increasing intrathoracic pressure and decreasing venous return. Therefore, unnecessary high ventilation pressure must be avoided. If you are using a sophisticated anaesthesia machine with a ventilator, avoid high PEEP (positive end-expiratory pressure). For most patients, a PEEP of just 5 cm H_2O is sufficient and is not causing decreased venous return. The effect of decreased venous return is decrease in cardiac output. If CO is decreasing markedly, arterial BP will also drop. Patients in the intensive care unit who are suffering from severe lung disease sometimes need high PEEP around 10 cm H_2O for sufficient and lung-protective ventilation. Because decreased venous return leads to decreased CO, they often need continuous drugs like adrenaline or noradrenaline to keep a sufficient CO and maintain BP.

Veins can easily be compressed. The possibility of compression of the inferior vena cava is of paramount importance during caesarean section when the mother is placed supine. The uterus can compress the inferior vena cava which leads to sudden and marked drop of cardiac output and may lead to life-threatening circulatory collapse. This vena cava compression syndrome can easily be prevented by a slight left lateral tilt of the operation table or putting a pillow under the right pelvis of the mother until the baby is delivered. A very big intra-abdominal mass like a large ovarian cyst can also lead to vena cava compression.

While the peripheral venous pressure is never measured, the central venous pressure (CVP) can be measured by using a central venous catheter and a special device connected to it. Usually, this is only performed in the ICU but central venous pressure can be estimated by observing the filling of the visible veins on the hand or the neck. When slowly elevating the head or the hand above the heart, the disappearing vein would indicate how high in cm H_2O the central venous pressure is. Normal CVP is 2–12 mmHg (3–16 cm H_2O).

Raised CVP can be a sign of right heart failure. It may be caused, e.g. by hypervolaemia (caused by over-infusion or renal failure) or lung embolism.

2.4 Body Water, Fluid Compartments, and the Role of the Kidneys

In adults, about 60% of the body mass is water. The body fluids are distributed between the different compartments, making up the intravascular (blood / plasma), the extracellular and the intracellular fluid compartment (ECF and ICF).

ECF in adults is normally around 20–25% of BW. In children, it is more; at birth nearly half the BW is fluid in the ECF (40–50%). Normal blood volume in adults is 70 ml/kg BW that means around 5 L in a 70 kg average adult. Small children have 80 ml/kg BW that means a term neonate of 3 kg has around 0.25 L total blood volume. A 70 kg adult has around 42 L total body water which is divided between the extracellular and the intracellular fluid (ECF and ICF). The ICF is with 28 L about two-thirds of the total body fluid compartment while the ECF has 14 L. The ECF is consisting of the plasma volume and the interstitial space that is the small space surrounding all cells and tissues. Water and electrolytes pass freely between blood vessels and interstitial space while larger molecules like proteins (albumin and other proteins) cannot pass freely unless there is a damage of capillaries. The volumes and the composition of the ECF and ICF are well balanced and regulated with the kidneys playing a major role. Not only the volume of fluid but also its composition needs to be maintained. The number of dissolved ions (like Na^+ and K^+, Cl^-, Ca^{++}, Mg^{++}, HCO_3^- or bicarbonate, and some others) and molecules (like glucose or creatinine, plasma proteins, or urea) per litre ((osmolarity) is kept constant = isotonic. That keeps the cells at the same size. Hyperosmolarity lets the cells shrink, while hypoosmolarity lets them expand, and if it is extreme, the cells would disrupt. Osmolarity depends partly on the amount of salt in the body. Infusion of dextrose without saline in huge amounts would decrease osmolarity and should be avoided. One of the normal post-operative infusion schedules is to give dextrose and Ringer's lactate alternatingly. If available, you can also administer dextrose 5% with normal saline (DNS) or any other type of infusion with some dextrose and some sodium chloride and potassium. Normally the ECR, including plasma, contains around 135–145 mmol/L Na^+ and 3.5–5.0 mmol/L K^+. Ringer's lactate (which is also called Hartmann solution) is containing approximately the same concentration of ions than plasma while normal saline (NS) is not physiological with higher sodium and Cl^- of 154 mmol/L each which is much more chloride than in plasma where Cl^- is only around 110 mmol/L.

Whenever Ringer's lactate, Ringer's acetate, Plasmalyte, or any other type of full electrolyte infusion is available this should be preferred perioperatively for fluid replacement as advantageous over NS or Dextrose (Glucose). Dextrose/Glucose 5% is not suitable as IV fluid to restore blood volume in case of haemorrhage or in conditions of extended vomiting, diarrhoea, or acute bowel obstruction since it contains only water and glucose, no salt.

The kidneys normally produce 1.5 L urine per day. Dependent on the amount of fluid intake and losses for example by sweating, the urine volume may vary between 0.5 L as the minimum and up to more than 3 L per 24 h. With less than 500 ml urine per 24 h (or <0.5 ml/kg/h in children), it is impossible to excrete enough waste products.

The kidneys are also keeping the concentrations of K^+ and Na^+ in the body normal by excreting more or less of them. They help to keep the blood pH normal by excreting more acidic urine in case of alkalosis or more alkaline urine in case of acidosis.

Kidney failure can lead to hyperkalaemia which may also be caused by acidosis or ischaemia in any part of the body and by severe muscle trauma.

K^+ >6.5 mmol/L may cause severe dysrhythmias and finally cardiac arrest which is hardly corresponding to resuscitation efforts.

Hypokalaemia <3.0, caused by diuretics or by insufficient intake of potassium over longer periods, is also leading to potentially life-threatening arrhythmia, may even lead to ventricular fibrillation which may be responding to resuscitation with defibrillation if K^+ concentrations in plasma are restored by infusion.

However, in many remote hospitals, it is not possible to measure concentrations of electrolytes in the blood, and there is often no fluid available with higher concentrations of K^+ to be infused. However, all vegetables and fruits are containing potassium. Patients who can feed orally or via gastric tube may receive vegetables or fruits to restore potassium. When vegetables are cooked, the fluid is containing a lot of K^+. Even that fluid can be useful to replace kalium losses.

IV fluid replacement during haemorrhage: it is good to know that crystalloid infusions, that is NS, RL (Ringer's Lactate), or other electrolyte infusions, are distributed in the blood vessels and in the interstitial space (in the whole ECF). Only around one-third of the IV fluids will stay in the blood vessels. One L of bleeding would need 3 L of RL for volume replacement.

Plasma expander, e.g. HAES (hydroxyethylstarch) or albumin 5% would replace a blood loss of the same volume. Albumin 20% (200 mg/ml) is a real plasma expander since it draws fluid from the interstitial space into the blood volume. 100 ml of albumin 20% would replace blood loss of almost 500 ml.

Fluid intake is around 30 ml/kg BW per day for adults and approximately double as much for children. Extraordinary losses, especially during surgery, must be replaced. Fever increases fluid loss through the skin, per degree of increased body temperature 500 ml/day. In a very hot environment, sweating leads to increased fluid requirements, around 1 L per day at temperatures above 30 °C and even more during exercise.

If the urine output per 24 h is less than 1 L and is looking concentrated, the patient needs more fluids by mouth or IV. On the other hand, fluid overload must be avoided, since too much IV fluids may lead to lung and peripheral oedema.

Fluid balance is difficult to obtain in patients with acute kidney failure (AKF) . If patients are anuric (less than 100 ml urine or no urine output per day) or oliguric (less than 500 ml urine per day, resp. <0.5 ml/kg/h in children), and in all severely ill patients, or after major abdominal surgery, careful monitoring of fluid intake and output on observation charts is vital. Losses from diarrhoea, sweating, vomiting, and so on need to be replaced. The best way to be sure about fluid balance is to check patient's body weight daily. Losses mean too little fluid intake and weight gain from one day to another means too much fluid intake. One litre of water is nearly equivalent too 1 kg weight.

2.5 Body Temperature Regulation

Body temperature is normally kept constant between 36.5 and 37.5 °C independent of ambient temperature. The temperature control centre is located in the hypothalamic area of the brain. Sweating and vasodilatation of the blood vessels in the skin are the mechanisms by which body temperature is not rising in a hot environment. Shivering and vasoconstriction of blood vessels in the skin are generating heat in a cold environment. These mechanisms are not well established in small infants who cannot shiver and are particularly prone to get cold at cold ambient temperature.

During anaesthesia, general anaesthesia as well as spinal anaesthesia, temperature control does not work. Patients are very quickly getting cold in operating theatre, especially if air condition is used and the temperature of the operating room is kept low.

Body temperature might drop to 33 °C which is dangerous. Have warming blankets for the patients and cover them as much as possible. Convince the surgeon of keeping room temperature >22 °C for adults and >25 °C for infants. Make efforts to have thermometers in each room to monitor patients' body temperature. Surgeons can easier be convinced by telling numbers (the actual body temperature of the patient).

Low body temperature is not only unpleasant when the patient is shivering during recovery or feeling cold during spinal anaesthesia, but it is even harmful. Blood is clotting less because the function of the thrombocytes is decreased by hypothermia. The immune system is also depressed by low body temperature, so that the risk for post-operative infection is increased. Patients with heart disease are at risk for cardiac failure or myocardial ischaemia during shivering. The effect of muscle relaxants may be prolonged.

Patients are also at high risk to drop temperature during anaesthesia and surgery when IV fluids are administered quickly at room temperature. It is much better to warm the infusions to a temperature of approximately 37 °C (hand-warm), e.g. by putting infusion bottles into hot water before administration. Make sure that they are not getting too hot!

Small children have a larger body surface area compared to adults and cool down more quickly. Very old patients are also prone to drop temperature more quickly and markedly.

During spinal anaesthesia, at least the patient's thorax, arms, and head should be covered with blankets. Highest losses of temperature occur during extended abdominal surgery. If patients are getting cold <35 °C, they should not be extubated immediately after surgery but kept sedated and be warmed until regained 36 °C.

Usually, body temperature during surgery does not fall below 33–34 °C in adults, but infants may get even colder if no measures are taken to avoid that.

It is recommended to monitor body temperature continuously during all major procedures. Many vital signs monitors are equipped with a temperature probe. You can insert the probe into the oesophagus in intubated patients under GA, otherwise the probe may simply be put under the shoulders in supine position or under the chest in prone position. The skin temperature is not so much lower than the core temperature and gives a good measure for changes of temperature. If such temperature probe is unavailable, get a simple fever thermometer from the store and have it in place on the anaesthesia trolley. It should be used for every patient if anaesthesia is longer than 1 hour. Of course, the probe or the thermometer must be disinfected between patients.

Keeping patients warm can be challenging. The ordinary theatre gowns and towels are insufficient, thicker blankets are needed, also in the waiting area before surgery and in the recovery area after surgery. Forced air warmers or heated mattresses are very nice but expensive. Simple blankets are inexpensive but must be washed regularly, and the theatre management team must agree from the hygienic point of view that they may be used.

Further Reading

Chambers D, Huang C, Matthews G (2019) Basic physiology for anaesthetists, 2nd edn. Cambridge University Press, Cambridge

3 Anaesthesia Equipment and Infrastructure

Abstract

Electricity: Health facilities where major surgery is performed should have a main source of electricity plus a backup source like a well-maintained generator.

Oxygen: Safe anaesthesia is nearly impossible without the continuous availability of oxygen. A major source of oxygen plus a backup source is mandatory. Small, remote health facilities may use oxygen concentrators which are "producing" oxygen from ambient air but need uninterrupted power, plus a number of filled cylinders. Larger hospitals may have their own oxygen plant with pipelines to major theatre, maternity, ICU, and emergency department plus a backup system like a cylinder manifold to bridge malfunction of the plant or long-lasting power cuts.

Anaesthesia machine: The more remote a health facility, the simpler the anaesthesia machine should be (non-rebreathing circuit open to room air); and it should be easy to maintain by local technicians with support by the distributor or the manufacturer (e.g. WhatsApp hotline where advice and instruction to repair a non-functioning machine is provided).

Vital signs monitor: Pulse oximeter, stethoscope, and BP machine are mandatory where anaesthesia is performed. ECG and capnography are adding a lot to patient safety during GA.

Suction machine: That device is mandatory even if only short GA without tracheal intubation is performed, as anaesthetised patients are at risk for aspiration of secretions.

Airway equipment: Face masks and oropharyngeal airways are minimum standard. A functioning laryngoscope (with spare batteries stocked), ETT all sizes, stylets and bougies for difficult intubation, and laryngeal masks are highly recommended for district and larger hospitals.

Keywords

Airway equipment for low-resource anaesthesia · Draw-over anaesthesia system · Minimum equipment for safe anaesthesia · Oxygen concentrators for anaesthetic machines · Pulse oximetry during anaesthesia

A hospital cannot be operating well in a place where basic infrastructure is missing. Roads which are trafficable all year round, ambulance cars and public transportation, e.g. by buses, are necessary for patients to reach the hospital in due time. Transportation on the backseat of a bicycle or a motorcycle is often practiced but can be dangerous and is very unpleasant for a sick or injured person. The hospital needs clean water, ideally running water from public pipelines. Large rainwater tanks may serve as a backup. It is very difficult to keep proper cleanliness without sufficient water. Electricity is getting more and more

D. Kietzmann, *Anaesthesia in Remote Hospitals*, Sustainable Development Goals Series,
https://doi.org/10.1007/978-3-031-46610-6_3

important, not only for light, but modern medicine is impossible without equipment which needs electricity. The hospital needs to have a reserve backup system for electricity in case the public or private main source of electricity fails. Operation theatres should be air-conditioned (if possible) for hygienic purpose and keeping a nearly dust-free environment, however, AC (air condition) needs a lot of electrical power. It is not impossible, but difficult to provide safe anaesthesia without electricity, especially if the only oxygen source is from a concentrator which needs power. Many anaesthesia machines are not running without electricity. Vital signs monitors, rechargeable pulse oximeters need power, and electrical suction machines are much stronger than manual suction devices. Surgeons need electrocautery (diathermy) for many major operations, and without a bright operation lamp, it is very difficult to perform surgery. All technical equipment needs to be maintained and serviced, either by a biomedical engineer or electrician with special skills on medical equipment, or at least the more basic tasks of maintenance of anaesthesia equipment, by the anaesthesia staff.

In remote places, it can be challenging to get equipment maintained since expert medical technicians and engineers may be lacking. However, it is always the responsibility of the anaesthetist to ensure all equipment being used is working without fault. In that case, I recommend that the anaesthetist has good communication with the most skilled electrician at the place and with the hospital administration for getting spare parts and having equipment repaired or replaced if necessary.

3.1 Electricity

Without stable, reliable electricity it is difficult to provide safe anaesthesia. Even small hospitals should make effort to have a power backup system, e.g. a well-maintained generator which is available 24 h a day 7 days a week. An increasing number of equipment needs electricity including even the computers of the administration office. For every operation, a good lamp is vital which needs electrical supply. It is quite unpleasant to operate in the light of a mobile phone although such way of working has saved many lives, e.g. during caesarean section when better light sources were not available. In theatres with frequent power failures, the surgeon would be well advised having a battery-driven forehead torch. During major surgery, an electrical suction machine is needed which is also important for anaesthesia staff, as we must be able to apply suction to the airways or the stomach. For many types of surgery, additional electrical equipment is used such as diathermy, patient vital signs monitor, anaesthesia machine with ventilator, and others. A bronchoscope/oesophagoscope for removing of foreign bodies is used with an electrical light source. There are many other examples, and most readers will have experienced difficulties with operating during electrical power failure (the author too).

New equipment: Ideally, a thorough device instruction for the users should be performed by the distributor. Ask for it if your equipment is bought from a store in your own country. After unpacking, check the power which the machine needs. It is not the same around the world. The power needed may be either 110 V at a frequency of 60 Hz or 230 V at a frequency of 50 Hz. The correct voltage and frequency of the alternating current (AC mains electricity) is mandatory for the machine to work. Whenever equipment is delivered by donation from abroad, ask in advance about the electricity required. If it is not the same as in your country, refuse to get that equipment since it is only producing costs for getting it transported, stored, cleared at the customs, and it will be completely useless. Even locally purchased equipment, although usually fitting for your type of mains AC, may be delivered with the wrong plug. There are many different plugs and sockets, unfortunately. Each continent has got at least one different, not compatible system, Europe has two. The African continent is so large that it has more than three different types of sockets and plugs. You may need to buy the local plug and ask an electrician to exchange the original plug with a local one if the plug is not fitting into your sockets. That does not do any harm to the equipment and is not expensive.

The voltage of the mains electricity should not be fluctuating too much. While a range of 220–240 V is okay for most machines, larger fluctuations would cause a shorter life span. Frequent power cuts can also damage sensitive electrical, especially electronic, equipment. In such environments, it is highly recommended to buy a *voltage stabiliser* (AVS) together with every new machine or even a UPS (uninterruptible power supply) device which has a battery for bridging power cuts. The extra costs make the equipment still cheaper since its life span will be much longer, and your patients will be treated much safer if you can rely on working equipment.

In very remote places where the power supply by public electricity companies is very unreliable or absent, it is on the long run better for the environment and cheaper to have a private electrical power plant, e.g. with solar power (or hydro power if a downhill running river with water during the whole year is located near the hospital for installation) for the whole hospital or at least for critical areas like operating theatre, maternity, neonatal care unit, emergency department, ICU/HDU or sick patients room, resp., and administration office.

3.2 Oxygen Supply

Oxygen is by far the most important "medicine" within anaesthesia and critical care. Unfortunately, the provision of continuous supply of oxygen is not easy and is rather expensive. Atmospheric air consists of 20.9% oxygen (O_2), 78% nitrogen, and 1% of argon and other inert gases. Many patients during and after surgery or with critical illness need higher concentrations of oxygen than in ambient air. Medical oxygen is available in two qualities: oxygen100 consists of 99.5–100% oxygen. Oxygen93 consists of 90–96% O_2, 4% argon, and a small rest of nitrogen. Oxygen93 is sufficient for medical use and much cheaper than medical oxygen.

There are three types of oxygen supply for hospitals: ***Piped oxygen*** from wall outlets (produced at the hospital's own oxygen plant or obtained as liquid oxygen), free standing or attached-to-anaesthesia-machines ***cylinders***, and small ***oxygen concentrators***. In many places, the cylinders are the property of the hospital which can make maintenance difficult. They need to be sent to far-away places for filling, and it is vital to have a sufficient supply of spare cylinders. The filling is usually expensive. This system can only work if the filling plant is not too far (not more than about 200 km), and the source of O_2 can be reached via all year-round trafficable roads. A piped gas supply is expensive to set up and needs a permanent technician/engineer to run and maintain it; but if well working, it is the best choice for larger hospitals. Power failure or any fault would stop the system and may lead to lack of oxygen in the whole hospital unless there is a good backup system (e.g. reservoirs and enough filled cylinders plus some small concentrators).

In remote places, small ***oxygen concentrators*** will usually be the best alternative. A concentrator is not so expensive, is obtainable in many countries, and its running costs are only for electricity. However, maintenance must be performed regularly to keep it working.

3.2.1 How to Assure Continuous Availability of Oxygen

Dependent on the size of the health facility, the amount of oxygen needed per day/month, and the geographic location nearby or far away from a city with a large oxygen plant and reliable cylinder filling station, the hospital needs to decide about the type of oxygen source and the backup. Additionally, a plan should be made for disaster or pandemic with markedly increased oxygen demand for the catchment area.

A smaller health facility with maximum two operation rooms and a maternity plus small neonatal unit and an intermediate care room for maximum 2–3 patients would need some oxygen concentrators for each of these places. At least one new oxygen concentrator in the main hospital store would be wonderful as spare. The best way is to buy only oxygen concentrators of the same brand with a detailed and comprehensive maintenance instruction manual and available spare parts. Avoid buying in an urgent need situation what you get instead of choosing what you want. Consider AVS for each concentrator to make them longer lasting especially if your electrical power is not so reliable and voltage fluctuations are common. All tools for corrective

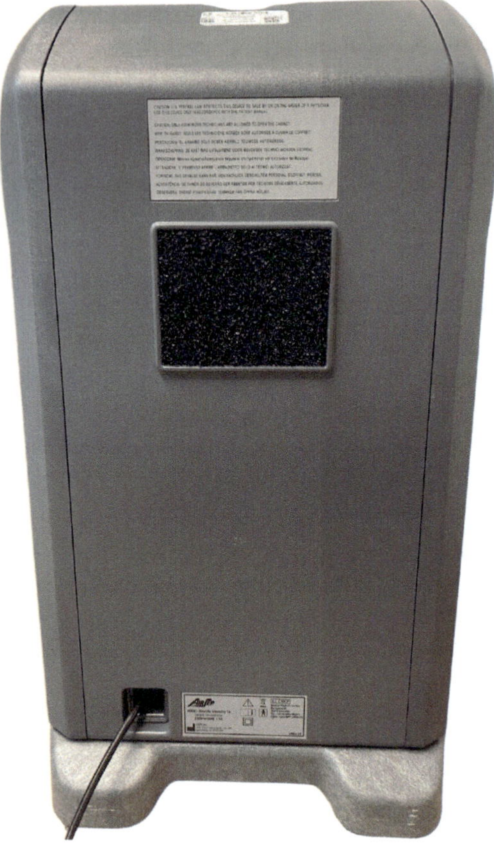

Fig. 3.1 The rear of an oxygen concentrator showing the gross particle filter which needs to be washed regularly (by hand in warm water with little soap, then put it back). From Diamedica (UK) Ltd. with permission

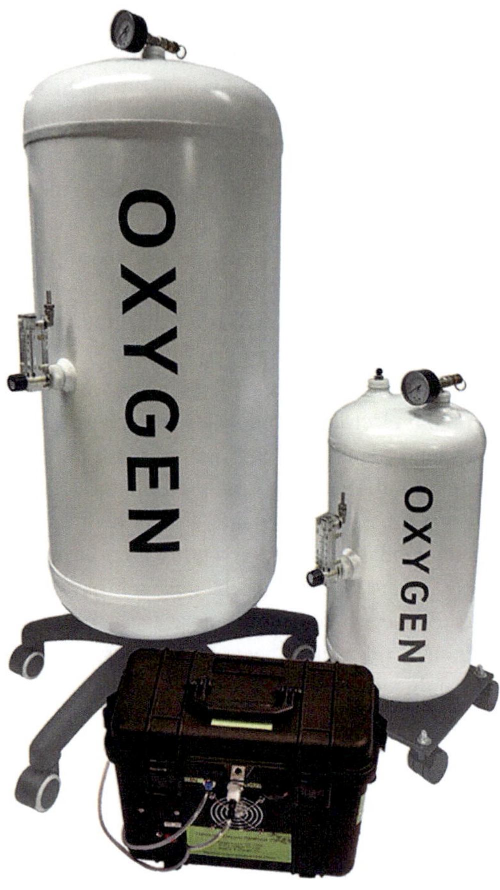

Fig. 3.2 Oxygen reservoir and compressor to be filled from a small oxygen concentrator at the local health facility. (From Diamedica (UK) Ltd, with permission)

maintenance and all spare parts should be stocked in quantities which are matching the number of concentrators. Donated equipment is often lacking instruction manual and contact to the distributor or manufacturer. Do not hesitate to ask the benefactor to provide you with spare parts and maintenance instruction. If these are not obtainable, do not assume that equipment to be very long-lasting. Aim for having a technician/engineer who is trained at maintaining oxygen concentrators since this requires some special skills and also special tools. If not possible, get a reliable contact to someone who is available to visit your place and perform maintenance. The users should be trained at doing the most important and easy-to-perform preventive maintenance that is cleaning the gross particle dust filter (Fig. 3.1) and to check the performance of the machine.

Identify a responsible person for that task and have a book-keeping list where the performed maintenance is recorded.

As a backup for the concentrators, especially during power failure, either cylinders or reservoirs can be used. It is much cheaper and makes the facility independent, if you have a technician/electrician who is able/trained to fill reservoirs with 5 bar oxygen from the concentrators to be stored to bridge power failures. Diamedica (UK) Ltd. is specialised for equipment for remote places worldwide and does provide such easy-to-use reservoir systems for small oxygen concentrators, see Fig. 3.2.

Large hospitals with more than three operation rooms plus intensive care unit, emergency unit and so on, may aim for a large Oxygen 93 concentrator unit which serves as the hospital's oxygen plant for a system with a pipeline distribution. Such a concentrator needs two well-trained persons (always one of them on-call) plus a well-kept store of all spare parts and tools and a maintenance protocol. As backup a cylinder manifold with a capacity to bridge several days of oxygen requirements for the whole hospital should be available and always kept filled (from the same concentrator unit). Even in such a facility, it may be very useful to have some small oxygen concentrators well maintained as reserve and for situations of disaster or pandemic with a much higher demand of oxygen than usual.

3.2.2 Piped Gas Supply

Piped gas supply is a system where oxygen, compressed air, and vacuum are delivered from a central supply with a strong compressor/oxygen concentrator and a storage system at high pressure. The oxygen may be produced on site. Alternatively, the oxygen is not produced at the hospital but delivered from elsewhere as a supply to a cylinder manifold at a special place on the hospital compound. Such a system is delivering oxygen continuously via copper pipelines and labelled wall outlet sockets. Anaesthesia machines with hoses with the correct matching probes can be connected to the wall outlets. Alternatively, a flow meter with a fitting connector for the wall outlet can be used from which the patient may receive oxygen via mask or nasal prongs. For larger hospitals with several operating rooms and intermediate or intensive care units, it may be the most reliable, and in terms of running costs, even the cheapest source of oxygen. Good communication is vital so that any interruption of the central oxygen supply will be reported to all units in the hospital which are dependent on oxygen.

3.2.3 Oxygen Cylinders

A recommended video for training is available about how to use oxygen cylinders safely (by the WHO): https://www.who.int/teams/health-product-policy-and-standards/assistive-and-medical-technology/medical-devices/management-use/trainings#.

Always make sure that the cylinder is closed properly when not used immediately to avoid leakage which is one of the most common problems with cylinders. A cylinder may become empty without having been used for any patient. Cylinders must be labelled to avoid mismatch; e.g. nitrous oxide or carbon dioxide instead of oxygen would kill the patient. Unfortunately, the colour code may vary in different countries. Often, oxygen has a white colour on top of the cylinder and may be white on the whole cylinder. In the United Kingdom, oxygen cylinders have a black body and a white shoulder. A series of pins which are fitting to the right place on the yoke of the anaesthetic machine are called the pin-index system which shall ensure the right cylinder is mounted. These pins must never be removed! In many countries, it is very expensive to get oxygen cylinders refilled, and their capacity is limited. Small hospitals with less than 10 major operations per week and without ICU can be using cylinders only, provided the filling plant is not too far away and logistics are sufficient. For larger hospitals with piped oxygen or small concentrators in operating theatre and some in the wards, cylinders should be the backup in case of failure of the primary oxygen source. Oxygen is stored at high pressure in the cylinder, usually 130 times atmospheric pressure (130 bar). That means, a full cylinder contains 130 times its volume. A pressure reducing valve needs to be mounted on top of the cylinder. The valve should be opened slowly when connected to the anaesthesia machine. Oxygen is highly flammable, and the high pressure inside the cylinders may cause hazards, in worst case explosion, if not handled carefully. Oxygen cylinders should be stored in dry, well-ventilated, and fire-proof rooms where temperature is not getting hot. They have a pressure release device which would reduce the pressure inside if it gets too high. Corrosion would produce leakage of the cylinder. Cylinders need a holder; they should not be just free standing to avoid hazards when they would fall.

Before using a cylinder, open the valve and check how much pressure is left. Never forget to close the valve after use. Be sure the cylinder is containing enough oxygen before you start an operation. The smallest cylinders, CD, have an internal volume of 2 L and contain 260 L at 130 bar/atm or 400 L at 200 bar. If a patient is receiving 3 L/min, the cylinder would be empty in less than one and a half hour if filled at 130 bar or within 3 h if filled at 200 bar. A full medium size E cylinder is containing 680 L at a pressure of 130 bar and would last for maximum 5 h if 5 L/min are administered shortly during anaesthesia induction and 2 L/min for maintenance. The cylinder would reach for only four patients with 1 h of general anaesthesia each. There is no warning alarm when the cylinder is getting empty.

The bulky size J cylinder contains around 6500 L oxygen at 130 bar. While this large cylinder may reach more than 1 week in an operating theatre with less than 3 h of GA per day, it would run empty within only 24 h in the ICU if a patient would need 5 L/min oxygen which is not very much in critically ill patients. This means, cylinders are quite impractical if oxygen is needed regularly. The smaller sizes are easier to transport but have poor capacity while the larger ones are bulky and not easy to transport to and from the filling plant.

3.2.4 Oxygen Concentrators

A recommended video for training is available for the use and maintenance of concentrators (by the WHO): https://www.who.int/teams/health-product-policy-and-standards/assistive-and-medical-technology/medical-devices/management-use/trainings#.

Or use (e.g. via Google) the website "WHO Trainings World Health Organization on medical equipment, choose trainings for medical devices", scroll down to the video you like to see, e.g. on preventive or corrective maintenance of concentrators.

Concentrators are by far the cheapest source of oxygen, but they need uninterrupted electrical power for operation and cannot store the oxygen they deliver (have reservoirs with oxygen or cylinders as a backup for electrical power cuts always stocked and ready to use). They also need regular preventive maintenance, without which they may stop working already within several months or, at best, a few years, while well-maintained they can be very long-lasting.

How they work: They produce oxygen by a pressure swing adsorption process. Two columns with zeolite are working alternatingly. Zeolite is a material which is capable of adsorbing nitrogen and water vapour from room air and releasing 95% oxygen to the patient.

The absorbed nitrogen then needs to be released back to the room which takes little time. Therefore, the two columns have a fixed time cycle. One is active while the other is releasing, then the other way round. The typical sound of a well working concentrator should be known by anaesthesia providers so to recognise if operation is not normal. Usually, alternating green lights somewhere at the back of the concentrator, maybe hidden by the dust filter, would indicate normal performance while a red light is a warning sign and means the concentrator cannot be used but needs maintenance/repair (for details check the instruction manual of your device which may be downloadable if not available as hardcopy).

Oxygen concentrators may last for 20,000 running hours but are sensitive to voltage fluctuations which may kill the electronic board inside. A voltage stabiliser is not expensive and should be obtained together with the concentrator and be permanently connected to it. Overvoltage is likely to overheat the compressor within the concentrator and can let it be damaged. Even low voltage can overheat the machine since the cooling fan in the machine wouldn't work properly at low voltage.

Spare parts may be difficult or impossible to obtain. The mainstay of maintenance is cleanliness since the concentrator is drawing ambient air together with dust particles inside and then separating oxygen from nitrogen. In dusty surroundings, the machine would be covered with dust inside which on the long run lets the compressor fail. Therefore, dust filters are vital, and they need to be cleaned regularly or exchanged as soon as they are looking dusty. While filters inside the machine need to be replaced at intervals (once per year if not stated differently), the outer filter sponge can be washed manually just with water and a little soap. In dusty environments, this needs to be done daily, otherwise weekly depending on how the dust filter is looking. If dust is entering the device, the concentrator will sooner or later break down. This basic maintenance of cleaning the dust filter should of course be performed by all anaesthesia staffs. There is no need to call a technician for that.

3.2.5 How to Assure an Adequate, Uninterrupted Supply of Oxygen During Anaesthesia

Before starting anaesthesia, check if your oxygen supply is working. In case of central gas supply check, the connection between the wall outlet and the anaesthesia machine and check if the flowmeters are working and delivering adequate fresh gas flow. Cylinders must have appropriate filling as indicated by the pressure gauge. Concentrators must be switched on, check if the sound is normal, and if the yellow light is switching off after some minutes, indicating that the O_2 concentration is >80%. Check if the rotameter bobbins in the flowmeters are moving properly.

There are three independent monitor systems existing which assure O_2 supply: Pulse oximeters which are monitoring the patients, oxygen analysers which monitor the oxygen concentration in the fresh gas of the anaesthesia machine or in the inspiratory patient limb, and oxygen supply failure alarm at the wall outlet for oxygen or in the oxygen concentrator. At least one of them should be available at all places where anaesthesia is performed, and the pulse oximeter is the most important of them, although the pulse oximeter is not measuring the oxygen concentration of the inspiratory gas, but it is assessing the patient's oxygenation state, which is the most important. If the patient's oxygen saturation does not rise although you administer what is supposed to be pure oxygen, you should assume low concentration in your oxygen device unless you find a reason for it in the patient.

The patient monitor should have a pulse oximeter, or in other words, a pulse oximeter is the most important monitor of the patient additionally to the AP as a "walking monitor" who would observe the colour of the lips, the tongue, or the nails.

While in some countries, e.g. in the United Kingdom and Sweden, an oxygen failure alarm of the oxygen delivering system is mandatory (a sound like a whistle which is unique and loud as soon as the oxygen pressure falls below a threshold value), this alarm may be absent in other countries. That is a potential danger since oxygen failure of the central delivery system would be recognised late. In the United Kingdom, anaesthesia machines open to atmospheric air in case of oxygen failure. The same is true for Gradian Universal anaesthesia machine series, a brand from the United States. Unfortunately, anaesthesia machines which are manufactured elsewhere (e.g. in Germany, India, or China) usually do not open to room air, so that in case of oxygen failure, the patient would re-breathe the exhaled air again and again without getting fresh gas. The exhaled air contains around 4% less oxygen than the inhaled air. Breathing 35% oxygen means approximately 31% of oxygen are exhaled. After one more breath concentration would fall to 27% and so on if no fresh oxygen would be added to the breathing circuit. Breathing 35% oxygen, when fresh gas flow supply is suddenly failing, would mean, after 9 times rebreathing that is within a minute, the exhaled air would not contain any oxygen. The patient might then die from hypoxia.

Many anaesthesia machines do have an oxygen analyser which is measuring the oxygen concentration of the inspired and expired gas (mandatory in most European countries). These O_2 analysers can increase patient safety but are expensive, and the oxygen sensor is often only lasting 1 year after which it needs to be replaced. In many countries, these exchange sensors are unavailable. The monitoring of the inspiratory oxygen concentration is fundamental and mandatory when using low flow anaesthesia with a re-breathing circuit because of high risk of delivering a hypoxic gas mixture (that is a gas mixture containing less oxygen than room air with its 21%). If you don't have a working oxygen analyser in your machine, you must not use low fresh gas flow. A fresh gas flow of at least 3 L/min may be regarded as safe in connection with the use of a pulse oximeter when using a re-breathing circuit and provided you have fresh soda lime for CO_2 absorption. If soda lime is out of stock, and your anaesthesia machine is not open to room air but has a re-breathing circuit, the fresh gas flow must be at least 5 L/min for adults to assure that the patient is not inhaling the CO_2 again. High fresh gas flow makes inhalational anaesthesia very expensive because a lot of inhalational anaesthetic is wasted. When using a draw-over anaesthesia device, there is no risk for hypoxic gas mixture, and an oxygen analyser is not mandatory since the concentration of oxygen in draw-over systems can never fall below that of room air. However, some patients really need high concentrations of oxygen, and it is always necessary to know if your oxygen source is working properly or not. Only with the help of an oxygen analyser you can be sure about the oxygen concentration. If oxygen analyser is not available, be aware if patient's oxygen saturation at the pulse oximeter reading is increasing when administering oxygen. If not, suspicion is needed to the quality of the "oxygen". Oxygen concentrators may be non-functioning in a way that gas is leaving them but at a lower oxygen concentration, sometimes only 21% as in air.

3.3 Anaesthetic Machine

Not all health facilities would need an anaesthesia machine which is only necessary for inhalational anaesthesia or for ventilating patients mechanically. At smaller hospitals where not more than approximately 100 major operations are performed per year and of which most cases are caesarean section or inguinal hernia, anaesthesia is usually performed as spinal anaesthesia or with ketamine. In those cases, you need a self-inflating bag and face masks for emergencies, may be a laryngoscope and ETT, but an anaesthesia machine is not mandatory. In bigger hospitals with up to 100 intubation anaesthesias per year, an anaesthesia machine is needed, but a simple model with manual and spontaneous ventilation would do. A device with a mechanical ventilator is almost double the price than without and is needed in referral hospitals or other hospitals with higher case load. On the other hand, even if not needed that often, a mechanical ventilator can be lifesaving in a situation with severe circulatory shock, e.g. due to ruptured ectopic pregnancy or complication during caesarean section which can happen even in a small health centre. With the ventilator connected to the intubated patient, the AP has the hands free and is more likely to be able to stabilise the patient. That means, if your health facility can afford, it is nice to have an anaesthesia machine with ventilator even if not needed daily. The machine will be more reliable if it can be used even in case of electricity or oxygen failure and in the absence of carbon dioxide absorber. Be familiar with your device and perform daily test procedures to keep it ready for use.

Inhalation anaesthesia needs a sophisticated device or machine. The anaesthetic machine can deliver gases and vapours in exact concentrations. Oxygen, compressed air, or nitrous oxide is delivered as gas, and dosage is via flowmeters. Halothane, isoflurane, sevoflurane, or other inhalation anaesthetics are liquids which are administered via calibrated vaporisers. Nitrous oxide is a gas delivered from cylinders by calibrated flow meters in the anaesthesia machine. Additionally, the anaesthetic device is consisting of pressure reducing valves, and one-way valves for separating inspiratory and expiratory limbs. The latter are consisting of corrugated tubing. A reservoir bag and a ventilation bellows are inserted in the breathing circuits. The corrugated tubes, reservoir bag, and the ventilating bellows are available in different sizes for adults and infants. Anaesthesia machines can be very complicated, expensive, and requiring regular preventive and sophisticated maintenance, or they can be rather simple, affordable hand-ventilation draw over apparatus. Note that for the patient it does not matter from which machine he/she gets the anaesthetic. Quality of anaesthesia is made by the anaesthesia provider administering the proper anaesthetic with proper doses which can be achieved with any functioning anaesthesia delivering system.

It is very important to understand the anaesthesia system before using it since the various types are different, and critical incidences may be caused by errors in handling them.

Follow the instruction of the manufacturer on how to perform the daily set-up test before starting anaesthesia. Instruction manuals are usually online available, and for some brands, videos can be watched online.

If no instruction manual is available, perform at least the following quick test: Connect the machine to the mains electricity and switch it on. Check if flow meters are operating and delivering fresh gas up to their indicated maximum flow. Inspect your oxygen source if it is working (cylinder filled, wall outlet functioning, or concentrator operating). Check the vaporiser. Is it filled? Is it easy to move the lever? Connect a reservoir bag as a test lung to the patient outlet and perform a few breaths manually. Is the test lung inflated and emptied accordingly? If not, something seriously is wrong, and you must not connect the device to a patient but perform troubleshooting. If the device has a mechanical ventilator, test if it is working with the test lung connected. Test the disconnection alarm. If the device has a soda lime canister, check when it was changed last time. All these tests can be performed within no more than a minute and should never be omitted.

The main difference of anaesthesia machines is between open and closed breathing systems. Draw-over anaesthesia systems are open to the environment both in the inspiratory and the expiratory part of the breathing system. Compressed gas machines can be used in different ways: The inspiratory tubing is not open to room air while the expiratory part of the breathing system can be open to the environment without allowing rebreathing of exhaled gas mixture or it can be a semi-closed circuit where patients are rebreathing exhaled gas mixture. In the latter case, it is vital to have a functioning, regularly refilled CO_2 absorber (usually filled with soda lime). Otherwise, the patient would rebreathe the CO_2, and within short time CO_2 in the blood would increase to dangerous concentrations. Of same importance is uninterrupted, reliable supply of oxygen, because the oxygen content in the exhaled gas mixture is lower and after several turns of rebreathing there would not be any oxygen left, the patient would die from hypoxia. The risk for hazards is higher with lower fresh gas flows, or in other words: The lower the fresh gas flow, the higher the risk of accumulating CO_2 and inhaling hypoxic gas mixtures.

3.3.1 Draw-Over System

In a draw-over anaesthesia system, the vaporiser is located within the breathing circuit so that room air and, if available, oxygen, are drawn over a low-resistance vaporiser (Fig. 3.3) into the inspiratory tubing by patient's effort to breathe or by pushing inspiratory gas with a ventilating bellows. During expiration, only little anaesthetic agent is wasted together with the oxygen which is often only 1–2 L/min. No re-breathing is possi-

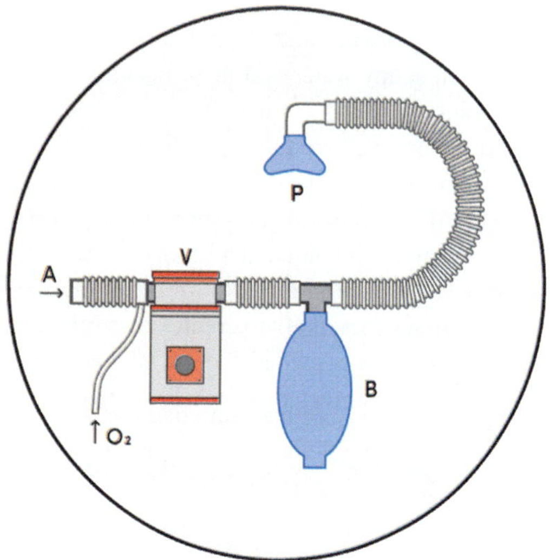

Fig. 3.3 Draw-over system. A = ambient air, B = self-inflating bag or bellows for manual ventilation, O_2 = oxygen added from any source of oxygen, P = patient, V = low-resistance vaporiser from which the spontaneously breathing patient can draw the volatile anaesthetic agent

ble, that means no risk for hypoxic gas mixture, and no need for soda lime, no need for continuously measuring the concentration of oxygen in the inspiratory gas. Draw-over systems are much easier and safer, especially in remote hospitals where regular maintenance of complicated equipment is not guaranteed. They are always using room air while the use of compressed gases is optional; however, an oxygen source should be connected to the device. That can be just the ordinary tube from a concentrator. Their running costs are much lower because neither soda lime nor expensive regular maintenance is needed. Some of these devices can be used for more than 20 years.

Examples for draw-over anaesthesia machines or systems are the Glostavent anaesthesia machine series (Fig. 3.4), the Diamedica ECO_2, the Diamedica portable (see Fig. 3.5), and the Gradian Universal anaesthesia machine series (UAM). At some places, even a Triservice apparatus or an old but still functioning OMV–OIB system might be used.

The anaesthesia devices can be used with different types of breathing systems. The breathing tubing systems should be in at least two sizes for the different age groups. Nowadays they are often made of light weight plastic rather than heavy rubber. They are not autoclavable and need to be cleaned in soapy water and disinfected in a suitable solution, then rinsed with clean water and kept dry. Very nice are tubing systems of silicone which can be autoclaved. They may or may not have an APL (adjustable pressure limiting) valve for choosing the intended inspiratory pressure for manual IPPV ventilation. Non-rebreathing systems are much less likely to create cross infection between patients provided face masks and connectors are disinfected properly between all cases.

Mapleson D or F systems are used for infants below 15 kg.

3.3.2 Draw-Over Vaporiser

Calibrated vaporisers are needed to convert liquid anaesthetic into a gaseous vapour which can be added to the gas mixture. Draw-over vaporisers have low resistance so that the patient can easily inhale the anaesthetic agent with normal breathing efforts. Exception is for children below 20 kg BW, so that in children the draw over vaporiser needs to be used with a continuous flow of compressed air and/or oxygen of around 3 L/min from cylinders or concentrator to ensure the child is getting the intended concentration of the anaesthetic. The amount of inhalational anaesthetic can be preset by moving the lever at the dosing dial and is given in Vol % saturated vapour as added to the gas flow. Examples for average adults: The patient is breathing room air plus 1 L/min oxygen which makes a concentration of around 35% O_2 and 1.5% of halothane, or the patient is breathing air plus 2 L/min oxygen and 2% isoflurane which makes a concentration of

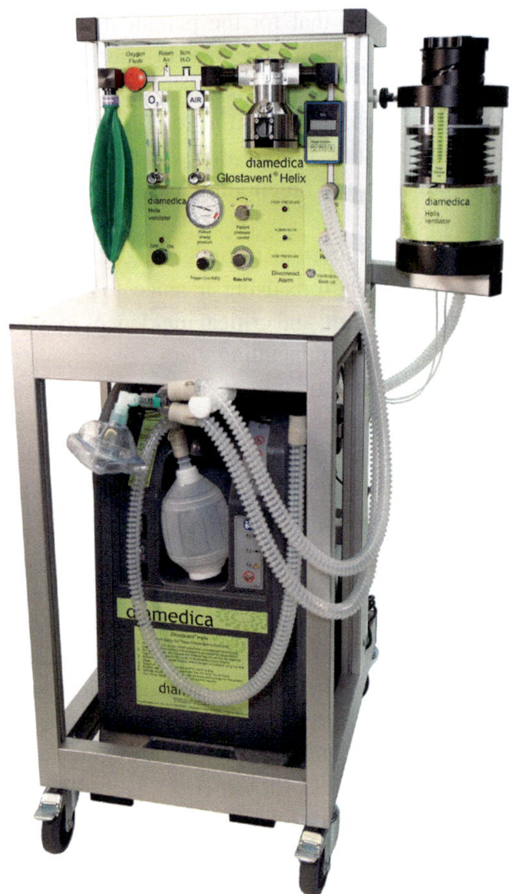

Fig. 3.4 Glostavent® Helix Anaesthesia system with integrated oxygen concentrator, non-rebreathing circuit with self-inflating bellows, low resistance vaporiser for draw-over anaesthesia, ventilator for mechanical IPPV ventilation, and vital signs monitor (from Diamedica (UK) Ltd, with permission)

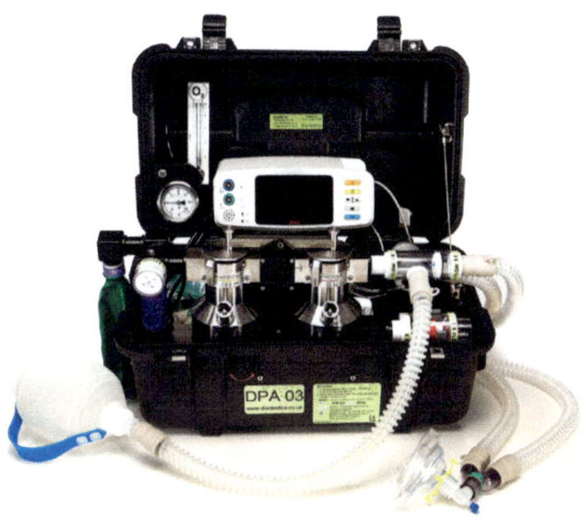

Fig. 3.5 Diamedica portable anaesthesia machine DPA03 with two low-resistance vaporisers for draw-over anaesthesia, capnography and pulse oximetry monitor, working even without electricity (from Diamedica Ltd. (UK) with permission)

about 45–50% oxygen and 2% isoflurane. They are calibrated for one agent, but halothane and isoflurane have the same boiling points so that the calibration is the same, while sevoflurane has a different boiling point and needs a different vaporiser. A halothane vaporiser can also be used for isoflurane and vice versa—but the two agents must not be mixed. Their mixture causes a poison-like substance which cannot be used for anaesthesia. Therefore, make sure that the correct agent is filled into the vaporiser. If a vaporiser is used for halothane but at another time the same vaporiser shall be used for isoflurane it must first be emptied, then cleaned, and before filling it with the new agent it must be labelled accordingly.

Vaporisers should be serviced from time to time—as all medical equipment. This is not so difficult. Most important is to empty the vaporiser completely. This should be performed when only little anaesthetic is left inside since the remaining drug must be discarded. While an isoflurane vaporiser might function long time even without cleaning inside for maintenance, a halothane vaporiser could get real problems because halothane is usually containing an additive, thymol, as stabiliser. 100 ml of halothane are containing 10 μl = 0.01 ml thymol. The problem with thymol is that it is not vaporised. Therefore, with time, thymol would accumulate in the vaporiser. After refilling a 150 ml vaporiser 100 times, it would contain about 1.5 ml of thymol. Thymol is not creating any pharmacological effect and does not do harm to the patient. However, when thymol concentration is increasing it may gum up the vaporiser dial and cause it to stick. Thymol is also changing the colour in the vaporiser. When it is looking yellowish it is the sign that you should empty the vaporiser completely, let it dry, and then refill it with fresh halothane. Vaporisers which are not used regularly should also be emptied. A completely stuck vaporiser can be filled with some new agent, be put upside down and back several times to get it less sticky, then be emptied, cleaned (never with water but with organic solvent like alcohol, ether or even with halothane itself) and afterwards be filled with fresh volatile anaesthetic. Then it should be working again.

A Triservice apparatus is a simple, portable draw-over device with two small vaporisers (OMV), sometimes with the same volatile agent, sometimes with different anaesthetics (usually halothane and isoflurane), a self-inflating bag and a non-rebreathing valve. It can be used for spontaneous or manual ventilation. The Triservice apparatus does not need electricity unless an oxygen concentrator is used together with it. In case of oxygen failure, the Triservice can function with room air provided the patient has acceptable oxygen saturation.

3.3.3 Compressed Gas Machines

Compressed gas anaesthetic machines are operating with continuous flow of compressed oxygen and air, or more seldom nitrous oxide at a pressure which is several times higher than atmospheric pressure, often 4 bar. See Fig. 3.6 for a typical compressed gas machine.

These machines cannot operate with room air as the draw-over devices can. An uninterrupted supply of pressurised gases is required, either from pipelines or from cylinders, and only for few types of these machines, from a modified 3.5 bar (older machines 1.5 bar) Staxel™ oxygen

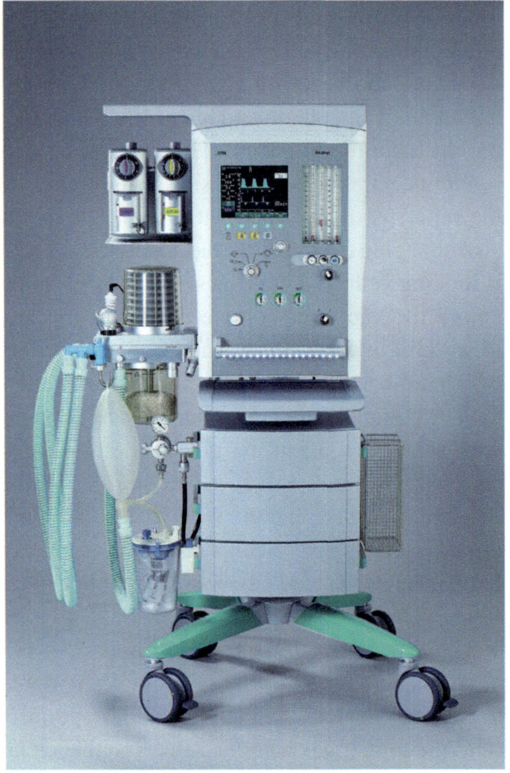

Fig. 3.6 Stephan Akzent Color®, a modern compressed gas anaesthesia machine, with two plenum vaporisers, ventilator for IPPV, and CO_2 absorber canister (with permission from Stephan Company, Germany)

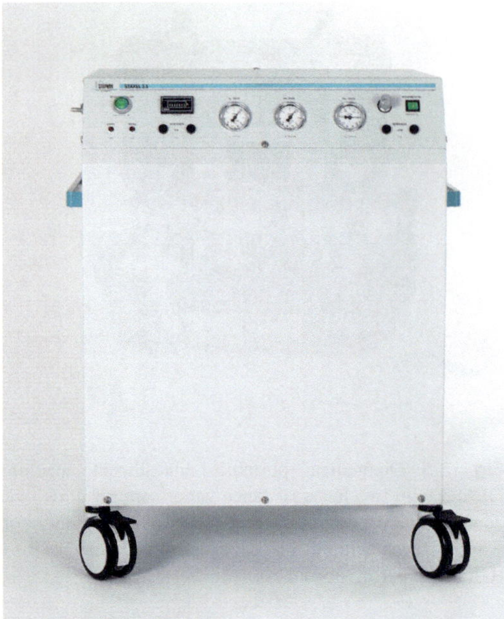

Fig. 3.7 Stephan Staxel® 3.5 bar oxygen concentrator for use with an anaesthesia machine or an ICU ventilator (from Stephan Company, Germany, with permission)

concentrator (Stephan Company, Germany), see Fig. 3.7.

Non-interchangeable special valves are inserted into the wall ports and connected to the anaesthesia machine (Schrader sockets and hoses). The valves are specific for each gas and the hoses are colour-coded. The gases flow to the rotameters where the flow rate of the gases is controlled. The flow rate is shown by a bobbin or float in the vertical column of the respective gas in the flowmeter which is calibrated to each gas. Rotameters need to be checked before starting anaesthesia, since they can get stuck, and the flowmeter can be non-functioning.

3.3.4 Breathing Circuit and CO_2 Absorption with Soda Lime

Before starting anaesthesia, check if the breathing circuit is assembled correctly. Open the oxygen source at about 5 L/min and check if gas is leaving at the connector of the tubing to the patient. Compressed gas machines have an adjustable pressure limiting (APL) valve which allows the exhaled gases and excess fresh gas flow to leave the breathing system and it prevents room air from entering the system. This is one of the most significant differences compared to the draw-over devices. For check, please close the APL valve at open fresh gas flow of about 5 L/min, then close the patient connector with your thumb and look if the ventilating bag is filling and the pressure gauge is indicating maximum pressure which typically is around 60 cm H_2O to ensure there are no leaks. Release the APL valve and try to squeeze the ventilating reservoir bag.

Whenever using a rebreathing circuit, that is, the patient would rebreathe the exhaled gas at least partly (depending on the amount of fresh gas flow), the exhaled gas must be cleared from carbon dioxide; otherwise, the patient would very quickly get poisoned with CO_2. Soda lime is used to absorb the CO_2. See Fig. 3.8 for the typical parts of a rebreathing circuit. The expired gas is directed through a soda lime canister for absorption of the CO_2, and then the gas is

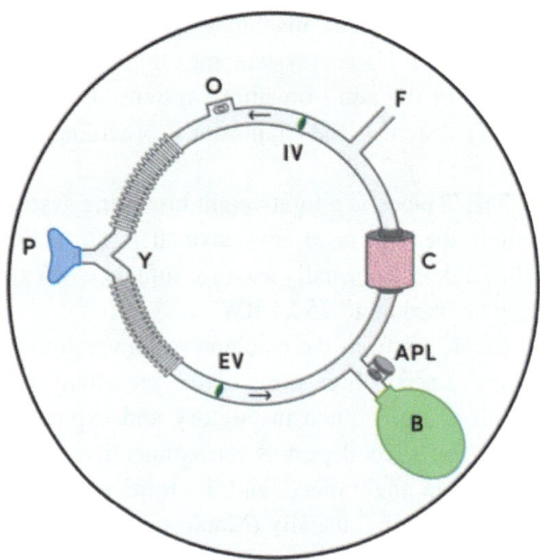

Fig. 3.8 Rebreathing circuit. APL = adjustable pressure-limiting valve, B = reservoir ventilation bag, C = CO_2 absorber canister, EV = expiratory unidirectional valve, F = fresh gas flow, IV = inspiratory unidirectional valve; O = optional oxygen sensor, P = patient, Y = y-piece connector which is together with face mask and volume of the airways adding to the dead space of ventilation

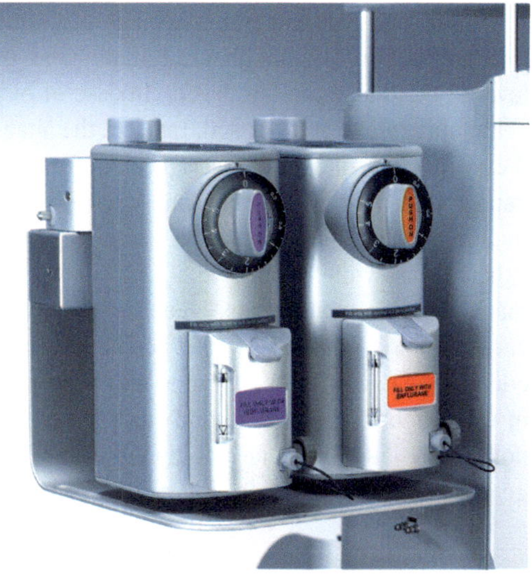

Fig. 3.9 Plenum vaporisers, calibrated for different anaesthetic agents (from Stephan GmbH, Germany, with permission)

rebreathed by the patient after some oxygen has been added as fresh gas. The advantage is that only a small amount of fresh gas is flowing through the vaporiser while the patient is rebreathing the exhaled volatile anaesthetic. A significant smaller amount of anaesthetic is needed if the FGF is <2–3 L/min. Very sophisticated machines with functioning electronic monitors for concentration of O_2, exhaled or end-tidal CO_2 (capnography) and anaesthetic gases need only less than 1 L/min FGF. If the oxygen monitor or the capnography are not working, low FGF must be avoided because it is dangerous if you cannot safely control the concentration of all gases (Oxygen, CO_2, and the volatile anaesthetic agent). Soda lime has limited capacity to absorb CO_2 and must be exchanged regularly depending on the hours of anaesthesia with rebreathing. After 10 h of anaesthesia, the soda lime may already be wasted. This may be indicated with colour change to lilac or purple. However, some products of soda lime do not have a colour changing indicator and then you do not see if the soda lime is still working or not. In that case, you should use capnography and exchange the soda lime if inspired CO_2 is >0.7% (normally, it is 0%). If capnography is not available, the FGF should not be lower than 3 L/min, and the soda lime canister should be labelled with the date of last refill. Depending on the number of general anaesthesias performed, soda lime needs to be changed once or twice per week. The disadvantage of high FGF is that you need more volatile anaesthetic which makes anaesthesia expensive.

3.3.5 Plenum Vaporisers

The vaporisers of compressed gas machines are called “plenum vaporisers” and have a high internal resistance so that they can only be used in continuous flow mode with pressurised gas supply, not with room air. Inside they are looking a bit different from the draw-over vaporisers, but they operate in the same way and need very little maintenance. These vaporisers (Fig. 3.9) need to be attached with the back bar locking mechanism fully engaged to operate well and to avoid leaks.

All vaporisers should be used regularly, otherwise they should be emptied. Maintenance is the same as for draw-over vaporisers, please read there.

Before each anaesthesia, check if the vaporiser is containing enough anaesthetic and the lever of the dial is moving freely. In case of oxygen failure, they can't be used. Instead, the anaesthesia machine must be disconnected from the patient and ventilation performed with a self-inflating bag. Otherwise, the rebreathing of exhaled gas while connected to an anaesthesia machine without fresh oxygen supply would cause hypoxia. The anaesthesia needs then to be continued IV, e.g. with ketamine and diazepam, or the patient may wake up and surgery be postponed. The latter of course is only possible if surgery was not yet started.

3.3.6 Catheter Mounts, Angle Pieces, Tube Connectors, T-piece System

The breathing tubes are connected to the patient via an angle piece with 90° angle and optional with a flexible, so-called catheter mount which is a short piece (5–15 cm) of corrugated tube. Some catheter mounts have the angle piece already integrated. They are used to stabilise the connection between the breathing system and the airway that is the endotracheal tube, the laryngeal mask or a face mask, and to increase mobility at the patient end of the circuit.

It is important to place the breathing tubing in a way that it is not pulling and twisting the patient's artificial airway. A fixation may be needed for the tubing especially if heavy silicon or rubber tubing is used. Some of these devices have a gas sampling port where the sampling line for capnography can be attached. Whenever no capnography is used, the sampling port must be closed to avoid a leak to the room air which would make controlled ventilation impossible. If the original sealing plug for closing the angle piece is missing, a spigot or similar plug can be used instead since their size is the same. Even the plug or spigot of venous cannulae can be used for that purpose. The angle piece and the catheter mount must be exchanged between patients, cleaned, and thoroughly disinfected (while in some places they are used as disposables).

Most anaesthetic machines can optionally be used with a T-piece system for children <15 kg instead of the adult breathing system. The most spread system is the Mapleson F breathing system, see Fig. 3.10.

The T-piece is a lightweight breathing system which does not need any valve. It is not bulky. Although it is normally used for infants <10 kg it may be used up to 25 kg BW.

Fresh gas from the machine is delivered via a tube to one of three ports of the breathing tube which is a combined inspiratory and expiratory limb. The second port is the connection to the patient via angle piece, and the third port is the reservoir tubing, usually (Mapleson F) equipped with an open-ended reservoir bag. The reservoir bag, 0.5 L for infants, has an open end or a hole so that exhaled gas can leave the breathing system and is prevented from being inhaled again. That works well during spontaneous breathing. During manual ventilation, that hole must be closed partly or fully. Remember to open that hole very frequently to avoid rebreathing and accumulation of CO_2. It is of paramount importance to use high FGF, at least 2.5 times the minute ventilation to avoid rebreathing. A thumb rule is to use 4 L/min which will be sufficient for almost all infants. A fresh gas flow of 4 L would even change a draw-over system into a continu-

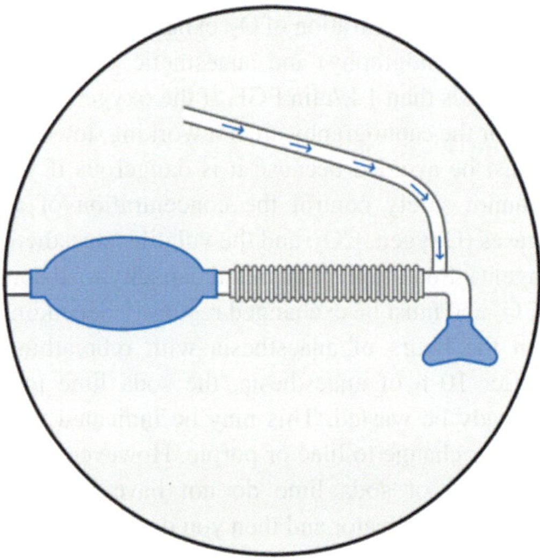

Fig. 3.10 Mapleson type F breathing system

ous flow machine which can be used for even the smallest patients.

Some hospitals have Mapleson D systems instead of Mapleson F or T-piece for infants. It is quite similar, but the reservoir bag is not open-ended since that system has an inner tube as inspiratory limb and the outer corrugated tube for expiration. It has an APL valve by which the ventilation pressure can be adjusted. Remember to never use a reservoir bag without open end or hole with Mapleson F since the patient would not be able to exhale CO_2.

Scavenging

Anaesthetic gases should not be inhaled by theatre staff. In ideal situation, the theatre would be equipped with a scavenging system which collects the anaesthetic gases and clears them to the outside of the building. If such a system is unavailable, the exhaust port of the anaesthesia system may be connected to a long tube which is placed on the ground. The anaesthetic would be diluted quickly, and no harmful concentrations would occur in the air of the operating room. If possible, the operating rooms should have outlets to the environment outside to which anaesthetic gases are directed via tubes.

3.4 Patient Monitoring Devices

Patients during anaesthesia need very close observation since they cannot move (spinal anaesthesia), often they cannot even breathe (deep general anaesthesia), and their circulation may be affected significantly by the anaesthetic drugs or by loss of blood and body fluids. While the best and most important patient monitor is the attentive, alert anaesthesia practitioner, some technical equipment is adding significantly to patient safety.

The absolute minimum needed is a stethoscope and blood pressure cuff. However, nowadays pulse oximeters are regarded as mandatory and are highly recommended for anaesthesia by the WHO as they make anaesthesia safer. Additionally, ECG, respiratory rate, capnography, automatic non-invasive blood pressure monitoring, temperature probes, or, in highly equipped hospitals with specialist physicians for anaesthesia, even invasive arterial and central venous pressure measurement and other additional functions may be used.

Patient vital signs monitors may include several or all the above-mentioned functions with the results visible on a single screen.

3.4.1 Pulse Oximetry

Pulse oximeters measure the percentage of oxygen binding sites in the red blood cells in pulsatile, arterial blood which are occupied (that is called 'saturated') with oxygen. The maximum is therefore 100%. Please refer even to Sect. 2.2 about physiology of oxygen in the body. Below a saturation of 90%, the patient would be hypoxic which is potentially dangerous. The oxygen binding sites are located on the haemoglobin molecules. Patients would also suffer from hypoxia if the haemoglobin level was very low, although the oxygen saturation in the blood might be normal but amount of oxygen carried by the blood would not be sufficient. Low oxygen saturation may be visible as bluish skin colour or bluish colour of the nails or the tongue. However, that is far from being a reliable sign since skin colour might not change if Hb level is low, or bluish skin may be invisible if skin colour is dark. On the other hand, cold fingers are showing blue nails even if oxygenation is normal. In other words, it is impossible to assess a patient's oxygenation state clinically. A pulse oximeter is very useful since it is measuring the oxygen saturation, SPO_2, and the pulse rate and displaying them continuously.

How it works: A visible red light in the probe is indicating that the pulse oximeter is working. Two light-emitting diodes produce beams of red and infrared light at certain frequencies, on one side, and there is a photodetector, on the other side. The saturation is estimated by measuring the transmission of light in pulsatile blood. Thereby, the saturation is measured only in the arterial blood but not in the venous blood which is not pulsatile. The probe is positioned on a finger, toe, or earlobe. In small infants, the probe may be put on the palm of the hand.

The pulse oximeter does not need maintenance; but handle the probes with care since they can easily break. The same is true for the cable. Avoid squeezing it while closing a drawer. Pulse oximeter cables should not hang on the ground; someone might step on the probe. Try to have a spare probe stocked since their life span is shorter than that of the pulse oximeter.

A sustainable and inexpensive brand with excellent sensitivity, robust construction, rechargeable batteries, and available spare parts is the Lifebox-Smile Train Pulse Oximeter™, manufactured in Taiwan by Acare Technology Co., Ltd., distributed worldwide via the global non-profit organisation Lifebox. Lifebox is devoted to safer anaesthesia and surgery in LMICs. The device can easily be ordered via email to oximeters@lifebox.org.

Alarm limits of pulse oximetry can be set for saturation <90 and for too low or too high pulse rate.

Sources of error: Cold fingers or toes may lead to false low S_PO_2 or no reading at all. Try to rub fingers and to warm them up or use a probe at the earlobe.

Intravenous injection of certain dyes, e.g. indocyanine green or methylene blue (administered during certain types of operations), can produce false low readings. Some sorts of nail vanish can produce false low readings as well, and carbon monoxide poisoning, e.g. caused by fire, is giving false high results.

Circulatory failure or shock makes pulse oximetry impossible, there will be no reading. That is really a critical situation since you cannot see if there is a pulse or not. Have the stethoscope in precordial position taped on the chest and listen continuously to the heart and breathing sounds, feel the pulse at the carotid artery, or, better, use an ECG monitor to see the heart beats.

3.4.2 Non-invasive Blood Pressure Measurement

As soon as there is an automatic blood pressure device, people would like it very much. However, it is good to know that they are not more accurate than a person who is measuring BP manually with a cuff and a stethoscope. The pulse oximeter is measuring saturation which cannot be assessed by clinical observation, while the automatic BP machine is not measuring anything better than the nurse can do. The only advantage of a NIBP monitor (non-invasive blood pressure monitor) is during anaesthesia that the anaesthesia provider keeps hands free for other tasks while the BP is displayed at intervals set by the anaesthetist, e.g. every 5 min or every 3 min or every minute in critical situations. The cuffs are available in several sizes, even for babies. It is good to stock at least 3, better 5 sizes, since readings are false low or false high if the cuff is too large or too small. The cuffs are not lasting more than a few years if handled with care. It is useful to stock spare. They should be washed and disinfected between patients but avoid soaking the connecting tubes of the BP cuff in disinfectant since that could kill it. No fluids must enter the connectors of the tubes. Bleach is not well tolerated by BP cuffs; alcohol-based disinfectant is more suitable.

3.4.3 Electrocardiogram (ECG)

ECG devices monitor the heart rate which is normally the same as the pulse rate. However, in arrhythmia or if pulse is weak, heart rate might differ from pulse rate. If no pulse can be detected but the heart is beating, ECG would still work and is thus adding to patient safety during and after anaesthesia and in critical care. It is working by detecting the small electrical potentials of the heart action which are transmitted to the skin surface.

Single-use ECG electrodes are expensive and may be out of stock. That is no problem since they are not needed. The ECG works very well with a little jelly/gel on the skin, then place the ECG cable with its metallic end (crocodile clip) on it and put adhesive tape to keep it in place. Alternatively, a little cotton wool soaked in saline can be put under the ECG crocodile clip which is taped on the proper places on the skin. Performance of the monitor is the same as with single-use electrodes. Old, expired ECG electrodes can be renewed with injecting a little saline into the foam.

3.4.3.1 Colour Code of ECG Cables

The colour code of ECG leads is different in Europe and the United States, and both types of ECG monitor accessories are sold on monitors in Africa and Asia. Therefore, it is good to know:

- 3-lead Europe: red—right shoulder; yellow—left shoulder; green—left abdominal wall or hip.
- 3-lead USA: white—right shoulder; black—left shoulder; red—left abdominal wall or hip.
- 5-lead Europe: red—right shoulder; yellow—left shoulder; green—left abdominal wall or hip, black—right abdominal wall or hip; white—middle of the chest.
- 5-lead USA white—right shoulder; black—left shoulder; red—left abdominal wall or hip, green—right abdominal wall or hip; brown—middle of the chest.

A 5-lead ECG can also be used as 3-lead just by omitting to use the extra leads on the middle of the chest and the right abdominal wall.

3.4.4 Capnography (CO_2 Monitoring)

Capnography is a plot of the partial pressure of carbon dioxide against time in exhaled gas. In many countries, capnography is regarded as mandatory during anaesthesia. Requirements vary between must-have for every GA with endotracheal intubation or LMA and capnography mandatory for certain procedures such as laparoscopy. CO_2 can only be exhaled sufficiently if patient is breathing or is ventilated adequately, and if the heart is pumping, the venous blood carrying CO_2 adequately through the lungs. Exhaled CO_2 is thus an indicator for ventilation and circulation.

The capnograph is using an infrared analyser since carbon dioxide is absorbing infrared light. Two different types of capnography sampling devices can be used: "main-stream" or "side stream analysers" dependent on the part of the breathing system from where the gas sample is taken. The main-stream analyser is attached to the breathing system close to the patient. CO_2 is measured breath to breath with instantaneous result. The more common side stream analyser uses a long sampling line which is connected to the catheter mount with or without an angle piece and connected to the gas sampling port. It draws a sample out from the breathing system for analysis which is a bit delayed.

Although capnography is highly recommended for general anaesthesia with endotracheal tube or laryngeal mask airway, and it is adding a lot to patient safety, in many places it is not used since it is quite difficult to establish and to keep running. Devices are expensive and sensitive for entrance of humidity into the sampling line which stops capnography from functioning. Sampling lines with water inside need to be exchanged. Some devices have even filters which need to be replaced from time to time. After a moist sampling line has dried it can be reused.

The amount of CO_2 in a gas mixture is measured as partial pressure. Normal values are zero for inspiration and 4.5–6 kPa = 34–45 mmHg at the end of expiration = end-tidal concentration.

3.4.4.1 What Can Be Monitored with Capnography?

Correct placement of ETT or LMA and assessment of ventilation (normo-, hypo-, or hyperventilation). Oesophageal intubation would mean that no or very little CO_2 is detected (remove the tube and re-establish ventilation of the patient). When there are regular capnography waves this means proof that the patient is breathing or is ventilated, see Fig. 3.11 for normal capnography trace. A sudden drop of the end-tidal concentration of CO_2 usually means either a disconnection of breathing system from the patient, or there is a sudden drop in cardiac output since CO_2 is not transported to the lungs when the heart does not pump sufficiently. The sudden heart failure may be caused by lung embolism or by anaphylactic shock or myocardial ischaemia. A steep wave form without a

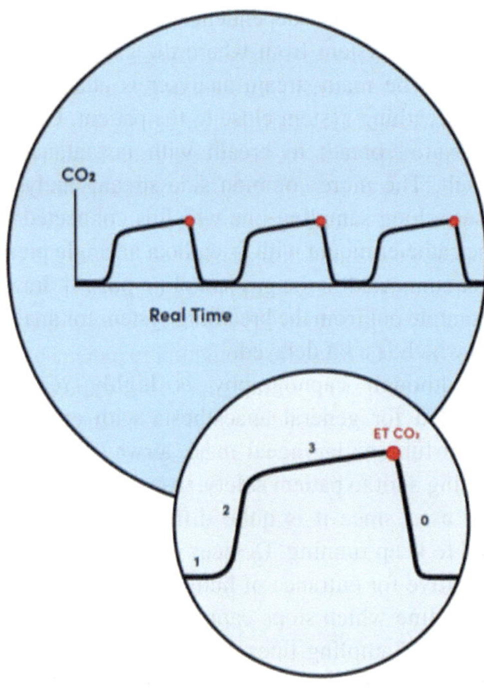

Fig. 3.11 Capnography traces. The four phase of normal capnography waveform: 1 = end of inspiration and beginning of expiration with dead-space expiration, 2 = alveolar gas exhaled, 3 = plateau with the end-tidal or ET CO_2 = end-expiratory level of CO_2 (red), 0 = inspiration

plateau is caused by airway obstruction and needs action (listen to chest sounds, rule out kinking ETT, consider suctioning the airway, consider laryngospam, or bronchospasm or foreign body in the airway).

3.4.4.2 Action to Be Taken If Capnography Is Giving the Following Results

$PaCO_2$ between 4.0–6.5 kPa or between 30–50 mmHg resp.: continue ventilation which seems being rather adequate.

$PaCO_2$ <4.0 kPa resp. 30 mmHg: decrease ventilation/resp. rate by 2/min so that CO_2 rises. Check if tidal volume is adequate or too large (chest excursions looking good? Avoid over-inflation of the lungs. Check if ventilation pressure <20 mmHg that is normal.

$PaCO_2$ >6.5 resp. 50: increase ventilation/resp rate by 2–4/min provided tidal volume is sufficient, otherwise increase it. Are chest excursions adequate? Is ventilation pressure >10 mmHg?

CO_2 suddenly decreasing: Check chest sounds. Are ETT/LMA still in place? Patient ventilated? If yes, assume sudden drop of cardiac output. Check heart rate, BP, and SPO_2. Take actions for stabilising circulation. Is the patient bleeding? Or does the patient get high dose of anaesthetic which needs to be decreased? Ephedrine needed? Adrenaline needed? CO_2 suddenly increasing: A rise in CO_2 which continues even after increasing ventilation may be an early sign for malignant hyperthermia, a complication which is very rare but life-threatening if not immediately treated (see under Sect. 15.7).

3.4.5 Body Temperature Monitoring

During anaesthesia, temperature regulation is not working so that body temperature follows passively the surrounding temperature. Air condition, exposure, laparotomy, long duration of surgery, and fluid losses may lead to temperature drop to 33–34 °C with harmful implications. On the other hand, warming devices can also overheat patients and body temperature may rise >37–38 °C. In rare cases, life-threatening malignant hyperthermia can develop with temperatures >40°C. Patients with low body mass index and children are most prone to temperature changes. Vital signs monitors often have a temperature probe which can be placed under the patient's back or, if disinfected sufficiently, into the oesophagus. Even ordinary thermometers as in the patient wards can be used in OR. Temperature should be monitored and recorded on the anaesthesia chart at least for procedures of >1 h duration.

3.4.6 Oxygen Concentration Analysers

Oxygen analysers are mandatory in some countries while in others they are not. There are two types: One is integrated in the anaesthetic machine, the other is a movable, hand-held device which can be used to check the concentration of oxygen of any source. In all cases, the oxygen sensor within the analyser is not long-lasting. After 1–2 years, the sensor is exhausted and needs to be replaced. That applies even if it was only used occasionally. In many remote hospitals, it is not possible to get spare analyser sensors regularly if at all. Safe anaesthesia without oxygen analyser is no problem if no nitrous oxide is used, and if rebreathing with low fresh gas flow (<3 l/min) is avoided.

If the oxygen source is from cylinders or from a well-maintained huge compressor, it is rather safe to use that oxygen even without analysers and monitoring the exact concentration. If the oxygen is from small concentrators, however, it is very good to check their performance regularly. At least once per month the oxygen output of the concentrator should be measured, since it is possible that a malfunctioning concentrator is just producing 21 or <50% oxygen while you assume it is delivering nearly pure oxygen. That can be dangerous for patients who need high concentration of oxygen. Low fresh gas flow with a rebreathing system may only be applied when an oxygen sensor is integrated and working.

If you are using nitrous oxide, you really should have an oxygen analyser to avoid the risk of giving a hypoxic gas mixture (that is, gas mixture containing less oxygen than ambient air, or <21%) to the patient.

How to perform a rough check of the oxygen output of a concentrator if you don't have an oxygen analyser: Have a pulse oximeter attached while breathing room air. If that SPO_2 is <98%, you apply 5 L/min O_2 via tight fitting mask. Observe if the saturation is rising. SPO_2 should rise to 100% within less than 5 min. If no rise in saturation, assume the concentrator is having a problem and let it be checked thoroughly. If SPO_2 with room air is already 100% that type of check is not possible.

Table 3.1 gives some examples for the approximate oxygen concentrations with mixture of oxygen and air: 100% oxygen is achieved with pure medical oxygen only (very expensive).

Table 3.1 Approximate concentrations of a mixture of O_2 and air

O_2 concentration in the resp. mixture (%)	Air (L/min)	O_2 100% (L/min)	O_2 95% (L/min)	O_2 90% (L/min)
100/95/90	0	5	5	5
84/80/76	1	4	4	4
68/65/62	2	3	3	3
53/51/49	3	2	2	2
37/36/35	4	1	1	1
21/21/21	5	0	0	0

Oxygen compressors usually produce 93–96% O_2 while small concentrators are regarded as well-functioning if O_2 is >90%. The difference of 90, 95, and 100% is clinically insignificant and does not change patient's outcome.

Pure oxygen is equal to 99 or 100% O_2 while a small concentrator can produce 90–96% O_2 at a rate of up to 5 L/min. The oxygen concentration from a concentrator is slightly decreasing at higher flow rates. Table 3.1 shows the concentration of O_2 in the mixture of air and 0–5 L/min oxygen. Depending on the oxygen source, the resulting concentration of the mixture does not differ significantly whether pure medical oxygen is used or 90 or 95% O_2 from a concentrator. If a patient is breathing/ventilated with 5 L/min and is receiving 2 L/min O_2, he will inspire around 50% O_2 if a non-rebreathing system or draw-over is used. In a non-rebreathing system, which is open to room air, the O_2 concentration will never fall below 21%.

3.5 Airway Equipment

3.5.1 Face Masks

Face masks are available in many different sizes since they must fit exactly to the face of the respective patient. Only with a tightly fitting mask positive pressure ventilation is possible. Masks are available of silicon, plastic, and rubber. Silicon is the best lasting material. The face mask is connected to the breathing system with an angle piece. Both face mask and angle piece must be cleaned and disinfected between patients. Silicon and rubber material, but not plastic, can be autoclaved.

3.5.2 Endotracheal Tubes

ETT are made of rubber or plastic, disposable, or re-usable and are available in many sizes from premature infants to adults. Adult women may be intubated with size 6.5, 7, or 7.5 ETT, and even number 8 ETT is often fitting if the woman is not small. Men may be intubated with ETT nr 7, 7.5, or 8. Big or tall men may be intubated with size 8 or 8.5, but even 7.5 would do. For children the correct size of ETT please find in Table 6.1. Paediatric ETT may be with or without cuff, please see Sect. 14.1.2.

Armoured endotracheal tubes are containing a metallic spiral which makes them non-kinking. They are useful for several types of head and neck surgery. An introducer stylet is always needed for intubation. An oropharyngeal airway is also mandatory to avoid that the patient might bite on it and destroy the tube so that air passage would become impossible.

RAE tubes are preformed for oromaxillofacial surgery. They are available for orotracheal and for nasotracheal intubation.

3.5.3 Laryngeal Mask Airways

LMA are also available in different sizes and types. No. 1 for neonates 2–5 kg, No. 1.5 for babies 5–10 kg, No. 2 for infants 10–20 kg, No. 2.5 for children 20–30 kg; No. 3 for small adults 30–50 kg; No. 3.5 for 30–70 kg; No. 4 for normal adults 50–70 kg; No. 5 for big adults >70 kg, and No. 6 (rarely needed) for very big adults >100 kg (while in most adults >100 kg even a No. 5 mask would fit). However, sometimes one size bigger or smaller than for the bodyweight is fitting better. Most LMA have a cuff which is inflated with air up to a pressure between 30–60 mmHg or (if no cuff pressure monitor available) inflated as little as possible just to keep the LMA tight that is without significant leakage. Too high cuff pressure can damage nerves in the throat. Other LMA have a channel for suctioning or placement of a gastric tube. A third type is called fast track and enables intubating the trachea through the LMA. That can be helpful in a condition of difficult airway where endotracheal intubation is required but laryngoscopy failed. LMA do not require laryngoscopy for insertion. Another type of LMA is called I-gel LMA and does not have a cuff. Same sizes as for other types of LMA are available.

How is the correct placement of the LMA assured? After insertion in deeply anaesthetised patients until feeling a resistance when it is not possible to insert it further, connect the breathing circuit and apply hand ventilation. Listen to the lungs and above the larynx on the neck of the patient. A correctly fitting LMA means there is a clear breathing sound. Light anaesthesia with vocal cords not completely relaxed, or wrong placement in the hypopharynx would sound obstructed or like wheezing, and there would be significant leakage.

3.5.4 Laryngoscopes

A laryngoscope is necessary to insert a tube into the trachea. Good quality with bright light is key, and the best quality is with cold light laryngoscopes. In hospitals where the laryngoscopes are used frequently (elective surgery several times per week), it is recommended to use a charging station for the laryngoscope instead of disposable batteries. There are different sizes of blades which can easily be exchanged. Unfortunately, blades from different brands are not fitting to the handle. Only the original blades would fit, no other products would. If possible, a hospital should have all laryngoscopes from the same manufacturer so that all parts are fitting everywhere. Have always batteries stocked in operation theatre (size C for most types) as you might need them during the weekend or night when the hospital store is closed. Without a sufficient light source, the laryngoscope is of no use. The light must be bright, of white or bright yellow colour. As soon as the light is looking dark yellow or orange or if it is flickering, the battery must be changed or put on the charger.

The sizes of the blades are: Size 0 for small neonates or premature; 1 for infants, 2 for children, 3 for most adults, 4 for large adults (>180 cm tall). While it is possible to intubate with a blade one size too large it is almost impossible to use a too small blade successfully.

There are two different types of blades: Miller and Macintosh. A Miller blade is straight while the Macintosh is curved. Both types are available in all sizes. However, it is advantageous to use Miller size 0 or 1 for infants <6 months or until the first teeth are visible. Thereafter, for most cases and especially those with normal anatomy, it is easier to intubate with a curved blade that is Macintosh for all patients older than 6 months. For more details, see Chap. 6.

In case of difficult intubation a ***stylet*** or gum-elastic bougie (Eschmann stylet) is helpful which is inserted into the tube or, if long enough, is inserted into the trachea first, then the ETT is put over the stylet into the trachea. Make all efforts to get one gum-elastic bougie for every OR and attach it to the anaesthesia machine so that it is always at hand. The plastic wrapping of suction catheters, fixed with adhesive tape to the anaesthesia machine, can be used as envelope to hold the bougie in place, so it is just to pull it out of that sheath when you need it.

In very difficult cases direct laryngoscopy may be impossible even for experienced anaesthetists. In those situations, either a LMA can be used or, if available, a videolaryngoscope can be helpful. For difficult airway management please see Sect. 6.6.

The monitor of a videolaryngoscope is also ideal for teaching as the instructor can guide the student while practising. Even fiberoptic intubation, FOI, usually through the nose, is an option in difficult airways, especially when the mouth opening is not sufficient for a laryngoscope to be inserted. Fiberoptic bronchoscopes, which can be used for intubation, need special skills and need to be handled with care and maintained well since they can easily be damaged and stop working. FOI is beyond the scope of a health centre or district hospital. Normally it should only be used by specialist anaesthesiologists or ENT doctors.

While videolaryngoscopes are expensive, stylets are not, and the stylets are sufficient to get most patients intubated successfully. Therefore, you should aim for stylets in different sizes. Thin stylets are needed for paediatric intubation. Stylets can easily be cleaned and disinfected. They are lasting many years if treated with care. You can even make them yourself using wire which is covered with rubber. The best stylets are the long gum elastic bougies. Be careful not to damage the patient's trachea with the tip of the stylet.

The use of fiberoptic intubation devices and of videolaryngoscopes is beyond the scope of this book for anaesthesia practitioners and left to specialist physicians. Textbooks and websites are describing these devices for readers who are interested.

3.5.5 Filters and Heat and Moisture Exchangers

Bacterial filters which are also protecting from viruses should be used between the airway device and the breathing system if available. They can only be used for one single patient preventing from cross-infection between patients in case a patient who is operated on has got airway or lung infection. Fortunately, infection from patients breathing systems are rare even if no filter is used. Heat and moisture exchangers (HME) are filters which also prevent from airway infection; and at the same time, the device is humidifying the completely dry medical gases. For longer operations with general anaesthesia (>2 h), it is highly recommended to use humidifying devices if available.

3.6 Other Equipment

3.6.1 TOF Monitors and Other Nerve Stimulators

TOF monitors are special nerve stimulators as a useful tool to assess remaining muscle relaxation at the end of surgery when the patient is expected to recover. It is used at the ulnar nerve, e.g. with the help of two ECG electrodes. A nerve stimulator is applying a small current at a frequency of about 50/min, usually as so-called train of four (TOF) that is four stimuli. All four stimuli must be answered with a strong and equal contraction of the muscle which adducts the thumb. A patient must not be extubated if there is residual neuromuscular block since he/she would not be able to keep a patent airway.

Other types of nerve stimulators can be used for facilitating regional anaesthesia. This type of device is using single-use special needles which are connected with the stimulator. With the help of the stimulator, the needle can be located close to the nerve which is to be blocked; then the local anaesthetic drug is injected. It is beyond the scope of this short book to describe any details for regional block with nerve stimulator, and it is uncommon that anaesthesia providers who are not specialist physicians for anaesthesiology are performing regional blocks for which a nerve stimulator is needed.

3.6.2 Suction Machine

Suction machines are using vacuum which is needed for suction. The device is necessary to clear the airway from secretion, to empty the stomach before anaesthesia or during laparotomy, and to clear the operation wound from blood or other fluids. Without effective suction a patient might die from pulmonary aspiration, or the surgeon might be unable to perform the planned operation because blood would blur the vision. Suction machines are simple apparatus but need to be handled with care as the vessels could break or the rubber sealing get damaged. Spare is often difficult or impossible to obtain.

Each operation room must have at least one suction machine. Additionally, the postoperative recovery area needs a suction device, the emergency department, the maternity and the ICU/HDU area need one. It is also very nice if the general wards have a suction device. Electrical suction units with vacuum are strong, but small suction devices can also be used with a foot pump and do not need electricity.

3.6.3 Soda Lime

Exhaled carbon dioxide can be absorbed by soda lime with a chemical reaction that requires moisture. The soda lime will get exhausted after some hours of use and needs to be replaced regularly. Soda lime makes anaesthesia more expensive. Unfortunately, many anaesthesia machines, especially all models with re-breathing circuits must not be used without soda lime and need regular supply of soda. The author does not recommend such type of anaesthesia machine for remote places where soda lime might be out of stock. Capnography is regarded as mandatory if re-breathing and soda lime are used.

How long is soda lime effective? That depends on the minute ventilation and CO_2 production of the patient and on the FGF. The lower the FGF the faster the soda lime is exhausted, sometimes already after 6 h of anaesthesia. If FGF is not below 3 L/min and general anaesthesia with re-breathing is performed only 1–2 h a day, the soda lime is often lasting a week. If supply is no problem it should be changed weekly in such settings. If soda lime is difficult to obtain or out of stock, FGF should be around 5 L/min in adults. After a maximum of 1 month, soda lime must be exchanged because it gets dry and does not function even if it was used less than a few hours. Label the containers always with the date of exchange. To protect yourself, it is wise to use face mask and gloves while handling with the soda lime which may be irritating for skin and eyes. It must be packed firmly but not too tight in the canister. If packed too loosely, the exhaled gas mixture would flow through the side channels without having the CO_2 absorbed. Don't overfill the canister but have around 1 cm on top empty. Dehydrated soda lime cannot change colour even if it is equipped with a colour indicator. If you are in doubt about the quality of your soda lime: Feel the canister during anaesthesia. If it is warm the soda lime is working, if it remains cold it is definitely exhausted and not functioning. Fresh soda lime is easily crumbled if you crush it between your fingers. If it is feeling hard it is probably exhausted.

Use capnography if possible. Aim at end-tidal CO_2 of 35–45 mmHg or 4.5–6 kPa. Functioning soda lime lets the inspiratory CO_2 be almost zero. Inspiratory CO >0.7 kPa or 5 mmHg is indicating exhausted soda lime. Increase fresh gas flow and exchange soda lime as soon as possible, usually after the on-going anaesthesia is finished.

3.6.4 Defibrillator

A defibrillator is used to treat severe, life-threatening arrhythmias, especially ventricular fibrillation with cardiac arrest. How it works: It delivers an electrical shock to the heart which causes a depolarisation of all myocardial cells leading to a synchronised contraction of the heart muscle. After the shock, in many cases but not always, the heart is beating with a stable rhythm again.

Three types of defibrillators are common: *Manual defibrillators* need the user to decide and choose the energy (150–400 J for defibrillation in adults; 50–200 J for cardioversion in adults), charge and apply shock. *Semi-automatic* or half-automatic *defibrillators* are analysing the heart rhythm automatically, choosing the energy, charging the pads and tell the user with a voice what shall be done, e.g. to put the paddles on the patient, and so on. The automated device is guiding the user, but the user is the one to start the shock. *Fully automatic defibrillators* also talk to the user when opened. The user is putting the paddles according to the pictures on the pads. The device is checking the patient's rhythm and will tell the user if a shock is needed. If the shock is needed, the device will warn the user not to be in touch with the patient and will then apply the shock automatically.

The device should be connected to the mains electricity when not used to keep the internal batteries charged. Then it is brought to the patient who is to be defibrillated. Switch it on and choose the energy (usually start with 150 J: maximum energy is 400 J at high voltage up to 5000 V). Place the paddles (apply jelly to them if required) on the sternum and the left midaxillary line (5–6th rib). Alternatively, instead of paddles adhesive defibrillator electrode pads can be used. Switch the charge button to charge the capacitor. After charging is complete, assure that no person is in touch with the patient or the bed, then apply the shock.

For details, please see Sect. 15.4 Advanced cardiac life support.

3.7 List of Minimal Equipment for Safe Anaesthesia

The three categories listed in Table 3.2 are approximately similar to the WHO international standards for safe anaesthesia from 2018. The three categories of the WHO are "highly recommended—recommended—suggested". If the standard does not even match "highly recommended", only emergency procedures with no option for referral may be performed while patients for elective operations should be referred to a better equipped facility. This category is called "mandatory" in Table 3.2. A torch is important if electricity is intermittent.

Please note that the more equipped the anaesthesia unit is the more educated the AP has to be. In the category "recommended", this means trained AP plus regular visiting anaesthesiologist are minimum; in the category "suggested", a permanent anaesthesiologist is desirable. If nurse anaesthetists or clinical officers have to work on their own, it is safer to have a small scale of simple anaesthesia methods and simple that is mandatory or recommended equipment than going for high tech and increased risk of avoidable complications. The official rules about anaesthesia staffing are different in all countries and have of course to be followed.

Table 3.2 List of minimal equipment for safe anaesthesia according to WHO international standard guidelines

Mandatory	Recommended	Suggested (nice to have)
Regular supply of oxygen (e.g. from small concentrators or cylinders)	Oxygen concentrators plus cylinders as back up	Piped oxygen from own oxygen plant; backup cylinders, reservoirs, or small concentrators
Suction device with foot pump	Electrical suction machine in OR, ICU and maternity	Suction machines in OR, maternity and all wards
Self-inflating bellows	Anaesthesia machine for spontaneous and manual ventilation with one vaporiser	Anaesthesia machine with ventilator and one or two vaporisers in all OR
Face masks, oropharyngeal airways	ETT different sizes, LMA different sizes, laryngoscope with different blades, bougie, pillow	Videolaryngoscope, fiberoptic intubation device
Pulse oximeter	Vital signs monitor	Temperature probe
Stethoscope	ECG	Capnography
Blood pressure device	Automatic blood pressure device (NIBP)	Nerve stimulator for TOF
Syringes and cannulae	3-way stop cock and extensions	Central venous lines
Spinal needles and local anaesthetics		Epidural anaesthesia sets Regional block equipment
Infusion giving sets	Paediatric infusion giving sets	Infusion pumps
NS, RL, Dextrose	Plasma expander like hydroxyethyl starch	Albumin, Ca^{++}, K^{+}, Na^{+} to add to infusions Dextrose 10%, Dextrose 40%
Blood for transfusion in emergencies	Some units of packed erythrocytes of different blood groups	Packed red cells, plasma and platelet transfusion when needed; blood bank
Essential anaesthesia drugs (ketamine, thiopentone, diazepam)	Volatile anaesthetic like halothane; propofol	Isoflurane, sevoflurane; strong opioid drugs like fentanyl, morphine
Analgesics like diclophenac, tramadol	Strong analgesic like pethidine; short acting muscle relaxant	Several muscle relaxants and reversal drugs
Atropine, adrenaline	Ephedrine	Phenylephrine, noradrenaline
Anaesthesia record form and pen,	Postoperative observation chart	ICU observation list
Blankets to keep patients warm	Body temperature monitor	

Links to Videos

Animation of the Universal Anaesthesia Machine and ventilator. https://www.youtube.com/watch?v=W4UVE3rQgn0

The Diamedica Portable Anaesthesia system. https://www.youtube.com/watch?v=a2ZxKNlkoqM

The Diamedica Glostavent® Helix Anaesthesia Machine. https://youtu.be/2rO1VIHstwU

Further Reading

Al-Shaikh B, Stacey S (2018) Essentials of equipment in anaesthesia, critical care, and postoperative medicine, 5th edn. Churchill Livingstone Elsevier, London

Dobson M (2017) The right stuff. Anaesthetic equipment and techniques that work best in low resource countries. MD Publications Oxford, Oxford

Gelb AW, Morriss WW et al (2018) World Health Organization – World Federation of Societies of Anaesthesiologists (WHO – WFSA) international standards for a safe practice of anesthesia. Anesth Analg 126:2047–2055

4 Preparing for Anaesthesia

Abstract

Preoperative evaluation of the patient, even in emergency cases, is mandatory. The patient needs information about the planned anaesthesia including possible risks. The anaesthetist needs to check the general condition, history, airway anatomy, heart and lung function, vital signs including body weight, present medication, lab results, and must plan the anaesthesia.

Patient preparation includes a shower or having the body washed, fresh bed linen, fasting food 6 h and water 2 h. Antihypertensives like β-blockers or calcium antagonists should be continued in the morning of surgery while diuretics or ACE antagonists should be omitted. Insulin dose is adjusted according to b-glucose; oral antidiabetics are omitted. Anti-asthmatic drugs, antibiotics, cortisone, and thyroxine are continued.

Preparing the anaesthesia working place according to the following checklist. Are electricity and oxygen available and stable? Perform a check of the anaesthesia machine for circuit leakage, performance of vaporiser (filled with proper anaesthetic agent?), manual/mechanical ventilation possible? SIB and face mask proper size, laryngoscope, tubes, stylets prepared and functioning? Suction machine and pulse oximeter are functioning? Prepare infusions and drugs in labelled syringes. Have emergency drugs such as atropine, adrenaline, and ephedrine prepared.

Perform a surgical checklist before starting surgery: Right patient, procedure, site of operation? Expected blood loss, possible complications? Antibiotic has been given before starting surgery? Are there any concerns about patient positioning on the table, e.g. prone position or lithotomy?

Anaesthesia and surgical checklists cost nothing and save lives.

Keywords

Patient positioning on the operation table · Preoperative anaesthesia assessment · Preparing equipment before anaesthesia · Preparing patient before anaesthesia · Safety checklist before starting anaesthesia

4.1 Preoperative Evaluation

4.1.1 Anaesthesia Assessment by Preoperative Visit

Preoperative evaluation has two goals: Informed consent must be obtained from the patient and information about patient's health and individual risk factors obtained for the anaesthetist. Information should be recorded on a special form by the AP (anaesthesia provider). An example of a preoperative evaluation form please see in the Appendices.

D. Kietzmann, *Anaesthesia in Remote Hospitals*, Sustainable Development Goals Series,
https://doi.org/10.1007/978-3-031-46610-6_4

The patient should be informed about the planned procedure, anaesthesia, fasting, postoperative care, and potential anaesthesia related risks. Patient concerns should be addressed. The rules about informed consent vary between countries. Local regulations are to be observed. In many countries, patients have to sign a consent paper while in other countries, e.g. in Sweden, patient does not need to sign. The anaesthetist should always inform the patient about the type of anaesthesia and about typical side effects or risks. In some countries, patients must be informed about all potential risks, even very rare ones like paralysis after spinal anaesthesia. This is not very helpful and adds to patient's anxiety but local law must of course be observed.

For spinal anaesthesia, patient information could be like that: The regional anaesthesia which I am going to give you with an injection at your back will paralyse your belly and legs during few hours. You will not feel pain but numbness. We will control your blood pressure frequently since it may drop somewhat. You might need a urinary catheter to get your bladder emptied. Some patients develop headache which may last some days after the operation. Other complications are unlikely to happen. On the other hand, if the patient asks for information the AP must provide them: Damage to nerves or spinal cord is very unlikely to happen.

Before GA it is always wise to state that anaesthetic drugs are very strong (otherwise they would not produce anaesthesia during painful surgery), and therefore, some side effects especially on respiration and circulation are common, but that the AP will do the best to care for the patient's well-being. Special risk factors that apply to the individual patient should be addressed, and at the same time the AP should aim for the patient feeling confident.

The anaesthetist will perform a short physical examination with respect to airway anatomy, heart and lung function, and inspection of sites where venous access is possible to be placed. A short history is taken about previous operations and anaesthesia (any complications?), any severe disease in the past or present, drugs taken regularly, and possible drug allergies. Depending on the planned surgery, some lab examination can be needed as Hb, b-glucose, serum creatinine. Always take the actual body weight of the patient to avoid wrong doses of your drugs. Patients with leg injury who cannot stand on a weighing scale should get their height measured to get an idea about approximate body weight. In the (hopefully very unlikely) event that there is no weighing scales, estimate BW of children with the formula (age + 4) × 2 = kg BW.

4.1.2 ASA Risk Classification

The ASA score is an assessment of the patient's physical status (overall health) that can be class I–V, and that is assessed by the anaesthesia provider. The ASA score should always be documented on the anaesthesia record or the pre-anaesthesia evaluation form.

- ASA I score means a healthy patient who is not on regular medicine.
- ASA II means a patient with mild systemic disease such as hypertension or diabetes which is well regulated with oral medication.
- ASA III a patient with severe disease such as compensated heart failure, patient after stroke who has neurological deficits, insulin-dependent diabetes mellitus, severe COPD but saturation >94% on room air, kidney insufficiency with creatinine >200 μmol/L (>2 mg/dl), severe hypertension which is not regulated, cancer patients with poor general condition, and so on.
- ASA IV would mean a patient with life-threatening disease independent of the cause for the planned surgery, however, a patient with late presentation of acute abdominal problem like bowel obstruction with peritonitis and dehydration who is in poor condition would also match ASA IV. Examples for chronic disease are decompensated heart failure, end-stage kidney failure, diabetes mellitus with severe organ complications and poorly controlled blood sugar, severe liver cirrhosis with oesophageal varices, and so on.
- ASA V is a patient in poor condition expected to die the same day but might be saved with emergency surgery.

General consideration: A patient with a potentially serious disease for elective surgery should be operated only if the hospital is able to manage that underlying disease and any complications which may arise during and after surgery and anaesthesia. Otherwise, those patients should be transferred. For emergency patients with severe chronic disease when referral is no option: try to get information on how the condition is to be treated and which complications can arise. If necessary, call a colleague in a tertiary hospital and ask for advice.

4.1.3 Fasting Before Anaesthesia

Before elective surgery patients are starved to make sure their stomach is empty at anaesthesia induction. While "fasting from 10 PM the day before surgery" was tradition up to recently that proves no longer adequate since patients would be fasting unnecessarily long and reach theatre in a dehydrated condition especially if they are not the first patients to be operated on. The 6-4-2-hours rule is nowadays recommended and means 6 h fasting solid foods, soup, yoghurt, porridge, formula milk, cow milk; 4 h fasting fluids like breast milk, energy drinks based on juice, coffee or tea with little or without milk; up to 2 h water only. Exemption is little water together with oral medicines which is allowed without restrictions. After breast milk gastric emptying is faster than with cow milk or formula so that babies can be breastfeeding up to 4 h before anaesthesia induction. The challenge with the obviously better rule is communication between theatre, ward, and patients including their relative-caretakers. It is not always easy to guess when it is "4 h before that scheduled operation" or "2 h before anaesthesia induction". However, patients who are not the first ones on the list could be allowed to drink as much water or tea without added milk as they like at 8 AM. Patients who are on the list for the afternoon could get a light early breakfast around 7 AM and water at 10 AM. Be communicative to create a schedule which is fitting best at your health facility and improving patients' wellbeing.

4.1.4 Patients with Chronic Disease Like Hypertension, Diabetes Mellitus, or COPD

Consultation with a physician for internal medicine may be required if a patient's condition with chronic disease should be improved before surgery, e.g. poorly controlled diabetes mellitus, hypertension, heart disease, COPD or asthma, kidney disease, liver disease, or other.

Check if patient is on regular medicine and discuss with the surgeon if drugs should be continued. Often antihypertensive drugs need to be continued even before surgery although the patient is fasting. ACE antagonists such as captopril or enalapril are not given before anaesthesia while β-blockers (e.g. atenolol, metoprolol) or calcium antagonists (e.g. amlodipine, hydralazine, nifedipine) should be taken with little water in the morning of operation day.

Acute operations, e.g. ORIF for treating a fracture, need to be performed within a short time frame even in patients with uncontrolled hypertension. If BP is >180/100, the patient should receive additional antihypertensive drug perioperatively. Anaesthesia is to be performed with caution, preferred as spinal or inhalation anaesthesia with deep anaesthesia before tracheal intubation (a sudden increase of already high BP can lead to heart failure or stroke). If GA is necessary, avoid ketamine in higher dose than 0.5 mg/kg for induction if BP is high but use propofol or thiopentone instead. Ketamine should not be used as sole induction agent but only in combination with other hypnotic-like thiopentone or propofol. After induction there is risk for hypotension which needs to be treated with ephedrine or other vasoconstrictor.

Oral antidiabetic drugs and diuretics are not administered in the morning of surgery.

Patients who are on insulin: Frequent measurements of b-glucose are recommended. As a rule of thumb, the ordinary dose in the evening before surgery and half the morning dose of long-acting insulin should be administered. Aim for target blood glucose between 6–12 mmol/l. A drip with 5% glucose should be given slowly if b-glucose is <6–7 mmol/l (or below around 100–

120 mg/dl). Control b-glucose regularly until the patient is eating after surgery. Have the surgeon prescribe how much insulin should be given at which b-sugar level. Avoid hypoglycaemia as it is more dangerous than high sugar. Glucose levels higher than 15 mmol/l (270 mg/dl) should be avoided if possible and must be treated. On the other hand, in patients for amputation or wound debridement of diabetic foot, b-glucose is often very high and may be impossible to control before surgery is performed and the site of inflammation removed. Remember that any inflammation or infection is making diabetes worse. High b-glucose may also cause forced diuresis with dehydration. Infusion with RL is required already before starting anaesthesia and surgery. In such cases, you may have to go ahead with anaesthesia and surgery, but have good communication with the surgeon.

Chronic lung disease and smoking are increasing the intra- and postoperative risk for respiratory complications and periods of hypoxia. Smokers should stop smoking for at least 2 months before elective operations. Patients with COPD and asthma should get bronchodilators (usually as spray) until the morning of surgery. Consider corticosteroids if patients are showing symptoms of their lung disease. Physiotherapy with breathing exercises before and after surgery may improve outcome for patients with lung disease. Patients with obstructive sleep apnoea should be nursed in lateral position during night and, if SpO_2 showing episodes of desaturation receive CPAP if available. Artificial ventilation during GA should include positive end-expiratory pressure (PEEP) of at least 5 cm H_2O if available. Avoid unnecessary high inspired oxygen since that facilitates atelectasis formation.

4.2 Anaesthesia Working Place, Trolley, Drugs, and Equipment

4.2.1 Anaesthesia Machine, Oxygen Source

Using an oxygen concentrator, remember that it takes at least 5 min until the oxygen delivered by the machine will have reached a concentration of >80%. In the very moment when the concentrator is started it just provides air. Therefore, the concentrator should be switched on a few minutes until you are about to start the anaesthesia. Cylinder oxygen: Open the cylinder by using the wrench to turn the valve and check if the pressure gauge is indicating sufficient capacity. Pipeline: check if oxygen from the wall outlet is showing up as fresh gas if the flowmeter of the anaesthesia machine is opened. Ideally, an oxygen sensor should be available to verify the concentration of oxygen.

If you have an anaesthesia machine or draw-over device in your operation room, check its performance and be sure it works correctly. The manufacturer's machine check according to the instruction manual is mandatory and must be performed regularly that is at the beginning of every working day and a shorter test before every patient. Instruction manuals are downloadable.

Short Test Have a bellows attached on the patient outflow as a test lung and inflate it with a fresh gas flow of around 5 l/min using manual ventilation (2 bag test). Look if the bellows is filling and emptying. With this simple test, you would also detect leaks of the breathing circuit. Check a T-piece or respective alternative system connected to the anaesthesia machine separately if planned to be used. Check the vaporiser: Is it connected, filled, and the lever freely movable? Have a SIB in the room with a connection tube to oxygen source in case anaesthesia machine stops working. Check the operation of the APL valve (if the machine has one), if it can be fully opened and closed and the pressure is obtained accordingly.

4.2.2 Essential Equipment Per Operating Room

The following list is an example. Create your own checklist which is matching the local requirements which depend on the types of surgery and patients for which equipment should be. The checklist can be printed and laminated and be one for each operation room. Before starting operations, every day the list should be used to check if everything is at hand. Equipment which is not often needed and not urgently required may be stored at a central place in the operation theatre, e.g. a store room.

Airway and Ventilation Equipment:

Oxygen source: Oxygen concentrator or oxygen cylinder with manometers or pipeline
Resuscitation (self-inflating) bag (with reservoir if possible), adult and paediatric size
Suction device with tube connected, checked for tightness
Oxygen nasal prongs, masks
Oral airways
Face masks and laryngeal masks different sizes
Laryngoscope set with checked batteries and light source
Endotracheal tubes different sizes with connectors
Stiff or gum elastic bougie or both
Breathing tubes/circuit
Angle piece, tube connector, catheter mounts to be connected at the patient end of the circuit
Magill forceps different sizes

Monitoring Equipment:

Stethoscope
Vital signs monitor if available, or
Pulse oximeter (with spare probe if available)
Sphygmomanometer or other BP device (adult, child, and neonate cuffs)

Disposables and Consumables:

Gloves, sterile and unsterile
Swabs
Adhesive tape
Disinfectant for hands and surfaces
Intravenous cannulae, needles, syringes size 2 ml, 5 ml, 10 ml, 20 ml, and, if available, 1 ml
Infusions (e.g. NS, RL, DNS)
Infusion giving sets
Spinal needles (multiple sizes if available, e.g. 22 g, 23 g and 25 g)
Electrocardiogram sticker electrodes if available
Nasogastric tubes and bags
Suction catheters size 10 Ch, 12 Ch, 16 Ch
Bladder catheters and urinary bags
Breathing circuit filters if available

Other:

Pressure infusion bag
Blankets to keep patient warm
Pillows, belts
Sharps disposal container for discarding needles

4.2.3 Essential Drugs for Anaesthesia Management

Although the list is for essential drugs, not all of them will be available and needed everywhere. Often it is sufficient to just have one or two of the suggested drugs per row. In some countries, other drugs instead of the listed ones are used. It is impossible to cover all drugs which are used worldwide here. For details of pharmacology please see Chap. 7. *Create your own list of essential drugs which should always be present in the OR,* and a list of the drugs which should be available at a central place of the operation theatre, e.g. anaesthesia office/store with a fridge/cupboard for drugs which ideally should have a lock and a defined person who has the key. Before starting the operation list of the day, and before starting emergency operation during on-call, check with the list if all essential drugs are at hand. After finishing a case, refill the anaesthesia working place since in very acute emergency there may be no time to check and fetch items.

Intravenous fluids: Normal saline, lactated Ringer's solution or similar, NS with 5% glucose, plasma expander like hydroxyethyl starch, Haemaccel®, or Plasmion®, 100 ml NS if available, water for injection

Sedatives: Diazepam or midazolam, promethazine or chlorpromazine

Hypnotics: Ketamine, propofol or thiopental, halothane and/or isoflurane/sevoflurane/or others

Vasoactive medications: Atropine, adrenaline (epinephrine), ephedrine or others, hydralazine

Analgesics: Ketamine (which is both, analgesic and hypnotic), opioids like fentanyl and/or morphine, pethidine or tramadol; optional IV paracetamol, NSAIDs like diclofenac or ketorolac ampoules; optional ibuprofen suppositories, or other analgesics

Opioid antagonist: Naloxone if available (only where opioids are used)

Neuromuscular relaxants/reversal: Succinylcholine, optional atracurium, pancuronium, or others; neostigmine for reversal

Local anaesthetics: Lidocaine, hyperbaric or isobaric bupivacaine, or other LA

Antibiotics: Amoxicillin + clavulanic acid, cefazolin, ceftriaxone, gentamicin, metronidazole

Cortisone: Dexamethasone or betamethasone, and hydrocortisone

Drugs for obstetrics: Oxytocin and ergometrine (if available) or misoprostol

Others: Dextrose 10%, calcium gluconate, potassium chloride if available, tranexamic acid, magnesium sulphate, furosemide, salbutamol or aminophylline.

4.3 Preparing the Patient in the Operation Room

4.3.1 The Anaesthesia Record

The anaesthesia record form is an important document which must be kept timely and carefully. Medical practitioners must keep records of all procedures, consultations, and, if they are anaesthetists, record all drugs administered and patient's vital signs during anaesthesia and recovery. It helps also to recognise any problems or deterioration of the patient better as it gives the trends of vital signs like heart rate or blood pressure. Please see an example for an anaesthesia record in the Appendices. Every hospital should create its own or adopt existing forms. The number of hours should be matching most of operations which are performed including time for anaesthesia induction and emergence, e.g. 3 h, but some hospitals would need 4 or more hours or an anaesthesia record on both sides of the paper. Even a "record No. 2" for the same patient may be required for very long procedures. In the recovery area either the anaesthesia record would be continued, or a special patient observation form would be used. The standard drugs which are very often used should be printed on the anaesthesia record form but leaving enough empty rows to add other medication. It is by convention that vital signs as pulse and BP are recorded every 5 min. However, in some situations, especially after anaesthesia induction or giving spinal anaesthesia, BP should be measured more frequently, and not all of these measurements can be recorded on the form.

Special events should be written as free text under "Remarks" or on the rear page, especially complications or cardiac arrest with subsequent resuscitation. In a situation like cardiac arrest, it is very helpful to start a timer, e.g. the stopwatch of your mobile phone if it is possible without delay. Some patient vital signs monitors and anaesthesia machines have a timer function, just to press a button to start measuring the elapsing time. That tool helps you, e.g. to administer drugs like adrenaline exactly every 3–5 min. The anaesthesia record can even be a document of importance if a patient or the relatives would go to court after severe complications. Therefore, thorough documentation is also protecting staff and helping to get a fair appraisal. Also for internal quality control and audits, anaesthetic records can be useful.

4.3.2 Patient Preparation, Venous Access, Monitoring, Preloading with Fluid

Place the patient on the operation table, check the patient's identity, introduce yourself with your name and function to the patient, insert an IV cannula and start a drip, usually Ringer's lactate, alternatively, NS. If patient was fasting many hours, consider around 500 ml as fast infusion for preloading. Apply monitoring: measure the BP and document it on your anaesthesia record. Attach the pulse oximeter and, if available the ECG, alternatively a precordial stethoscope. If ECG monitor is available but no disposable electrodes use little jelly or moist cotton wool (with NS) on the skin, attach ECG cable and use adhesive tape for fixation. Document the heart rate/

pulse rate on your anaesthesia record. It is very important to do this before giving the GA or spinal anaesthesia, because if you start writing later, you might have forgotten the exact time and values to be recorded. It is much easier to keep up with all this if you are a team of two persons.

Ask the surgeon if the patient should receive antibiotic prophylaxis. If yes, prepare the drug and inject it before starting anaesthesia, since the antibiotic will be most effective if administered 20–30 min prior to surgery.

If the patient is to get general anaesthesia you need to preoxygenate him/her for 3 min. You may save time by asking the surgeon or runner or anaesthesia assistant to hold the face mask with oxygen while you are preparing the anaesthesia record and the monitoring. If you are planning laryngeal mask (LM) or endotracheal intubation, set the timer of your mobile phone or at the patient monitor, if available, to 3 min so that you are sure to have preoxygenated adequately. Of course, in life-threatening bleeding or other high urgent situation, the procedure may be shortened. Then start giving anaesthesia drugs.

After induction and securing the airway devices, protect the eyes with adhesive tape. The cornea can easily be damaged because the eyelid reflexes are absent during GA.

Before spinal anaesthesia, no preoxygenation is necessary but check your concentrator before taking the patient to the OR to be sure it is working. If you are preparing for caesarean section, switch the concentrator on immediately before you are starting to give the spinal, because you should apply oxygen via nasal prongs until the baby is delivered.

4.3.3 Prevention of Wound Infection During and After Surgery

4.3.3.1 Patient Hygiene

It is particularly important and should be mandatory everywhere that the patient has a shower/the whole body washed with soap and water and gets a fresh gown and fresh bed linen before going to theatre to reduce the risk of wound infection. Sometimes, trauma patients are brought to theatre still covered with the dust from the road accident (of course, the patient with severe bleeding should immediately be brought to theatre, but all other patients should be washed first). If the surgeon then is just painting the dirt with disinfectant instead of first washing the leg/arm to be operated on with soapy water, let it dry, and thereafter using fresh linen and disinfectant, a surgical site infection is more likely to happen. Disinfectants need a minimum of time to kill the germs. Methylated spirit and chlorhexidine are effective within 1 min while povidone-iodine would need 3 min. Please use a timer (mobile phone) or observe a clock. Povidone-iodine is contraindicated in patients with allergy towards iodine and with risk for thyroid storm before goitre surgery.

4.3.3.2 Hand Hygiene

With good hand hygiene, we can prevent cross infection between patients. Be aware of the risk that germs are surviving on surfaces as anaesthesia machine, monitor, trolley, and so on if we touch them after we have touched patients or our own face (which we should not do). Hand disinfectant must be available at every anaesthesia working place, and it is the responsibility of the AP to always have a bottle with it ready. Wearing gloves does not reduce the need for hand disinfection, and gloves cannot be disinfected. Before putting on gloves, you need to sanitise hands. After touching the patient with gloves you need to remove them before touching clean surfaces. After removal of gloves hand disinfection is necessary again.

4.3.3.3 Antibiotic Prophylaxis

To give a single dose of IV antibiotic is standard for operations with a significant risk for infection. It is necessary before all kind of orthopaedic surgery, plastic surgery, skin grafting, neurosurgery, colorectal surgery, and gynaecological operations, as well as caesarean section. It is optional for gastric surgery and gall bladder operations unless the patient has a perforated ulcer or acute cholecystolithiasis with fever. Inguinal hernia, breast surgery, thyroid surgery, or haemorrhoidectomy are also examples of operations where antibiotic is not mandatory. Although it is the responsibility of the surgeon to prescribe antibiotics, it is wise as AP to remember the surgeon and ask if antibiotic should be administered and which kind, because surgeons in some hospitals tend to forget about antibiotic prophylaxis, and in operation theatre we always act as a team.

The antibiotic must be given shortly before surgery is starting. It is not effective to begin the antibiotic after operation. A single dose is often sufficient.

Cloxacillin or Ampiclox®, cephazolin or cefuroxime are effective first-line drugs as antibiotic prophylaxis. Patients with known penicillin allergy should receive clindamycin instead. In colon surgery, metronidazole needs to be added. Ceftriaxon in combination with gentamicin is an alternative where the first-line drugs are unavailable. Gentamicin may cause rare but devastating side effects on kidneys or the inner ear especially if given in overdose. The correct dose is 3–6 mg/kg, not more, IM or IV with infusion over approximately 30 min. Avoid fast IV injection since a high peak plasma concentration is more likely to cause tinnitus or even irreversible loss of vestibular function including sense of balance.

4.4 Positioning on the Operation Table

4.4.1 Supine Position Flat, with Head Up or Head Down

Patients who are anaesthetised cannot move, and they cannot feel numbness or pain. That implies risk for damage from position on the operating table. Even persistent paresis is possible if nerves are damaged.

Supine flat: Avoid damage of the brachial plexus by keeping the arms not more than 90° abducted from the body. Avoid damage of the ulnar nerve caused by compression of the elbow against the operating table or arm holder. Patients with large abdominal mass can develop aortocaval compression syndrome with decreased venous return and cardiac failure. Obese patients get impaired lung function because their functional residual capacity is decreasing markedly. They are prone to deoxygenate fast during apnoea.

Head up position, e.g. during laparoscopic procedures, is likely to cause significant decrease of blood pressure. It may be difficult to keep a sufficient blood pressure. The patient must be fixed well to avoid sliding on the table.

Head down position, also called Trendelenburg position: this position is used for elective operations, usually laparoscopic procedures. The diaphragm is moved upwards, the functional residual capacity of the lungs is markedly decreased. Ventilation should be with PEEP (positive end expiratory pressure). If the anaesthesia machine does not have a PEEP valve, surgery in Trendelenburg position should not be performed. The risk for brachial plexus damage is increased. Padded holders for the shoulders are needed to prevent the patient from sliding.

4.4.2 Lateral Position

After turning an intubated patient, listen to both lungs and confirm that the ETT/LM is still in place. Have a plan for the event of airway dislocation. Lateral position is used by orthopaedic surgeons for some types of ORIF of the femur, and for other types of surgery which are uncommon in remote hospitals (like kidney or lung surgery). Ventilation problems can occur as the lower lung is well perfused but not so well ventilated while the upper lung is well ventilated but not so well perfused. That leads to ventilation-perfusion mismatch, and in patients with impaired lung function, this may leads to desaturation. Have oxygen ready even if the patient has spinal anaesthesia. Wait at least 10 min after bupivacaine injection before the patient is turned into lateral position, otherwise the upper leg which is to be operated on may not be anaesthetised. In the lateral position, the brachial plexus of the lower side can be damaged. Even the upper arm must not be stretched too much. A pillow for the head is essential.

4.4.3 Prone Position

Prone position is not uncommon, e.g. for lipoma resection on the back, or for certain type of humerus ORIF. Turning a patient into prone position is not without risk. Have a plan for cardiac arrest in prone position. A stretcher should be available outside the room so that the patient in such situation can quickly be turned for resuscitation. You need enough persons to do put patients in prone position. All cannulae, airways, and so on need to be fixed particularly well. Beware of accidental extubation and of losing intravenous access! Before turning the patient, extra doses of IV anaesthetics should be given to avoid light anaesthesia or arousal. Remember, that muscle relaxants are not anaesthetics. A relaxed but insufficiently anaesthetised patient might wake up but cannot move which is a terrible experience. Before turning the patient, disconnect BP cuff, ECG and pulse oximeter, infusion and finally the breathing tubes. Be careful with the patient's neck when turning him/her. Also the eyes and the lower ear need to be protected. Have a soft ring to put the head in a lateral position with the ear being protected, or use special face down pillows designed for prone position. After turning, connect breathing tubes again, confirm the patient is ventilated, the anaesthetic is continued and start the infusion again. Attach pulse oximeter and ECG and take BP. Listen to both lungs. Aim to make the phase without vital signs monitoring as short as possible, normally not more than 2 min. Pulse oximeter is always the last to disconnect and the first to connect. To feel the pulse is also a useful measure to quickly know if BP is probably adequate. Before turning a patient, all team members should know their roll and task.

4.4.4 Lithotomy Position

Around 90° flexed hips and knees with the legs in a higher position than the trunk. This position is common for haemorrhoidal operations, anal fistula or urological surgery, for gynaecological procedures at the vagina, and for vaginal hysterectomy. Anaesthesia is usually with spinal. Wait at least 10 min after giving spinal anaesthesia before putting patient into lithotomy since there is risk for too high spread of the spinal anaesthesia before it is "fixed". Risk for damage of the peroneus nerve and other nerves in direct contact with the leg holders should be addressed and the leg holders should be padded. Elevate both legs simultaneously to avoid back pain. Make sure that the patient's pelvis and sacrum have direct contact with the table and avoid them slipping off the table edge. In patients under GA, hold the head and the tube or laryngeal mask, resp., while moving the patient.

4.5 Patient Safety and Checklists

A list with phone numbers should be available and updated, so that in difficult situation—several injured patients brought to the hospital and the like—even someone who is not on call could be called from home. The hospital should find a way to reward such extraordinary commitment.

The heads of the hospital departments should meet regularly and discuss issues of patient safety and how it can be improved.

All staff must follow the principle "**Call for help**, then check **A**irway **B**reathing **C**irculation **D**isability **D**rugs" during any critical incident. It is under no circumstances safe to have one single anaesthesia provider being alone with nobody available to be called for help. Consider patient transfer and perform only lifesaving, necessary operations if situation is like that. If there is only one trained anaesthetist at the whole health facility, at least two more persons should be trained on the job thoroughly to act as professional assistants. Unfortunately there is shortage of trained anaesthesia providers in many countries.

The WHO created a globally adopted checklist for safe surgery (see under further reading, can be downloaded). They recommend a "time out session" before starting surgery. That procedure has saved a lot of lives worldwide and helps preventing avoidable complications such as amputating the wrong leg, operating the wrong eye, giving an antibiotic the patient is known to be allergic to, and so on. To do a briefing with anaesthesia checklist is preventing many avoidable anaesthesia complications.

Create a mandatory scheme to be followed at your health facility, print it and laminate it, have it in every theatre.

Please adopt/change phrases in the example given here to your facility and create your genuine *Name (of the health facility) Hospital Safe Surgery Checklist*. The checklist consists of two to three parts. If anything is unavailable which is listed, discuss in the team and with the surgeon if you should go ahead with the patient or postpone/transfer the patient because of too high risk.

Before starting anaesthesia, the anaesthesia team should always perform the following briefing:

Anaesthesia Safety Checklist before Starting Anaesthesia:

- Electricity—stable or unreliable, generator available?
- Oxygen—concentrator working and switched on, or cylinder turned on and filling pressure sufficient for the planned anaesthesia, or piped oxygen available?
- Anaesthesia machine—check performed, circuit no leakage, vaporiser filled and working?
- Self-inflating bag and face mask proper size?
- Suction machine working and suction catheters available?
- Patient monitor working/pulse oximeter, stethoscope, BP cuff?
- Laryngoscope with proper size blade functioning?
- Endotracheal tubes plus laryngeal mask correct sizes and stylet/bougie for difficult intubation at hand?
- Drugs prepared in correctly labelled syringes?
- Emergency drugs like atropine, ephedrine, adrenaline, prepared?
- Infusions, syringes, cannulae, adhesive tape?
- Critical moments expected during the planned anaesthetia?
- Patient has known allergy? Difficult airway anticipated? Fasting? Aspiration risk?
- Mobile phone number of the one we may call for help?

After anaesthesia is completed and before starting surgery, the whole theatre team including the surgeon is performing the following time-out procedure:

Surgical Checklist Before Starting the Operation:

- Name of the patient
- Procedure planned
- Site of the procedure (check with X-ray if applicable)
- Expected blood loss >10–15 ml/kg BW? If yes, is blood available?
- Antibiotics administered (if applicable)?
- Do all team members know each other? If not, everybody is presenting himself by name and function/roll
- Scrubb nurse: is sterility confirmed? All equipment/instruments ready?
- Anaesthetist: any problems anticipated?
- ICU place available in case of anticipated problems during recovery?

At the end of surgery, a short debriefing of the whole surgical team with everyone in theatre present is also recommended:

Sign-Out Debriefing List:

- Was the conduct of surgery as planned? Any complications?
- Scrubb nurse: Instrument, needle, sponge/swabs counts are correct?
- Anaesthesia went well? Any problems? Have long acting muscle relaxants been reversed?
- Recovery period: Any problems are to be expected? How are they to be dealt with? Where should the patient be observed and for how long? Analgesics are already administered/prescribed? Any other drugs/infusions prescribed?

Further Reading

Ariyo P, Trelles M, Helmand R, Amir Y, Hassani GH, Mftavyanka J et al (2016) Providing anesthesia care in resource-limited settings. A 6-year analysis of anesthesia services provided at médecins sans frontières facilities. Anesthesiology 124(3):561–569

Bashford T, Morriss W, Roques C, Shamamba N, Wilkes M (2020) Perioperative care. In: Craven R, Edgcombe H, Gupta B (eds) Global anaesthesia. Oxford University Press, Oxford, pp 77–91

Kirkbride D (2019) The practical conduct of anaesthesia: preparation for anaesthesia. Patient positioning for surgery. In: Thompson J, Moppett I, Wiles M (eds) Smith and Aitkenhead's textbook of anaesthesia, 7th edn. Elsevier, London, pp 441–455

The WHO surgical safety checklist. From: safe surgery saves lives - WHO/IER/PSP/2008.07 © World Health Organization. 2008; Reprint 2009

Woodman N, Walker I. World Health Organization Surgical safety checklist. Anaesthesia tutorial of the week. WFSA. Feb. 2016:Tutorial 325

5 Post-anaesthesia Care

Abstract

Patients after major surgery with spinal or general anaesthesia should continuously be observed by a qualified nurse until all vital signs are stable and the patient has regained consciousness, or, after spinal anaesthesia, the block has begun to wear off. They should not be transferred to the peripheral ward too early.

Avoidable complications and even death in the early postoperative phase are likely if patients are left unattended, or resuscitation equipment, oxygen, or suction device are unavailable.

On arrival in the recovery area, the nurse should assess the patient with the ABCDE approach after having received a short report by the anaesthesia provider about the anaesthesia and surgery. An observation chart must be kept, or the anaesthesia record may be continued for postoperative monitoring.

Airway: check if the patient needs an oropharyngeal or nasopharyngeal airway after extubation, and check the ability to cough and swallow sufficiently. Have a suction device ready.

Breathing: look at the chest excursions, count respiratory rate, and measure oxygen saturation (aim for >94) with a pulse oximeter. Give oxygen if required.

Circulation: take BP and pulse, continue infusions. Check Hb if bleeding was huge and give blood if required.

Drugs and disability: are analgesic and antiemetic drugs prescribed? Adjust drip rate. Check consciousness level and pain intensity.

Exposure: check body temperature and keep the patient warm. Check wound dressings, drainages, and urine output.

Criteria for discharge and transfer to the peripheral ward should be defined clearly.

Keywords

Delayed extubation · Discharge criteria · Post-anaesthesia care · Post-anaesthesia complications · PACU · Postoperative analgesia

5.1 Recovery Area, Equipment

Many severe anaesthesia-related complications worldwide could be prevented by continuously observing patients after surgery until they are able to keep their airway patent and breathe sufficiently, have stable blood pressure and pulse rate, and are able to communicate. Post-anaesthesia care should be performed in a specially designated recovery area or recovery room close to the operation rooms. In larger hospitals with several operation rooms, a post-anaesthesia care unit (PACU) should be integrated in the theatre complex and have trained nursing staff. The recovery area should have good lighting, stable electricity, oxygen, suc-

D. Kietzmann, *Anaesthesia in Remote Hospitals*, Sustainable Development Goals Series,
https://doi.org/10.1007/978-3-031-46610-6_5

tion device, and monitoring equipment. The patients can be lying on padded stretchers with protection from falling off, or they can be lying in their own, cleaned beds with fresh linen. The wheels of the beds are not increasing risk for infection when moved to inside the theatre building. For the patients, the bed is more comfortable and should be preferred. If possible, stretchers and beds should be adjustable for head up position. If more than one patient is in the recovery area at the same time, a separation screen between beds is recommended for keeping privacy, but that screen must not hinder the nurse from seeing the patients. Blankets to keep patients warm are mandatory, particularly if room temperature is not high since patients might have got cold during operation and need to be warmed up. Drip stands must be available for every patient.

Most important monitoring "equipment" is of course the nurse who is present and alert without interruption and observing the patient carefully. Observation of patient's breathing cannot be replaced by pulse oximetry, and pulse oximetry cannot be replaced by just the person who is observing the patient; both are complementary. Ideally the staff in the recovery area is a trained nurse anaesthetist, alternatively a nurse who has been trained on the job by the anaesthetists and has basic knowledge about anaesthesia, Advanced Life Support, and about recognising and managing possible complications after surgery. Two persons staff are required if more than two patients are to be cared for at the same time. A patient who is still intubated, unconscious after extubation, or circulatory unstable would need a nurse on a one-to-one base.

A stethoscope, BP device, pulse oximeter, and thermometer are highly recommended and should not be missing. A ventilation bag (SIB) with face masks multiple sizes must be available. A laryngoscope, defibrillator, or resuscitation cart is also recommended. Rescue drugs, syringes and needles, swabs, sharps disposal container, hand disinfectant, gloves, adhesive tape, nasal prongs for application of oxygen, suction catheters, some infusions, and a phone for communication are essential. If available, a glucose meter is useful as quite many patients are diabetics.

The findings are either recorded on the anaesthesia record (just as continuation sheet), or a special observation list is started for the postoperative period. The latter is preferred if the patient needs prolonged observation and intermediate care. The observation list can later be continued by the staff in the HDU or ICU or the critical patients' area in the surgical ward. Example of an observation record form, please see under Appendices.

5.2 Admission to Recovery Area, ABCDE Assessment, Managing Complications, Discharge

Do never send a patient to the general ward immediately or just few minutes after finishing GA and performing extubation. A hospital is responsible to provide adequate staffing. If recovery staff is unavailable, the anaesthesia provider is responsible for the patient until he/she has regained airway control, consciousness, and stable circulation, even if that is causing delay to start the next patient who may need anaesthesia. The patient must be breathing sufficiently and showing stable vital signs before transfer from the OR to the recovery area. Long-acting muscle relaxants should have been reversed, and the patient should be able to lift his head and to keep eyes open.

As soon as the patient is arriving in the recovery area—whether it is improvised on the corridor or in an indicated separated and equipped room or area—the nurse who is to take over the patient needs to get a systematic, short report for handing over the patient by the anaesthesia provider: Patient's name, age, operation performed, type of anaesthesia, previous disease, drug allergies, complications if any, amount of blood loss, analgesics already given or not yet, need for blood transfusion, lab checks like Hb or b-glucose, and the last vital signs should be included in the report. The anaesthetist should also inform the recovery nurse about discharge criteria and be available on phone.

After admission and taking over the patient in the recovery room the nurse should immediately check ABCDE and record these vital signs and other findings on the post-anaesthesia form or on the anaesthesia record if there is no separate form for the post-operative period. **A** means *airway*, **B** *breathing*, **C** means *circulation*, **D** *disability* (consciousness) and *drugs*—is there any need for analgesic or antiemetic drugs? **E** *exposure* means body temperature and wounds/dressings/drains.

- A—check if the patient is keeping a patent airway. Maybe he/she is still needing a Guedel oropharyngeal airway, a nasopharyngeal airway or needs to keep the ETT or the LM until awake.
- B—count the respiratory rate during one minute using the timer of your mobile phone. Check oxygen saturation with a pulse oximeter. Listen to the breathing sounds and look if the thorax and the diaphragm are moving adequately.
- C—feel the pulse and measure the BP.
- D—continue with the infusion at appropriate drip rate and ask the patient if he is feeling pain, how much the pain is (little—moderate—severe—very severe—unbearable) and administer antipain medicine if necessary. Record the level of pain before and after treatment. Ask the patient if he is feeling unwell—nauseating and have a kidney dish available in case of vomiting. If needed ask the responsible surgeon to prescribe an antiemetic drug. Patients who are restless but don't respond to verbal command may need analgesia or, if pain is unlikely, a sedative drug like small dose of diazepam, promethazine, chlorpromazine or, if available, clonidine.
- E—check patient's body temperature, apply warm blanket if low or patient is shivering, check wound drains, urine bag, nasogastric drainage bag, and the dressings for postoperative bleeding.

5.2.1 Complications in the Early Post-Anaesthesia Phase

Airway obstruction due to loss of pharyngeal muscle tone is a common cause for hypoxia which may cause death if unobserved and untreated. Patients after major abdominal surgery are at highest risk. Even after patient's emergence from anaesthesia with regaining consciousness, residual effects of inhalational anaesthetics, opioids and muscle relaxants are lasting up to several hours. While the diaphragm is recovering early after muscle relaxation so that the patient can breathe, the muscles in the pharynx for swallowing, coughing, and keeping the airway patent are still weak for a longer period. This applies even for patients who have received reversal agents like neostigmine. Neostigmine is not reversing the effects of MR completely although muscle tone will be better than without antagonising non-depolarising MR at all. Nursing patients in a lateral position with the head being the lowest part of the body may be helpful. In patients who were alert but fall asleep again and seem to have airway obstruction, a jaw thrust manoeuvre, oropharyngeal airway device, or applying continuous positive airway pressure (CPAP) via facemask can be lifesaving. Consider re-intubation in patients who are not recovering within short time. Patients are at risk to be extubated too early. With the ETT in place, breathing may seem adequate, but shortly after extubation, when the stimulus of the ETT, and of being moved from operation table to stretcher or bed is absent, patient may be unable to clear upper airway secretions. Even after short-acting MR and ketamine GA there is risk for aspiration of secretions. Clinically, the patient's pharyngeal muscle strength can be assessed by the ability to strongly oppose a tongue depressor. A less reliable test is the ability to lift the head off the bed for 5 s. If the patient cannot do that, assume a non-patent airway! Patients with residual paralysis who are surviving the early postoperative phase are at significantly higher risk to get pneumonia as complication after surgery, a complication which is normally not related to anaesthesia but may be caused by inappropriate anaesthetic and post-anaesthesia management.

Laryngospasm (see Sect. 15.4.1), a sudden occlusion of the vocal cords, can occur in the early post-extubation phase upon awakening and is triggered by secretions in the airway. A small amount of saliva can already cause laryngospasm. Risk is highest in children. It is recognised by continuous observation of chest movements (never leave a patient alone, not even a minute, before fully awake and with patent airway). Paradoxical movements of the diaphragm are indicating laryngospam already before saturation is dropping and require immediate action. Unrecognised, the patient may die. Treatment is suctioning secretions and applying jaw thrust with positive ventilation pressure via ambubag/SIB. If available, attach oxygen at high flow rate to create a high ventilation pressure to break the laryngospam. If laryngospasm persists, succinylcholine is required. That situation is difficult to manage if you are working alone which is not regarded as safe. An assistant who is preparing a syringe must always be immediately available, even during night and public holidays if operations with GA are performed. In severe cases, intubation may be required.

Hypotension and oliguria are often caused by volume deficiency and require fast infusion of 500–1000 ml RL. Check Hb and consider BT if below transfusion threshold. If no improvement, call the surgeon, consider vasopressor, and aim for patient care in a high dependency or intensive care unit. Check if the abdomen is tense if urine production is inadequate and inform the surgeon if elevated intraabdominal pressure is suspected.

Hypothermia is common after major surgery and more likely in cold operation rooms with poorly adjustable AC. Patients after spinal and general anaesthesia are at risk and would feel unwell if body temperature is <36 °C. As platelet function is impaired with hypothermia, wound healing is delayed, and shivering may increase the risk for myocardial ischaemia, it is not just unpleasant but potentially hazardous. Apply warm blanket, have the room as warm as possible, give warmed infusions. Shivering can be treated with drugs: pethidine 25 mg or clonidine, 60–75 μg IV is usually effective within minutes. If both drugs are unavailable, morphine 2–5 mg is an alternative while tramadol is a bit less effective.

Nausea and vomiting can be treated with antiemetic drugs, see Sect. 7.10. In patients at risk for PONV, antiemetic drugs should be given as prophylaxis. If nausea or vomiting occurs, a different antiemetic must be given since additional doses of the same agent would not be effective before at least 6 h after the last dose have elapsed.

Emergence agitation early after awakening is transient, common after ketamine GA and in children after inhalation anaesthesia. Do not leave the patient alone, prevent him/her from falling off the bed, and exclude pain as a cause. Most patients will be calm again after a short while.

Discharge criteria: vital signs stable, breathing with patent airway and oxygen saturation >94% on room air; patient is awake and able to communicate, or easily arousable by voice; pain is treated, patient is not vomiting, and there are no obvious surgical complications like bleeding. In patients where SpO_2 is not rising >94% with air but is at least 94% with breathing oxygen, consider transfer to a ward with prepared oxygen source for the patient. Beware patient getting hypoxic on the way to the ward. Ideally, a transportable oxygen cylinder should be available for such cases. Pulse oximeters are essential; without which it is extremely difficult and often impossible to assess patient's oxygenation. Avoidable deaths are likely to occur if such a small device is missing in a hospital. AP must be in constant contact with the administration if essential equipment for patient safety is unavailable.

5.3 Postoperative Analgesia

Pain must be treated, and postoperative pain is common so that standards for postoperative analgesia are required in all hospitals.

Different analgesic drugs and local anaesthetics have different mechanisms of action. If combined, the total effect is more than additive. The combination of different types of analgesics or of systemic analgesics with local anaesthetics is called *multi-modal analgesia*. This way to treat pain should be preferred since side effects would be minimised while analgesia would be optimised with the multimodal approach. If the surgeon or the anaesthetist is trained and skilled to perform regional blocks, equipment and drugs for that purpose are available, postoperative pain relief can often be provided in excellent way using regional anaesthesia. However, that is beyond the scope of this handbook.

Wound infiltration with LA, on the other hand, is a simple, cheap, and effective option which is easy to perform and appropriate for, e. g. hernia repair, laparoscopy, caesarean section, abdominal hysterectomy, colon resection, breast surgery, and many others. Encourage your surgeons to perform wound infiltration whenever possible. Addition of 5 μg adrenaline per ml to the local anaesthetic (0.2 mg adrenaline = 0.2 ml adrenaline 1 mg/ml plus 40 ml LA) increases duration of action and decreases LA toxicity.

The required dose of analgesics is lower if pain level is lower and is increasing more than linear with increasing pain level. Therefore, it is advantageous to start treatment before pain levels are severe or more than severe. The next dose of analgesics should be administered when pain level is moderate. Regular assessment and documentation of pain intensity is important. In adults, either a numeric rating scale may be used where 0 means no pain and 10 would mean worst possible pain, or a descriptive scale can be used: 1-3 on the numeric scale corresponds to mild pain, 4–6 to moderate pain, 7–8 means severe pain, 9 is very severe pain, 10 is maximum pain. Pain scores are recorded on the patient observation chart, e. g. under "comments, interventions": pain score 6 → 5 mg morphine IM.

Pain before surgery, e. g. after trauma requires analgesic before operation. Postoperative analgesia with analgesic drugs can be performed as follows:

- Paracetamol may be given orally with premedication to prophylactically reduce perioperative pain.
- Intraoperatively, analgesics are part of anaesthesia. Ketamine or opioids like fentanyl, morphine, pethidine are commonly used as the analgesic component of GA. Good intraoperative analgesia usually decreases pain level after surgery.
- The first dose of postoperative analgesic should be given before the patient feels pain. Postoperative analgesics are administered by IM or IV injection during the first hours post surgery and should be given orally as soon as the patient is able and allowed to swallow water and drugs.

Average doses of common analgesics slowly IV (only in the postoperative recovery area by the AP or in the ICU, not in the general ward), IM, or later orally, for adults:

Paracetamol 0.5–1 g QDS, and diclofenac 75 mg BD, or ketorolac 30 mg TDS, or ibuprofen 400–600 mg TDS (not available for injection). This combination would be sufficient to treat mild to moderate pain. Remember that patients with renal impairment, asthma, or gastric ulcer should not receive NSAID (diclofenac, ibuprofen, ketorolac) but may get paracetamol.

For severe pain one opioid analgesic is added as a stronger component of multimodal analgesia: Tramadol 50–150 mg QDS, or pethidine 50-100 mg QDS (not available for oral administration) or morphine 5–10 mg QDS, or pentazocine 30 mg IM or 50–100 mg orally QDS, or buprenorphine 0.3–0.6 mg IM or 0.2–0.4 mg sublingually TDS.

Before and after each dose, pain intensity is assessed. Opioid drugs are stopped when pain levels decrease below 4–5 on the numeric scale or are mild to moderate.

For same type of injury or surgery, individual patients may require quite different amounts of analgesics and experience different intensity of pain.

Monitor conscious level and pulse oximetry closely. Also monitor respiratory rate (breaths per minute), pulse rate and BP after opioid drugs. In patients at high risk for respiratory depression, tramadol may be used instead of morphine as it is weaker and causes less respiratory depression.

Analgesics should be prescribed according to the severity of pain anticipated from the surgery and the anticipated, appropriate, postoperative route of administration.

Pain should be assessed at regular intervals postoperatively in the recovery area and after transfer of the patient on the general ward. Pain scores should be recorded with other routine postoperative observations. Prescription of analgesics should be adjusted to the individual requirements of the patient. The surgeon or assigned medical officer in the surgical ward should perform at least two rounds daily during the first two postoperative days after major surgery and additional rounds on request by the responsible nurse.

5.4 Intermediate or High-Dependency Care Unit

High-dependency care is improving the outcome of sick patients significantly. Since patients with acute impairment of vital organs are admitted to almost all health facilities, even a small hospital should have at least an improvised area or room for intermediate or high-dependency care of sick patients. Even without high-tech equipment like artificial ventilators such intensive care is making difference. The most important factor for improving outcome is the continuously present, alert, and observing nurse 24 h 7 days a week who is recording vital signs, fluid intake and output (infusions, urine output, losses from drains, and so on) and interventions like giving oxygen on an observation chart (see example in the Appendices).

When it comes to equipment, the most important one is available and affordable oxygen.

Oxygen can be delivered via nasal prongs or, in more difficult to oxygenate patients, a face mask connected to a reservoir bag. A CPAP/PEEP valve between a tightly fitting mask and SIB would further improve ventilatory support. Electricity 24/7, sufficient light, and a suction device are also very important. Oxygen concentrators are by far the cheapest tool to deliver oxygen but need stable electrical power and regular maintenance (see Sect. 3.2). Drugs and disposables approximately the same as in the recovery unit, see Sect. 5.1. A functioning suction device with large bore suction catheters is essential for removing secretions from the airways. Minimum monitoring is pulse oximetry which is not that expensive, and blood pressure machine plus stethoscope. A traditional sphygmomanometer for manual measurement of BP is as exact or even superior to automatic BP devices. A vital signs patient monitor is nice to have but not mandatory for improving outcome. An observation chart for vital signs and interventions is essential and findings must be recorded at least once per hour and at any time if patient is changing condition. A plan whom to call if patient deteriorates is necessary. Sick patients after abdominal surgery often need intensive nursing care for several days until they are starting oral feeding and ambulation. Physiotherapy with focus on breathing and encouraging coughing is also particularly helpful. Patients must not be lying flat supine 24 h but be turned every few hours and kept half sitting several hours per day if possible. Infusions should be monitored and fluids matching requirements.

5.4.1 Criteria for and Management of Delayed Extubation

Patients for acute abdominal surgery who are presenting late after several days history and who undergo GA with intubation, especially those who received a non-depolarising MR like pancuronium or atracurium, and those who were circulatory unstable perioperatively should not be extubated immediately at the end of operation. They may breathe spontaneously with a simple T-piece attached to the ETT and oxygen connected.

A PEEP valve, adjustable and reusable, which can be attached to the T-piece or any SIB (e. g. ambubag) would help to decrease atelectasis and improve oxygenation. The SIB is connected to the ETT. Make sure it would not pull at the tube. For most patients, a PEEP of 5 cm H_2O is sufficient. Obese patients should receive PEEP 7–8. If $S_pO_2 <$ 94% with PEEP, give oxygen 1–6 l/min. In patients with poor oxygenation despite regular spontaneous breathing with PEEP and oxygen, use a reservoir bag attached to the SIB to increase FiO_2.

If patient is showing respiratory insufficiency even then, perform assisted manual ventilation with the SIB or put the patient on ventilator if available. If mechanical ventilation is no option, you might need a caregiver 24 h at the bedside to assist ventilation. Aim for having pulse oximeter attached, at least intermittently. If the caregiver/health assistant/nurse who would ventilate the patient is not trained for that and not used to that particular job, close supervision is essential. The person who is delegating ventilation remains fully responsible and must be continuously available. Vital signs are checked and recorded on the observation list at least every hour, including respiratory parameters and interventions.

Additionally, assessment by responsible medical officer at least three times per 24 h is recommended for all patients in HDU or ICU. Extubation is performed by the AP when the patient is responsive, breathing sufficiently and keeping patent airway.

Further Reading

Bashford T, Morriss W, Roques C, Shamamba N, Wilkes M (2020) Perioperative care. In: Craven R, Edgcombe H, Gupta B (eds) Global anaesthesia. Oxford University Press, Oxford, pp 77–91

Braehler MR, Mizrahi I (2023) Postanesthesia recovery. In: Pardo MC (ed) Miller's basics of anaesthesia, 8th edn. Elsevier, Philadelphia, pp 697–715

Breivik H, Borchgrevink PC, Allen SM, Rosseland LA, Romundstad L, Hals EK, Kvarstein G, Stubhaug A (2008) Assessment of pain. Br J Anaesth 101(1):17–24

Shaw I, Drinkwater J (2019) Postoperative and recovery room care. In: Thompson J, Moppett I, Wiles M (eds) Smith and Aitkenhead's textbook of anaesthesia, 7th edn. Elsevier, London, pp 617–636

Whitaker DK, Booth H, Clyburn P, Harrop-Griffiths W, Hosie H, Kilvington B et al (2013) Guidelines immediate post-anaesthesia recovery 2013. Association of Anaesthetists of Great Britain and Ireland. Anaesthesia 68:288–297

6 Airway Management

Abstract

This chapter provides an overview for the management of patients' airways with affordable devices, suitable for most situations during anaesthesia and emergency.

During anaesthesia, patients often lose a patent airway and the ability to breathe sufficiently. The chin lift manoeuvre is described as well as the use of simple airway devices such as oropharyngeal or nasopharyngeal airways. A face mask must be fitting tightly. The proper size is vital for mask ventilation with the lowest possible airway pressure (max 20 cmH2O) to avoid inflation of the stomach and regurgitation of stomach contents.

For endotracheal intubation a laryngoscope with correct size of blade for the patient and a bright light is needed together with a pillow under the head dependent on the patient's anatomy, and several stylets and bougies to manage difficult intubation. Intubation should be performed by sufficiently experienced anaesthesia providers only, as failed intubation attempts may cause more damage than benefit. Supraglottic airway devices such as laryngeal masks in different sizes are easy-to use alternatives for endotracheal intubation but not suitable for all kinds of surgery. They can only be used in deep anaesthesia with strong anaesthetics, not with ketamine as the sole anaesthetic. A table with the correct size of airway devices is provided in this chapter.

Rapid sequence induction is described in detail and is performed for patients with a full stomach, e.g. with bowel obstruction or any kind of emergency surgery with a patient who is not fasting or who is undergoing laparotomy.

Keywords

Difficult airway management in resource-limited settings · Laryngeal mask airway · Performing endotracheal intubation · Rapid sequence induction

6.1 General Considerations

Anaesthetic drugs are necessarily very strong drugs; otherwise, they would not make patients tolerate even the most painful procedures without waking up and reacting. One of the most obvious side effects of these drugs is the loss of a patent airway and the ability of sufficient breathing. Ketamine is an exception, but even under ketamine patients may need artificial ventilation. Therefore, the anaesthetist must be able to secure the airway of the patient and ventilate him/her until recovery is achieved. A huge range of airway equipment is used all over the world.

D. Kietzmann, *Anaesthesia in Remote Hospitals*, Sustainable Development Goals Series,
https://doi.org/10.1007/978-3-031-46610-6_6

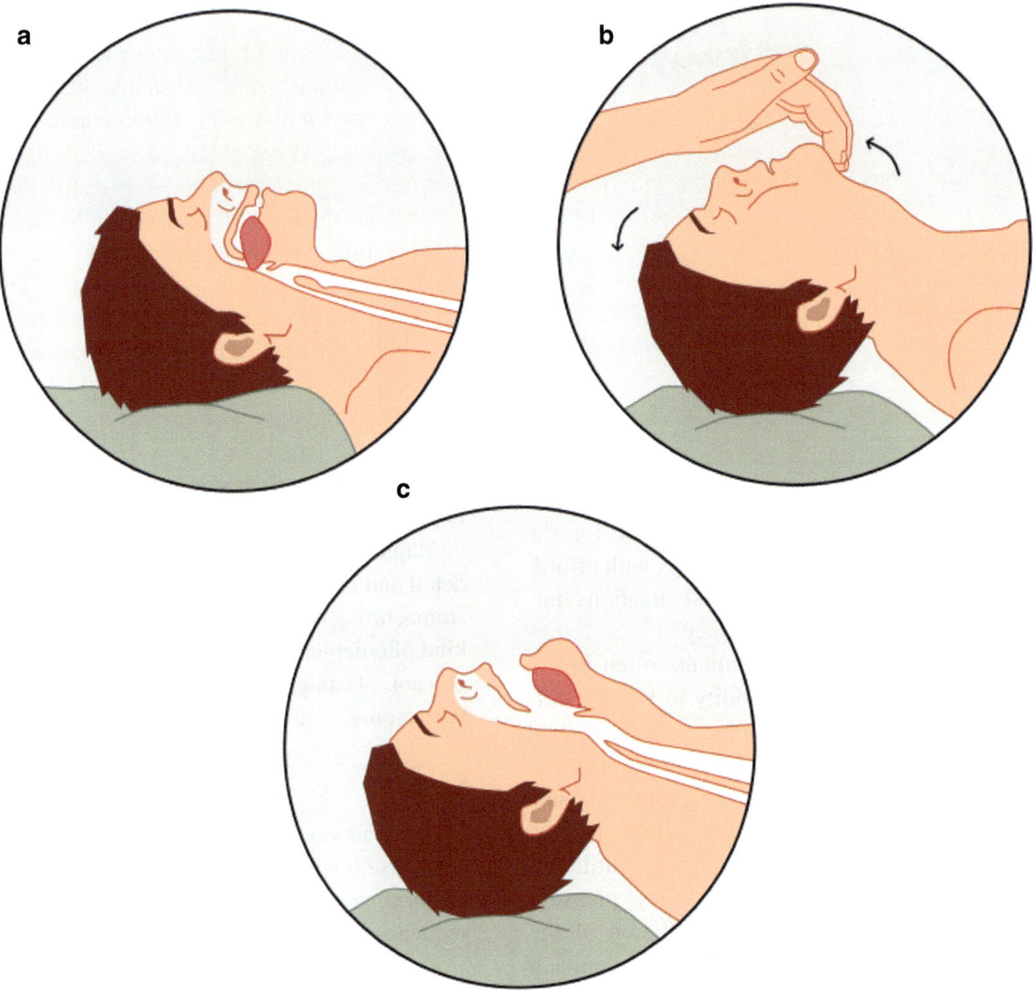

Fig. 6.1 Chin lift to keep the airway patent; (**a**) airway obstructed by tongue falling backwards; (**b**) chin lift and head tilt; (**c**) free, patent airway. Note the head being in the sniffing position

In this book, only the most relevant overview is given with affordable devices that would be sufficient to deal with most airway situations. However, the AP must be aware that nobody is able to manage every airway. It is vital to assess the airway before giving anaesthesia and to avoid anaesthetising somebody whose airway is likely to be unmanageable. Instead, such patients should be referred.

In unconscious persons, the tongue may fall backwards and obstruct the airway. Figure 6.1 shows the chin lift and head tilt manoeuvre.

6.2 Guedel Oropharyngeal Airway (OPA)

The Guedel oropharyngeal airway is a flattened tube, straight in the beginning and curved distally, keeping the tongue in place and facilitating mask ventilation, as well as spontaneous breathing in patients who are not fully conscious. It is possible to perform suction through the airway. Figure 6.2 shows the OPA and its position in the patient.

It is a simple oral or oropharyngeal airway that helps preventing the tongue from obstructing

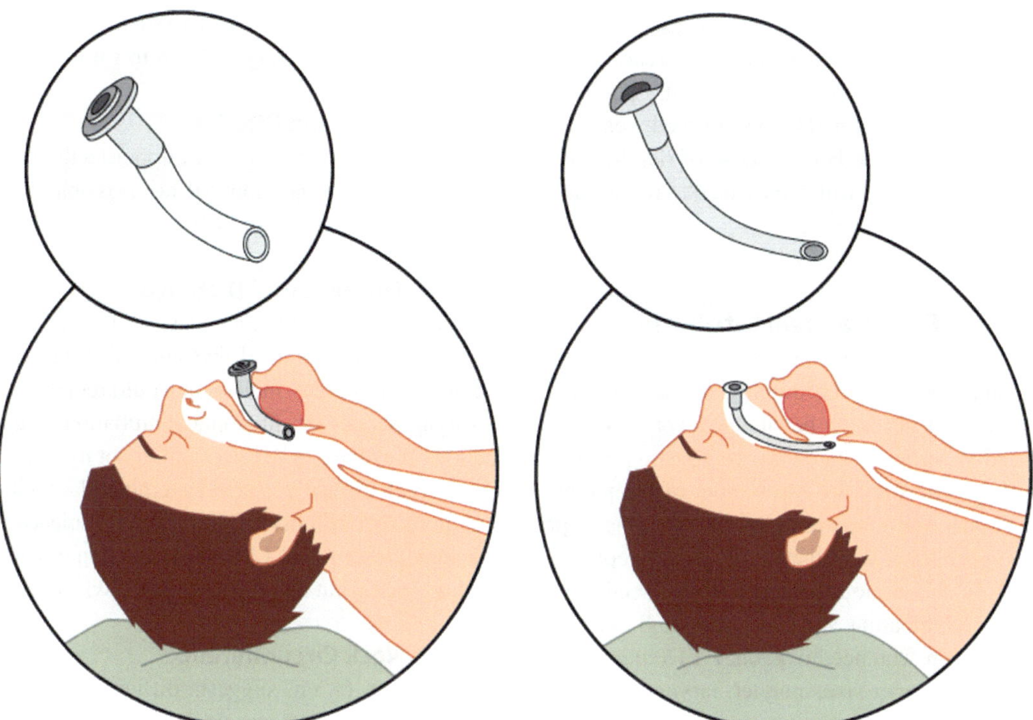

Fig. 6.2 Guedel airway (oropharyngeal airway, OPA) keeps the tongue in place

Fig. 6.3 Nasopharyngeal airway (NPA). Watch the video on youtube which is showing you how and when to insert a NPA www.youtube.com/watch?v=gVgAlWRCZBs

the pharynx and thus maintaining a patent airway. It is tolerated only in deep anaesthesia or in unconscious patients. Available in different sizes; and it is necessary to insert the correct size (approximate length is like the distance from the centre of the mouth to the angle of the mandible); otherwise, it will not be effective. Too large OPA may obstruct the airway. Do not leave the OPA several days in place as it can cause damage of soft tissue. Other side effect: may induce vomiting.

6.3 Nasopharyngeal Airway (NPA)

This device is also called nose hose or nasal trumpet. It can even be homemade of an ETT which is a bit shortened. It is gently inserted through the nostril after putting a little jelly on the tip. The correct length is measured before: From the nostril to the ear lobe is the approximate length needed to be inserted to reach correct position shortly before the entrance of the larynx. Figure 6.3 shows the NPA and its position in the patient. It helps keeping the airway patent in unconscious but spontaneously breathing patients. Confirm its correct position by feeling breath coming from the device. Indications are the same as for Guedel airways. The NPA is better tolerated by a patient who is not deeply unconscious. Complication: bleeding from the nose. Have suction at hands. Contraindication: patients with trauma of the base of the skull since the NPA could enter the brain through a hole in the dura (the outer layer of the protective meninges, tissue that protects and covers the brain and spinal cord).

6.4 Face Mask

Face masks are available in many shapes, materials, and sizes. Silicone is the best and most long-lasting material available. The best fitting device is used and must be held tight with elevated jaw in sniffing position. This device is used for anaesthesia induction, for spontaneous breathing during general anaesthesia, or for gently performed manual ventilation. Do not exceed ventilation pressure > 20 cm H_2O because of risk for inflating the stomach, which may lead to regurgitation and pulmonary aspiration.

6.5 Endotracheal Intubation

Intubation is a procedure which needs special skills and needs to be planned very well. You need to form a team of two persons to perform it safely. The steps are assessment of the patient's anatomy, the preparation of the equipment, preoxygenation, anaesthetic drugs (exception: a deeply unconscious patient does not need drugs), go for intubation and have a plan B for failed intubation. You need oxygen, ETT (endotracheal tube) of proper size, a stylet, laryngoscope with proper size blade, suction equipment, anaesthetic drugs, stethoscope, pulse oximeter, if available even capnography, and a device for ventilating with intermittent positive pressure (IPPV).

Recommended trainings video on https://www.youtube.com/watch?v=8AOB2PtHfVM

6.5.1 Assessment Before Planned Endotracheal Intubation with Direct Laryngoscopy

6.5.1.1 Mouth Opening

Incisor distance of >3 cm in adults is needed. Ask the patient to pull out his tongue fully and check Mallampati classification (see Fig. 6.4), the teeth and any abnormal findings which might interfere with the planned airway management.

6.5.1.2 Ability to Move the Neck

Ask the patient to extend and to flex his neck. At least some flexion and extension of the neck is needed in most cases for direct laryngoscopy unless a videolaryngoscope is used. Patients with unstable fracture of the neck are at risk to develop injury of the spinal cord when the neck is not strictly kept in a neutral position. Patients with rheumatoid arthritis are likely to suffer from neck stiffness and can be very difficult to intubate.

6.5.1.3 Upper Lip Bite Test

Lower teeth brought in front of upper teeth to test the motion of the jaw joint; if not possible difficulties for intubation are likely.

6.5.1.4 Thyromental Distance

Greater than three fingerbreadths is necessary in adults, four is optimal. If thyromental distance in adults is below 5 cm, intubation would require videolaryngoscope or fiberoptic intubation. Such patients may have to be referred. Do not try intubation in such cases if you are in a remote place without those special tools and sufficient experience to use them. Insertion of LM airway is often possible in those cases, but no guarantee that it will work.

6.5.1.5 Neck Circumference

Greater than 68 cm suggests difficulty in mask ventilation and laryngoscopy.

6.5.1.6 Mallampati Classification

The greater the tongue obstructs the view of the pharyngeal structures, the more difficult is intubation, see Fig. 6.4.

6.5.1.7 Pregnancy

Pregnant women may develop some oedema in the oropharynx which can cause difficulties with intubation. LMA is possible in most of these cases.

The Cormack and Lehane grades are indicating difficulties of inserting the ETT into the trachea. They are showing the view while performing direct laryngoscopy, see Fig. 6.5. ***Bougies or stylets facilitate intubation***. You should have several of them and at least one attached to every anaesthesia working station, e.g. a gum elastic (Eschmann) bougie.

The laryngoscope is available with blades of different sizes for infants and adults. The most common and universal one is the curved Macintosh blade, available in sizes 1–4. Size 1 is for infants, size 2 for children of 2 up to around 8 years, size 3 for children from around 9 years and small to medium size adults, size 4 for tall adults. Make sure that the light bulb is working,

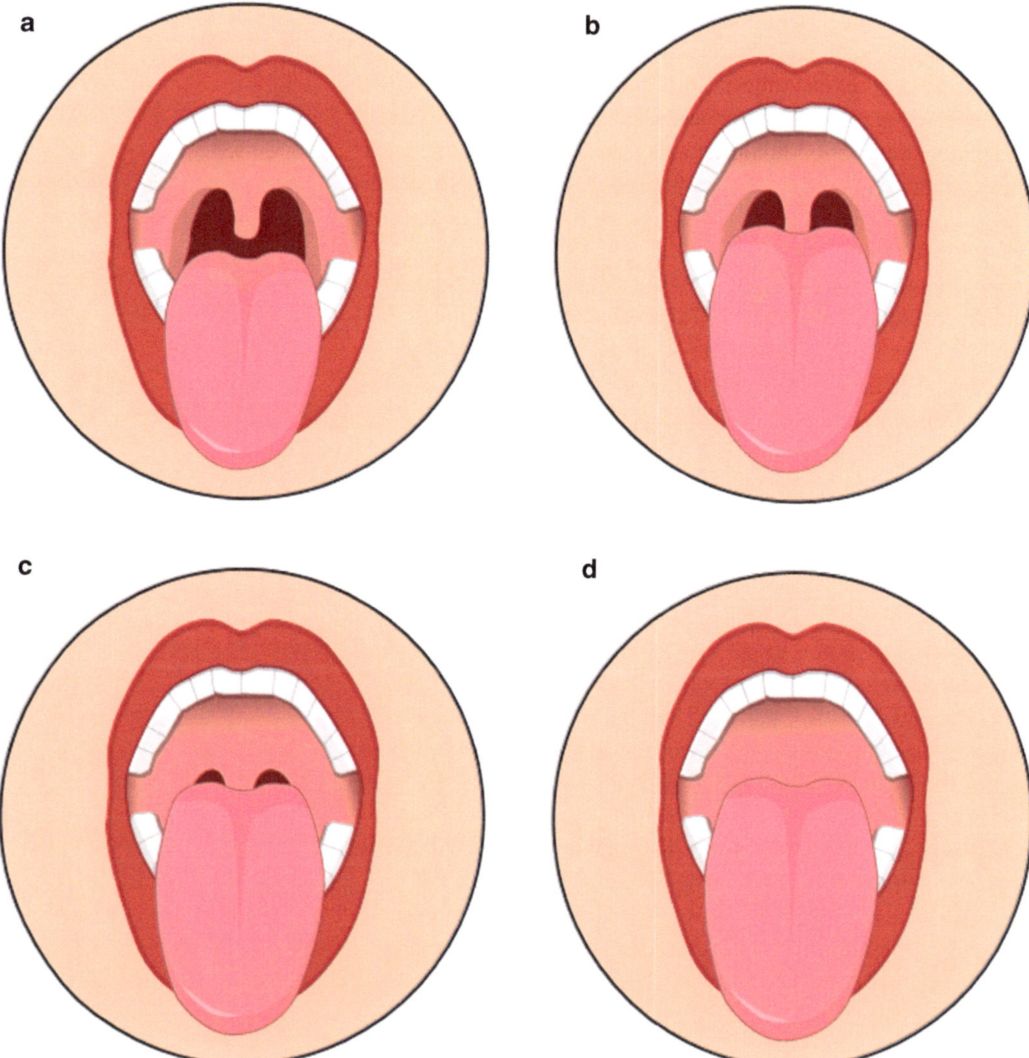

Fig. 6.4 Mallampati classification of the view of the pharynx: (**a**) refers to class I when soft palate, uvula, and pillars are visible; (**b**) to class II when soft palate and uvula are visible; (**c**) to class III, when soft palate and the base of the uvula are visible; and (**d**) refers to class IV when only the tongue and part of the hard palate are visible

and the battery is charged! It is impossible to intubate with insufficient light. The correct size of the endotracheal tube please find in Table 6.1.

6.5.2 Preoxygenation

This procedure must always be performed before intubation unless in emergency when time would not allow for it, e.g. massive bleeding. The procedure leads to the replacement of the lung's nitrogen volume with oxygen to provide a reservoir for diffusion of oxygen into the alveolar capillaries after the onset of apnoea as associated with endotracheal intubation or insertion of LMA.

Breathing room air (that contains 21% O_2) will often result in desaturation to <90% after 1–2 min of apnoea. Breathing oxygen for 5 min will usually maintain saturation at >90% for up to 6 minutes and may prevent the patient from life-threatening hypoxia thus buying time for establishing the airway, especially the endotracheal tube (ETT).

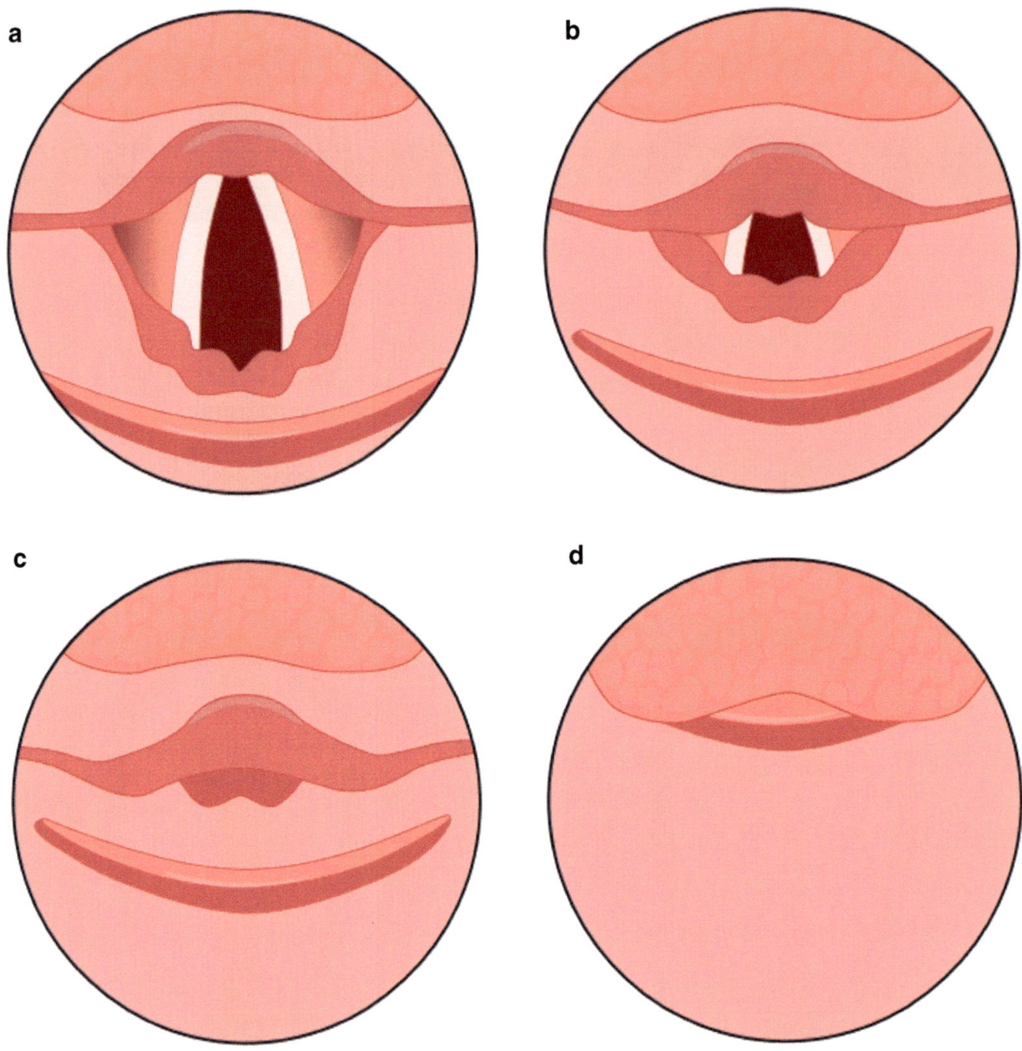

Fig. 6.5 Cormack Lehane classification of laryngoscopy. Cormack and Lehane grade I (**a**), grade II (**b**), grade III (**c**), grade IV (**d**) No laryngeal structures visible; only epiglottis visible

6.5.3 The Technique for Endotracheal Intubation

A Macintosh laryngoscope is used for adults and infants >6 months of age. Its blade has a curved shape, see Fig. 6.6. Blade size 3 is used for most adults, size 4 for tall adults (> 180 cm), size 2 for children, and size 1 with a Miller blade for smaller infants. The Miller blades are straight instead of curved. Specialised blades as McCoy or videolaryngoscopes can facilitate difficult intubation. They are beyond the standard equipment which should be available in every health facility where major operations are performed.

Figure 6.6 shows laryngoscopy and the view corresponding to Cormack Lehane grade 1.

Make sure the battery is charged and the laryngoscope is showing bright white light. Nobody is able to intubate successfully with poor light. Safe, successful intubation in almost all patients requires sufficient practical training with many attempts under supervision before any AP is sufficiently skilled for it. Always be a team of two persons. Watch the above recommended trainings video on YouTube repeatedly, espe-

Table 6.1 The correct sizes of ETT and LMA, the cm of the ETT at the teeth, the volumes of each breath, and the respiratory rate for average patients

Age [years]	BW [kg]	Size ETT	Intubation depth [cm length from teeth]	Size LMA	Tidal Volume [mL]	Breaths per min. Approx.
Premature	<1 <2	2 2.5	7 8–9	None 1	7 15	50
Neonate	2.5–3.0	3–3.5	8–9	1	20–30	40
1–3 months	3.5–5	3.5	9	1	25–50	30–40
3–6 months	6–8	3.5	9–10	1.5	50–60	25–30
6–12- months	7–10	3.5–4	10–12	1.5	60–80	24–28
1–2 years	10–12	4	11–13	2	70–90	20–26
2–3 years	12–14	4–4.5	12–13.5	2	90–110	18–24
3–4 years	14–16	4.5–5	13–15	2	100–120	16–22
5 years	15–20	5–5.5	14–16	2–2.5	120–160	15–20
6 years	18–24	5.5	15–17	2.5	140–180	15–20
7 years	20–26	5.5–6	15.5–17	2.5	150–220	14–18
8 years	22–30	6	16–18	2.5	180–240	14–16
9–11 years	25–50	6–6.5	17–19	3	200–300	14–16
12–15 years	30–60	6.5–7	18–21	3	250–400	12–15
>16 years	>35 kg	7–8	18–22	3–4	300–400	11–15
Female adult	> 35 kg >50 kg	6.5–7.5 7–7.5	18–22	3 4	300–400 400–500	10–14
Male adult	> 50 kg >100 kg	7–8 8–8.5	20–24	4 5	500–600 700	10–14

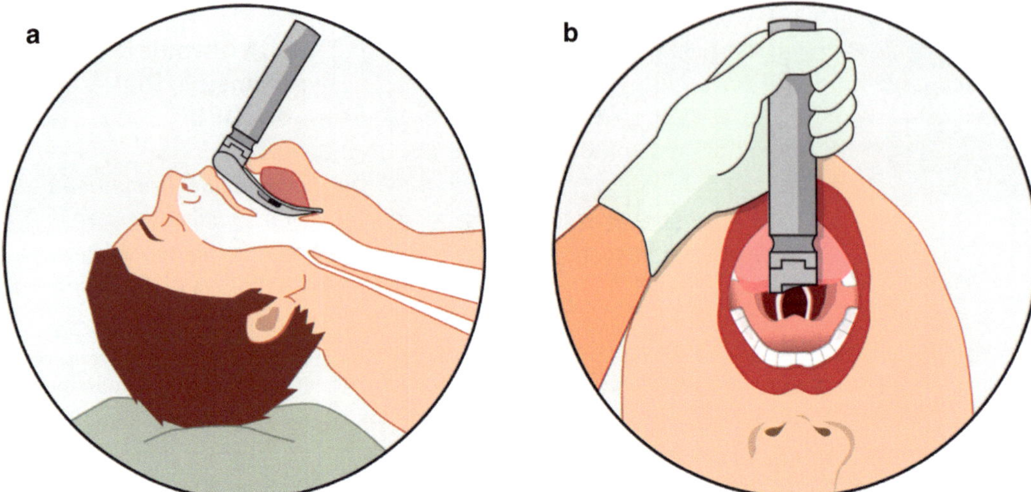

Fig. 6.6 Direct laryngoscopy. The left picture (**a**) shows the laryngoscope inserted, while the right picture (**b**) shows the view to the vocal cords and the entrance of the trachea

cially if you are performing intubation not so frequently. When the patient is anaesthetised and the muscle relaxation achieved, open the mouth with the second and third finger of your right hand while the thumb is kept on the nose. With the left hand insert the laryngoscope carefully (avoid damage of the front teeth), pushing the tongue to the left side and advance it until you see the epiglottis. Advance the laryngoscope into the vallecula and carefully lift the shaft at a 45° angle without putting pressure to the front teeth. Be also careful not to damage the lips. Sometimes you need your assistant to put external force on the neck over the larynx to get structures visible. You should at least see the arytenoid cartilages, better the vocal cords. Insert the ETT with your right hand while the left hand is strictly keeping its position with the laryngoscope. The ETT may need to be rotated anticlockwise to enter the trachea until it has passed the vocal cords between the two black lines. Inflate the cuff (assistant) gently (in most adults, around 6 cc of air are needed). Firmly hold the tube with your right hand while you remove the laryngoscope. Check the correct position and fix the tube carefully with adhesive tape or gauze bandage. Start ventilation and add inhalational anaesthetic if planned, otherwise continue with IV anaesthetics. Don't let anaesthesia get too light. Remember that a tube may be in the oesophagus although you had a good view while intubating. Always check according to the following criteria the ***correct position of the ETT***:

"***Looks good*** (symmetrical chest excursions), ***feels good*** (hand ventilation), ***sounds good*** (bilateral auscultation of the chest), ***saturation is good*** (or rising), ***and*** CO_2 ***is visible on the capnograph*** (if available)". Avoid unilateral/bronchial intubation by carefully adjusting the correct depth of intubation. The cuff of the tube should be palpated in the sternal notch.

6.5.4 Complications of Laryngoscopy/Intubation

The forces of laryngoscopy and intubation can easily cause damage. Special care is necessary to avoid breaking front teeth. Dental damage is more likely if laryngoscopy is difficult or if the one who is performing laryngoscopy is inexperienced. Avoid any rotational force with contact to the front teeth (upper incisors) during attempts to lever the tip of the laryngoscope blade. Call for help if more experienced colleague is available and apply force to the laryngoscope blade in a movement upwards and away from you without any leverage on the upper teeth. If still poor view with the laryngoscope, ventilate via face mask, make sure anaesthesia is still deep enough, optimise position of the head and neck, use bougie, special laryngoscope like McCoy or videolaryngoscope if available, and think if intubation is really necessary. Many operations can be performed with laryngeal mask airway which may be easily inserted in patients who are difficult to intubate. Even removal of ETT or LMA may cause dental damage if the patient is biting during extubation attempts. Wait until patient is opening the mouth and don't apply too much force. Check dental status preoperatively and inform the patient about risk for dental damage. If a tooth gets lost, spare and return it to the patient.

The mandibular joint can be dislocated during forceful laryngoscopy causing long-lasting pain after operation. Damage of the mucosa in the throat is painful after surgery. Swelling of the laryngeal structures and the trachea is possible after several attempts of intubation or if the cuff of the ETT is inflated too much. Vocal cords can be damaged, and patients get a hoarse voice. Patients may develop difficulties swallowing after intubation anaesthesia. Usually this is temporary but may cause risk for aspiration of secretions.

Table 6.1 Sizes of endotracheal tubes or laryngeal masks, tidal volume, and respiratory rate (breaths per minutes) for patients under general anaesthesia.

The numbers in the table are valid approximations for the average patient. Always have one size bigger and smaller prepared.

Always adjust ventilation parameters to the individual patient.

Below the age of 8–10 years, an ETT without cuff may be used when cuff pressure measurement is unavailable or the cuff be inflated as little as possible (tight <20 cmH_2O airway pressure). Tubes without cuff do not prevent pulmonary aspiration very well, and they can easily dislocate. Therefore, they can be combined with a throat pack.

A cuffed tube should be half a size smaller than a tube without cuff. Tidal volumes at all ages are 7–8 mL/kg BW, 5–6 mL/kg in obese patients. Breaths per minute (RR = respiratory rate) should be adjusted after end-tidal CO_2. The table is especially useful if end-tidal CO_2 monitoring is absent.

6.6 Laryngeal Mask Airway (LMA)

Laryngeal mask airways are supraglottical airway devices (SAD) since they are not passed through the vocal cords. Figure 6.7 shows the supraglottic airway device in place.

The **laryngeal mask airway (LMA)** is composed of a small "mask" designed to sit in the hypopharynx with an opening (aperture) overlying the laryngeal inlet. The rim of the mask is comprised of an inflatable silicon cuff that fills the hypopharyngeal space, creating a seal that allows positive-pressure ventilation with limited (<20 cm H_2O) pressure. Other types of LMA (i-gel®) do not have inflatable cuffs. However, I-gel masks are not so suitable in hot and humid environments since their special plastic material can become sticky.

The following links are for excellent training videos, part I and part II by the same authors:

https://www.youtube.com/watch?v=4cV3iRlzeRs and https://www.youtube.com/watch?v=pr9rWBmL0zE

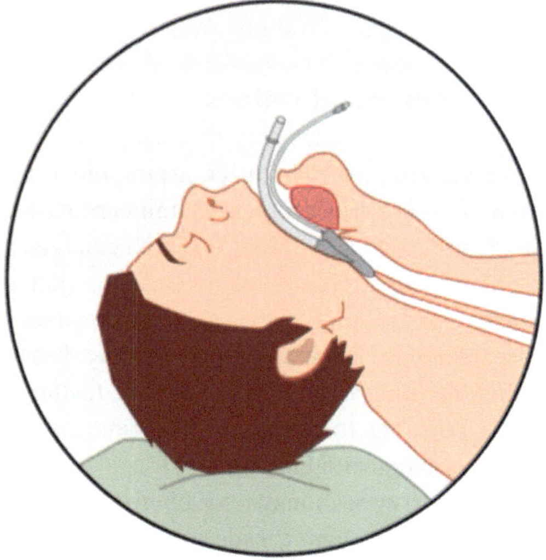

Fig. 6.7 LMA in correct place

Insertion of LMA may be facilitated with lubrication gel or just water or NS.

Advantages: you don't need a laryngoscope for insertion. LMA is much easier to insert than ETT. Disadvantage: Not possible in all patients; and deep anaesthesia is needed uninterruptedly, otherwise patients would cough, thereby letting the device dislocate, or they would get a laryngospasm. The LMA is also prone to dislocate by twisting. Always keep the ventilation tubes fixed without any pulling.

6.6.1 Size of the LMA

For details see Table 6.1. Size depends mainly on body weight but also a bit on body length.

6.6.2 Indications

General surgery of the limbs, inguinal hernia (if spinal is not the first choice, e.g. in children), breast surgery; spinal anaesthesia planned but failed and changed to general anaesthesia; patients planned for endotracheal intubation if intubation fails.

Positive-pressure ventilation can be safely accomplished with the LMA if airway pressure is limited to 20 cmH_2O.

6.6.3 Contraindications

Increased risk for pulmonary aspiration*:* ("full stomach"); hiatal hernia with significant gastroesophageal reflux; morbid obesity; emergency abdominal surgery, intestinal obstruction (ileus); delayed gastric emptying, e.g. during pregnancy; poor pulmonary compliance (severe lung disease or COPD); increased airway resistance (asthma); glottic or subglottic airway obstruction; limited mouth opening <1.5 cm.

However, even in a case of contraindication, the LMA may be used if endotracheal intubation fails and the patient must be ventilated in order to prevent hypoxia.

6.6.4 Practical Considerations and Complications

Unnoticed dislocation; gastroesophageal*:* reflux and aspiration; laryngospasm; coughing; bronchospasm; sore throat (less than after endotracheal intubation); transient changes in vocal cord function; cuff over-inflation may lead to nerve injury (recurrent laryngeal nerve, hypoglossal nerve, lingual nerve); nitrous oxide should not be used with LMA, because it may diffuse into cuff and increase the cuff pressure.

Insertion of the LMA is easier if it is moistened with water or normal saline and with the cuff half-inflated. While inflating the cuff further after insertion, it must not be hold, so that the LMA can place itself into the optimum position. Inflate the cuff only gently. Aim is just to avoid leakage. A little leakage may be tolerated. The cuff must feel soft. If you have a cuff pressure monitor, adjust it to a cuff pressure below 60 cmH_2O. Thereafter it is fixed with a tape. The ventilation tubes should be held in a hand until they are fixed in such a way that they cannot twist or pull at the LMA which can very easily be dislocated.

Neither laryngoscope nor muscle relaxation is required for insertion of LMA but really deep anaesthesia is needed. Propofol combined with fentanyl will result in the best conditions for LMA insertion. If fentanyl is unavailable, ketamine can be used to be combine with propofol. Alternatively, a combination of atropine, diazepam, and high dose thiopentone (7 mg/kg BW) may be used. Immediately after IV induction inhalation, anaesthestic agent is needed in high inspiratory concentration until anaesthesia level is sufficient, then in maintenance concentration.

With ketamine alone, it is very difficult to insert the mask because the mouth cannot be opened easily after ketamine. In that situation, you would need a muscle relaxant (suxamethonium 0.5–1 mg/kg) or let the patient breathe spontaneously without artificial airway. Inhalational induction is also possible. Usually, after 5 minutes with sevoflurane or 10–15 min with halothane until a deep level of anaesthesia is achieved, the LMA can be inserted while the patient is continuing breathing unless anaesthesia gets too deep.

The LMA always requires deep anaesthesia in the beginning, otherwise the patient would cough and the LMA would dislocate, or he/she would bite on the LMA. If that happens, additional IV anaesthetics need to be given instantaneously, often plus increasing the inhalational concentration at the vaporiser. Sometimes, the LMA needs to be removed and reinserted when anaesthesia is sufficient. Even suxamethonium is sometimes needed, especially in situation with severe laryngospasm and desaturation.

With LMA it is usually not possible to insert an oropharyngeal airway (Guedel tube) or a nasogastric tube. If the patient needs *a gastric tube*, then it should *be inserted before* the LMA. Nowadays there are special LMA available with a channel for oral gastric tube or suctioning.

After insertion of the LMA and fixation with tape, the head of the patient should be turned onto the side very carefully to avoid dislocation of the LMA. Alternatively, it may be placed on a ring (e.g. made from a piece of cloth in form of a donut) in order to lie stable during anaesthesia. The ventilation tubes must be fastened very carefully in order to prevent them from pulling at the LMA.

The patient should be allowed to breathe spontaneously as soon as possible. If spontaneous breathing is insufficient, the patient may be ventilated manually or by the mechanical ventilator. The maximum airway pressure must not exceed 20 cmH_2O (25 cm for LMA with integrated gastric drain tube), since with higher airway pressure the seal of the LMA is not tight and the stomach would also be inflated.

Therefore, a maximum ventilation pressure should be preset at 20 cmH_2O at the anaesthesia machine. To avoid ventilation with too high airway pressure or to prevent high pressure alarm of the ventilator, in some patients the tidal volume needs to be set a bit smaller than with an endotracheal tube. Approximately 6 mL/kg bodyweight is recommended and a respiratory rate of 12–15 breaths per minute.

6.7 Difficult Airway Management

Problems with airway access may cause severe anaesthesia complications. (A) cannot ventilate—cannot intubate situation is one of the major causes of anaesthesia-related death.

The AP should consider:

- difficulties mask ventilation—yes/no,
- difficulties of laryngoscopy,
- difficulties inserting the ETT although laryngoscopy is presenting a sufficient view,
- difficulty inserting a LMA—yes/no,
- any difficulty oxygenation via nasal prongs/ tight face mask.

Concerns about 1–5 would mean you should avoid intubation/GA with mechanical ventilation if possible and no emergency or you need to be prepared for tracheostomy or coniotomy (which normally should be performed by a surgeon). However, before elective operations, the patient needs to be informed about the option for tracheostomy and informed consent is vital. Without consent, the patient should be allowed to wake up instead. Additionally, the risk for regurgitation and aspiration of gastric contents needs to be considered before starting attempts to anaesthetise and intubate a patient.

If difficult intubation is anticipated, different techniques can be used depending on the case, equipment, and experience of the anaesthesia provider. Make a plan, have a plan B and consider referral of the patient or performing the operation with regional anaesthesia or without intubation if safely possible. Always form a team and have the most experienced AP at hands. Always have your equipment checked and at hands.

In spontaneously breathing patients with stable oxygen saturation under GA or sedation, a *blind nasal intubation* with a well-lubricated ETT may be tried but only by experienced anaesthetists. Main risk is bleeding from the nose followed by losing the airway and inability to ventilate. Apply some drops of vasoconstrictor as diluted ephedrine or adrenaline (a dilution of

0.5 mg per 100 mL) into the nose 1 min before. Give oxygen through the other nostril. Put the patient's head in a good sniffing position with a pillow under the head. Blind nasal intubation is not a method to try in an emergency if you never did it successfully before. It is neither part of the difficult airway algorithm.

Another option which also requires experienced anaesthetist is *intubating through a correctly inserted LMA*. You need a long bougie or tube exchanger which is first inserted through the LMA. Then the LMA is removed and the ETT is railroaded over the bougie. A laryngoscope is facilitating the procedure even if full view of the glottis is not achieved. This method is only indicated if ventilation through the LMA is working perfectly, and oxygenation is good. Many operations can be performed with LMA instead of ETT, so consider to just using the LMA instead of trying intubating through it which also might cause complications and finally losing the airway.

In ***obese patients*** and patients with short neck, the airway management can be facilitated significantly by creating a ramped position of the upper part of the body. The goal is to create a horizontal line from the ear to the sternal notch in obese patients. The more the airway axis is deviating from the horizontal line, the more difficult any airway management will be. Even mask ventilation may be impossible if obese patients are just placed supine without pillow or only with a pillow under their head. Youtube video: https://www.youtube.com/watch?v=IqToNS6rjaA. Ideal is the Oxford HELP® pillow or similar device. You can also improvise creating a ramp with some blankets or a wedge and a pillow as the following video is showing: https://www.youtube.com/watch?v=OO9o7EMzrRQ.

6.7.1 Intubation with a Gum Elastic Bougie (Eschmann Stylet)

When only a Cormack grade 3 view is achieved, a gum elastic bougie is a very good device to enable intubation. An excellent free trainings video was produced by the NPO "HQ Medical Education" in Minnesota, USA. The video is not available on YouTube but directly via: https://hqmeded.com/the-bougie-2/. Perform laryngoscopy. If you cannot introduce the tube but can identify at least the epiglottis, try to lift the epiglottis from the pharyngeal wall and insert the gum elastic bougie (Eschmann stylet). In some cases, the stylet needs to be preformed to create a 60° bend to be introduced successfully some centimetres past the line of the assumed larynx entrance. Leave the laryngoscope in place and ask your assistant to put the ETT over the bougie. Rotate the ETT counterclockwise 90° to prevent the tip from getting stuck on laryngeal structures during passage. After the ETT is in place, hold it firmly with your right hand, keep the laryngoscope still in place and ask your assistant to remove the bougie. Then remove the laryngoscope and try to ventilate the patient and confirm correct placement of the ETT. Although nowadays these bougies may be declared "single use", they can easily be cleaned and disinfected. Although inexpensive they are extremely precious, and you should never be without one.

Endotracheal intubation may prove to be more difficult than anticipated. Remember: No patient is dying from not being intubated but from not being ventilated! Avoid many attempts of intubation which would cause bleeding, swelling, and even may cause mask ventilation or LMA to be impossible. After two fruitless attempts, think before going on. Ventilate the patient with oxygen. Call for help. And follow the approach for difficult airway:

Always have all airway equipment well maintained and ready for use. A senior anaesthetist should be called for help in all difficult airway situations. Remember that for intubation always a team of two AP is necessary. Being alone is not safe.

6.7.1.1 Difficult Airway Algorithm

Difficult airway ➔ recognised in advance

➔ Proper preparation ➔ IV induction with low doses of anaesthetics without muscle relaxants followed by inhalational anaesthesia in spontaneously breathing patient ➔ position the patient in sniffing position so that the external auditory meatus (ear canal) is in the same horizontal plane as the sternal notch (use a wedge under the thorax, a cushion under the head if necessary).

➔ Try mask ventilation. ***If mask ventilation is not possible***, do one attempt to intubate without muscle relaxant, or to insert LMA, if that fails, wake the patient up.

In case of acute emergency operation, inform the surgeon and consider anaesthesia with spontaneous breathing (ketamine, moderate dose inhalation, no opioids, no muscle relaxants; *high risk!*);

➔ ***if mask ventilation possible***, then ***try to intubate*** using a stylet, or a bougie or a special long introducer (airway exchange catheter) and the best suitable laryngoscope blade. Avoid force and avoid causing any damage and bleeding. If available, use McCoy blade or a videolaryngoscope;

➔ ***if first attempt of intubation fails***, mask-ventilate and think. Call for help. Consider second attempt to intubate with optimised position and equipment. ***If two attempts to intubate fail*** and a more experienced anaesthetist is not available, ***insert LMA***, preferably an intubating LMA or an LMA with integrated gastric drain tube;

➔ ***if LMA fails*** then ventilate via face mask and consider waking up the patient or to perform operation under spontaneous ventilation dependent on the indication of surgery, that means discuss with the surgeon if to proceed or not.

➔ ***if mask ventilation fails*** and patient desaturates before waking up declare ***"cannot ventilate – cannot intubate"*** and prepare for emergency front of neck access (coniotomy or tracheotomy).

Difficult airway ➔ unrecognised in advance➔.

Patient anaesthetised and paralysed, failed intubation ➔ mask ventilation➔ call for help and second attempt to intubate➔ failed again➔ mask ventilation ➔ more propofol/ thiopentone or inhalational agent➔ LMA. Discuss with your fellow colleague/the surgeon if the operation can be performed with LMA.

If LMA fails➔ perform mask ventilation. Discuss with your assistant/fellow colleague/the surgeon if the operation can be performed with mask ventilation/spontaneous breathing or not.

➔ If mask ventilation, intubation and LMA fail declare "cannot intubate, cannot ventilate situation". Emergency coniotomy or tracheotomy must then be performed immediately unless the patient has started to breathe spontaneously again and keeps acceptable oxygen saturation. Follow the approach for emergency surgical airway:

6.7.2 Emergency Surgical Airway with Front of Neck Access (FONA)

Check the anatomy of the patient's neck before starting anaesthesia and identify the cricothyroid membrane so that you would localise that structure easily. Front of Neck access to the airway is often performed in "cannot intubate—cannot ventilate" situations. The video is showing how to establish a surgical airway quickly and without the need of special equipment. You need skin disinfectant, a surgical knife size 10, gauze, artery forceps, long bougie, and ETT 1–2 sizes smaller than for endotracheal intubation with laryngoscope plus a syringe to inflate the cuff. Adhesive tape for fixation and a ventilation device will be needed when the surgical cricothyroidotomy or coniotomy is done successfully. If a long bougie should be unavailable although it is recommended as mandatory equipment, aim to directly insert a small-sized ETT after having opened the cricothyroid membrane with a scalpel blade which is firmly held in position perpendicular to the skin until the bougie or the tube is inserted. Difficult Airway Society - FONA Training video https://youtu.be/B8I1t1HlUac All surgeons should be able to do it, and you might assist and guide them if they have little or no experience yet. Watch the video at the link above or any other suitable video on YouTube at least once per year and be mentally prepared to perform this procedure if situation is demanding it.

The front of neck access (FONA) to the airway can also be performed electively if the difficulty/impossibility of intubation/LMA are known in advance. Local anaesthesia and light sedation are recommended.

6.8 Rapid Sequence Induction

Anaesthesia induction of a patient with a full stomach is a procedure with high risk for regurgitation and aspiration of gastric contents into the lungs. All patients who need to be operated as emergency case without having starved at least 6 h are at risk. Patients for caesarean section, patients with acute abdominal problems, e.g. obstructed inguinal hernia, and all patients after trauma must be regarded as if they had a full stomach. After a trauma, the stomach may be paralysed and keeping its contents for much longer than 6 h. The anaesthesia provider must take preventive action to minimise the risk of aspiration and subsequent pneumonia. ***Patients with ileus/intestinal obstruction have the highest risk and should receive a nasogastric tube before being anaesthetised.*** Apply suction to the NGT and try to empty the stomach immediately before anaesthesia induction.

6.8.1 Indications for RSI

Patient with a full stomach who needs general anaesthesia. The decision to employ RSI balances the risk of losing control of the airway against the risk of pulmonary aspiration. This applies to all pregnant patients after week 12 of pregnancy, especially caesarean section when general anaesthesia is needed. RSI needs also to be performed in emergency patients who are not fasting >6 h, and in all patients for acute abdominal surgery.

6.8.2 Procedure

Before induction, the anaesthetist must carefully assess if difficult intubation is anticipated. *There must be a plan for management of the patient should intubation fail.*

The anaesthesia machine and vital signs monitor, all drugs, tubes, stylets, suction apparatus, large-bore suction catheters, laryngoscope (sufficient light?) with different blades, and so on must be prepared and checked in advance. Equipment for difficult airway must be ready and close at hand.

For RSI induction agents are combined with a fast-acting muscle relaxant like suxamethonium or, if suxa is contraindicated, with rocuronium. Mask ventilation is omitted as long as the patient is not getting hypoxic. If none of these MR is available, use vecuronium with its onset of 1.5–2 min or atracurium with an onset time of 1.5–3 min. If pancuronium is the only available MR, a real RSI is impossible since it takes at least 3 min for sufficient effect. During this time, the patient with a full stomach is at risk to regurgitate and aspirate. In such a situation, a relatively high dose of propofol of 3 mg/kg may be used as induction agent combined with a strong analgesic like ketamine 100 mg or fentanyl 0.1 mg, then pancuronium is injected but intubation already performed 1 minute after propofol injection. Pancuronium may even be the first drug to be injected, immediately followed by ketamine and propofol. These methods are not ideal but will probably work.

The fastest effect is achieved with the combination of thiopentone and suxamethonium. Remember that thiopentone and suxamethonium are pharmaceutically incompatible. Always flush the venous cannula with NS between different drugs or have infusion running fast.

The patient's head should be in the classic "sniffing position" with the head extended on the neck and the head elevated so that the earlobe is at the same level as the jugulum (sternal notch). Obese patients need a wedge-shaped bolster under the thorax and one or more pillows under the head to achieve a ramp position.

RSI must never be performed alone. The anaesthetist needs a skilled assistant.

- Check equipment and prepare drugs.
- Assess the patient, put IV line, and give infusion (RL or NS).
- Position the patient in sniffing position. If necessary, put NGT and apply suction.
- Preoxygenate 3–5 min with 100% oxygen.
- Monitoring with SPO_2, ECG, NIBP.
- Drugs for average adult: e.g. atropine 0.5 mg, ketamine 100 mg, thiopentone 250 mg, suxamethonium 100 mg are injected quickly. Alternatively, fentanyl 100 μg, propofol 150 mg, suxa 100 mg. Patient in poor condition: ketamine, fentanyl, suxa combined, no thiopentone or propofol. Other combinations are possible for individual cases. Caesarean section: No fentanyl, no diazepam before the baby is delivered. In case suxa is contraindicated, rocuronium or other muscle relaxant may be used. Pancuronium: Give 0.5 mg, wait 3 min on oxygen, give hypnotic drugs, give 3.5 mg pancuronium, then the effect will be after 1 min.
- Cricoid pressure (Sellick's manoeuvre) is no longer regarded mandatory. Therefore: If you are used to it, do it, otherwise leave it.
- Immediate intubation as soon as mouth opening is easily possible. Use a stylet/bougie to facilitate intubation. Inflate the cuff immediately, ventilate, use stethoscope (auscultation of both lungs) and endtidal CO_2 (if available) to ascertain correct placement of the tube.
- Start mechanical ventilation with the anaesthesia machine. Give anaesthesia drugs for maintenance, e.g. halothane/isoflurane or other anaesthetics.
- Check vital signs: RSI often causes severe hypotension, hypoxia, circulatory collapse or hypertension and tachycardia which need adequate intervention.

Further Reading

Apfelbaum JL, Hagberg CA, Connis RT, Abdelmalak BB, Agarkar M, Dutton RP et al (2022) 2022 American Society of Anesthesiologists Practice guidelines for management of the difficult airway. Anesthesiology 136(1):31–81

Cook T (2019) Airway management. In: Thompson J, Moppett I, Wiles M (eds) Smith and Aitkenhead's textbook of anaesthesia, Seventh edn. Elsevier, London

Crawley SM, Dalton AJ (2015) Predicting the difficult airway. Br J Anaesth 15:253–257

7 Basic Pharmacology for Anaesthesia Providers

Abstract

Most drugs can be stored at ambient temperature. Inhalational anaesthetics, muscle relaxant drugs, and oxytocin are exceptions and need storage in a fridge. Dilutions in syringes may be used 12–24 h. While thiopental and many other drugs remain sterile and stable for several days, diluted adrenaline loses its effect within 24 h. Open ampoules with local anaesthetics for spinal anaesthesia or propofol should not be used longer than 12 h due to risk of infection. Germs can multiply in open propofol ampoules or vials and cause life-threatening sepsis.

Syringes must be labelled clearly with name and amount/concentration of the drug and the date. Strong drugs should be titrated, injected in small portions until the desired effect is achieved.

The most commonly used drugs during anaesthesia are listed with a brief pharmacology, preparations, indications, effects, doses for adults and children, onset and duration, side effects, and contraindications.

Anaesthetic drugs: ketamine, thiopentone, propofol, etomidate; *opioid and non-opioid analgesics:* morphine, fentanyl, pethidine, tramadol, codeine, naloxone, pentazocine, buprenorphine, diclofenac, ketorolac, ibuprofen, paracetamol, metamizole; *sedatives:* diazepam, midazolam, lorazepam, chlorpromazine, promethazine, clonidine; *muscle relaxants and reversal agents:* suxamethonium, pancuronium, vecuronium, atracurium, rocuronium, neostigmine, pyridostigmine, sugammadex; *local anaesthetics:* lidocaine, bupivacaine; *cardiovascular drugs:* adrenaline, atropine, ephedrine, noradrenaline, dopamine, phenylephrine; *antihypertensives and diuretics:* furosemide, glyceryl trinitrate, hydralazine, labetalol, nifedipine, mannitol; *antiemetics:* ondansetron, metoclopramide, droperidol, promethazine; *antibiotics:* cloxacillin, flucloxacillin, ampicillin, amoxicillin, clindamycin, gentamicin, ceftriaxone, cefuroxime, metronidazole; *hormones:* hydrocortisone, dexamethasone, insulin, oxytocin; *bronchodilators:* salbutamol, aminophylline; *agents for treatment of acute coagulation disorders due to bleeding:* tranexamic acid and aminocaproic acid.

Keywords

Antibiotic prophylaxis before surgery · Antiemetic agents for perioperative care · Basic pharmacology for anaesthesia providers · Cardiovascular drugs during anaesthesia · Essential drugs for anaesthesia and perioperative care · Muscle relaxants (neuromuscular blocking agents) and reversal agents · Pharmacology of perioperative analgesics · Pharmacology of anaesthetics · Pharmacological treatment of severe bleeding

D. Kietzmann, *Anaesthesia in Remote Hospitals*, Sustainable Development Goals Series,
https://doi.org/10.1007/978-3-031-46610-6_7

7.1 General Considerations

Drugs need to be effective, safe, continuously available, and affordable for the patients and the hospital. This chapter gives a summary of the most important drugs which are used by anaesthetists globally. However, some drugs which are commonly used by anaesthetists in parts of the world could not be covered here and can be checked via internet or textbooks of anaesthesia. The safe management of drugs used during anaesthetic practice in hospitals is of particular importance. Reading the "Guideline for the safe management and use of medications in anaesthesia by the Australian and New Zealand College of Anaesthetists" may be helpful in that purpose; it is found via the link: bit.ly/3bFD5Ex.

7.1.1 Storage of Drugs

Always observe the expiry date of the drugs and don't use them after that, at least not long after that date. The expiry date does not mean that the drug is unsafe from 1 day to the next, but that date is a warranty for the drug to be effective. Most drugs are still of good quality within at least 10–20% longer period than stated as expiry. However, it is not recommended to take a chance; it is better not to use drugs after expiry.

Most drugs are recommended to be stored at room temperature below 25 °C. In many tropical countries, pharmacy stores and operation rooms have higher temperatures at least part of the day. Most drugs tolerate that well, but there are some exceptions for drugs used in anaesthesia, so that a fridge is really a recommended invention for anaesthesia store in operating theatre:

Inhalational anaesthetics should be stored dark and < 25 °C. A fridge will always meet these requirements. Muscle relaxants and oxytocin need to be stored in the fridge. At temperature above 8 °C, even at cool room temperature, oxytocin as well as suxamethonium, pancuronium, and other MR lose potency continuously. They should not be stored in larger quantities in the OR, but only one ampoule of each should be in the anaesthesia trolley, or the amount which is likely to be used during 1 day.

Adrenaline is light sensitive and needs to be stored dark at room temperature. A dilution of adrenaline in a syringe or infusion is only stable for 24 hours, thereafter it wouldn't be effective. Commercially available ampoules or syringes with adrenaline 1:10000 (1 mg in 10 mL) are more stable and can be stored several months until their expiry date.

7.1.2 Drugs for Injection Must Be Kept Sterile

Otherwise, there is risk that germs would enter the patient together with the injection. Especially intrathecal injection (spinal anaesthesia) may lead to spinal abscess or meningitis, an avoidable complication. Opened ampoules should be used only during the same day. That means sharing between patients is limited. While most drugs remain sterile after opening, propofol is sold in a fatty emulsion in which germs can grow and multiply very quickly. An *opened propofol vial, ampoule, or syringe must only be used within 12 hours*. Thereafter, it must be discarded. That can prove difficult if you get propofol in a 50 mL vial but need only 5 mL for one patient, and the next patient at your small hospital would need propofol first several days later. However, even in that situation you must not keep that propofol vial longer than 12 hours but discard the remaining 45 mL. Propofol is much more expensive than thiopentone if you need to discard most of it. Thiopentone is stable for some days and remains sterile after solution is made with water for injection or NS. An opened vial with thiopentone could be stored in the fridge until you need it next time. Write a date on it and use it during not more than a week. If you don't have a fridge, you cannot use it more than very few days but still longer than propofol. Discuss that with the storekeeper/the responsible person for the pharmacy and, if necessary, with medical officer I/C and administration. *If a propofol vial is used several days after opening the vial or ampoule that may kill patients by causing sepsis.* Deadly complications after injection of unsterile propofol have happened all over the world and are still occurring. In hospitals with limited use of induction agents, thiopentone vials (powder to be diluted) may be a better choice compared to propofol, since the vial with thiopentone would remain sterile even after dilution. Ketamine also does not show these problems. The vial can be used until it is finished provided sterility is kept when drawing portions from it.

7.1.3 Anaesthesia and Hospital Pharmacy

Anaesthetists should keep good communication with pharmacy staff. In smaller hospitals and health centres without qualified pharmacist, information about potentially dangerous anaesthetic drugs are important. The anaesthetist I/C should take initiative to inform the pharmacy keeper about most important effects and side effects of anaesthesia drugs, especially if a new drug is added to the list. The pharmacy keeper can inform the anaesthetist about drug prices and discuss which drug of a group should be preferred. It is not recommended to prefer a drug which is several times more expensive over a drug which is nearly as effective and safe as the more expensive variant.

Personnel without formal training as dispensing chemist or equal need to get on-job-training on drugs as adrenaline, suxamethonium, thiopentone, pancuronium. Unfortunately, several avoidable tragedies happened when untrained dispensing personnel handed out pancuronium instead of oxytocin to staff in the labour ward. The midwife believed it was a new sort of oxytocin and injected pancuronium to a mother after childbirth. Several deaths have occured in recent years in remote hospitals due to that misunderstanding of drugs. In remote health facilities, the AP is sometimes the most skilled person when it comes to drug effects. Have communication and provide training for hospital staff about avoiding those potential hazards. Pancuronium and oxytocin have in common that they need to be stored in the fridge, and they are "neighbours" in alphabetical order. The packages of these drugs may look alike if the manufacturer for them is the same.

7.1.4 Variability of Drug Response and Titrating a Drug to Effect

The response to anaesthetic drugs is showing great interindividual variability. Different patients may need different doses to achieve the same effect. As anaesthetics are strong drugs, they also exert potentially serious side effects. A dose which is necessary and well-tolerated by one person may exert dangerous overdose in another person. Therefore, drug doses must carefully be adjusted to patient's body weight, but also height and age must be considered. A 20 year old tall woman with 60 kg BW at 175 cm height would probably need a higher dose of anaesthetics or opioid analgesics than an 80 year old woman with the same BW of 60 kg but only 155 cm height to achieve the same effect. Many drugs which are used during anaesthesia and postoperatively need to be titrated because the individual dose which would produce the required effect cannot be known in advance. "Titrating" means the average predicted dose is divided into small portions, and a small portion is injected at a time. After a few minutes, the effect is assessed, an additional small portion is injected and so on, until the effect is reached.

7.1.5 Labelling Syringes

During anaesthesia, a number of syringes with different drugs are administered to the patient. Additionally, rescue drugs are prepared to be immediately ready in case of severe adverse events. Mistakes by giving the wrong drug, or giving the wrong dose, are amongst the leading causes of avoidable anaesthesia complications. The risk is higher if the person who injects the drugs is not the same who has prepared them and drawn them up into syringes. Therefore, correct labelling is of paramount importance. The anaesthetist I/C must design a standard of practice which is used same way by all staff involved. Ideally, all syringes in the whole hospital would be labelled the same way: The name of the drug or a short form known to everybody, its concentration per mL, the date and hour and a signature (2 characters will do) must be written on the syringe. Either a permanent pen for plastic can be used or adhesive tape attached on the syringe on which the labelling was written. Some manufacturers provide their ampoules with prepared printed labels which are easy to use.

In Sects. 7.2–7.12 the most important drugs for anaesthesia and perioperative medicine are listed with their pharmacology. The drugs are not listed in alphabetical order but in a hierarchic order starting with the most important and commonly used drugs. In this book, it is not possible to list all drugs which are used by anaesthetists worldwide. If a reader is missing a drug, check in one of the textbooks or via internet. The most common preparations relevant to the anaesthetist are mentioned; however, in some countries, the concentrations and amounts of drug in one ampoule or tablet may differ. Always read the label of ampoules/vials/packages for drugs thoroughly. When the pharmacy would buy a drug from a different manufacturer, concentration and amount per ampoule may be different. Avoid errors of dosing and adapt the local drug dilution scheme accordingly.

7.2 Anaesthetic Drugs

Inhalational anaesthetics are covered in Chap. 8.

7.2.1 Ketamine

Ketamine is an anaesthetic drug with widespread use.

Preparation: usually 10 mL vials with 50 mg/mL; even 10 mg/mL and 100 mg/mL preparations in some countries.

Indication: general anaesthesia, especially for emergency procedures, even for patients in circulatory shock; analgesia for painful procedures. Can be used as sole anaesthetic for patients in circulatory shock but should be combined with at least 2.5–5 mg diazepam as single dose to avoid awareness and nightmares.

Effects: amnesia, analgesia, dissociative anaesthesia (the communication within different parts of the brain is interrupted while signals from hearing or seeing still reach the cortex but without being able to recall or to react; no muscle relaxation. No deep hypnosis means combination with sedative/hypnotic/opioid/inhalational anaesthetic is usually required. Bronchodilation makes it useful for patients with history of asthma and can be part of treatment of status asthmaticus.

Dose: 1–2 mg/kg IV or 5–7 mg/kg IM for anaesthesia induction, 0.5–1 mg IV increments for analgesia or maintenance of anaesthesia. Infusion, e.g. with 500 mg/500 mL: adjust drip rate to effect, 100–300 mg/h depending on type of surgery and combination with other anaesthetic drugs or not. Ketamine 0.2–1.0 mg/kg IV given pre-incision may be a part of balanced anaesthesia in combination with inhalational anaesthesia and may even reduce persistent post-surgical pain. Ketamine orally: 10 mg/kg for children or 500 mg per adult with little sugar and water or syrup.

Onset and duration: IV within 1–2 min, IM 3–5 min, orally 15 min; anaesthesia lasting 10 min (20 min after IM or oral administration), some analgesic effect can last longer.

Side effects: unpleasant dreams and agitation, which can be avoided by combination with other general anaesthetics, e.g. propofol, halothane. Sedatives like diazepam or midazolam and a calm environment during recovery without waking/disturbing the patient are also helpful to avoid unpleasant dreams. Nausea and vomiting may occur. Hypertension and tachycardia are common. No muscle relaxation but increased muscle tone and sometimes jerking movements of the limbs may occur when used as sole anaesthetic. Respiratory depression may occur but unlikely at average doses. Most patients keep a patent airway but not all. Increased salivation can be prevented by adding atropine.

Contraindications: marked hypertension. In hypertensive patients, ketamine as sole anaesthetic should be avoided or doses be reduced to avoid extreme high blood pressure. In combination with vasodilating anaesthetics as propofol or thiopentone, or in combination with inhalational agents, BP usually is not rising markedly. Patients with head and brain injury may receive ketamine only if they are intubated and on controlled ventilation since it would increase intracranial pressure in spontaneously breathing patients.

7.2.2 Thiopentone

Thiopentone is a strong hypnotic drug exclusively for IV administration.

Preparation: vials with 500 mg or 1 g powder to be dissolved with 20 mL of water for injection. If water for injection is unavailable, it is possible to use NS. The solution is stable for many days and bacteriostatic that means it can be used for several patients provided a new syringe is used every time a portion out of the vial is withdrawn. Within the same hospital, always the same concentration should be used, e. g. 25 mg/mL. That means using a 1 g vial with a 20 mL solution of 50 mg/mL thiopentone in the vial would require one more step of dilution in the syringe to make 25 mg/mL.

Indication: Anaesthesia induction but not maintenance since repeated doses would lead to accumulation and prolonged effect; treatment of generalised epileptic convulsions. A small dose of 50–100 mg in adults may be used if anaesthesia is too light. In patients on ventilator in the ICU, repeated doses can be used for sedation or treatment of raised ICP in patients with brain oedema.

Effects: strong hypnotic drug with anticonvulsant effects, amnesia, no analgesia.

Dose: 5–7 mg/kg, 3 mg/kg may be sufficient if combined with 1.5 mg/kg ketamine or with 2 μg/kg fentanyl in elderly patients.

Onset and duration: within 30–45 s after IV bolus injection, duration 5–10 min after single dose, unpredictably longer after repeated doses which should be smaller than the first dose.

Side effects: decreasing BP by vasodilatation (pronounced in combination with hypovolaemia), tachycardia, cardiac depression especially in patients with cardiac disease; short lasting respiratory depression; occasionally laryngospasm. Bronchospasm is also possible and may be a problem in patients with history of asthma. Anaphylactic reactions are rare but can be severe. Extravascular injection may cause painful tissue necrosis. Inadvertent arterial injection may cause ischaemia with tissue necrosis.

Contraindications: acute asthma, barbiturate allergy; congenital porphyria, rare but absolute contraindication since use of barbiturates would cause severe disease.

7.2.3 Propofol

Propofol is an intravenous agent for induction and maintenance of anaesthesia and for procedural sedation as well as sedation in the intensive care unit.

Preparation: white lipid emulsion for exclusively IV administration. Available at 10 or 20 mg/mL concentrations in 20 mL ampoules or 50 mL vials – risk for wrong dose if different concentrations are mixed up. Very important: Bacteria grow quickly and multiply in the emulsion, therefore the syringe, opened vial or ampoule must not be used longer than 12 h. The remains must be discarded to avoid septic shock.

Indication: intravenous anaesthesia and sedation (not recommended longer than 10 days in adults) in combination with a strong analgesic, e.g. fentanyl, ketamine, or nitrous oxide.

Effects: amnesia even after low doses, hypnosis, some muscle relaxation which facilitates insertion of laryngeal mask and intubation (even without muscle relaxant), antiemetic and antiepileptic, no analgesia, pleasant and fast recovery.

Dose: 1.5–2.5 mg/kg for induction in adults, 3–4 mg/kg for children and young adults, 4–10 mg/kg/h for maintenance TIVA, 2–3 mg/kg/h for sedation.

Onset and duration: 1–2 min, after high doses 30–60 s; duration 5–10 min after single bolus.

Side effects: pain on injection especially into small veins is short-lasting but may be severe; therefore, it is of limited use in infants and toddlers where thiopentone is a more pleasant induction agent. Pain of injection can be reduced by mixing 1 mL of lidocaine (without adrenaline) into 10 mL of propofol. Propofol immediately injected after fetching it out of the fridge would also cause less injection pain. Vasodilatation and cardiac depression may lead to marked hypotension, worse in patients with dehydration; respiratory depression (less pronounced with sedative dose). Long-term sedation with high doses may cause the life-threatening propofol-infusion syndrome caused by fatty acids and leading to metabolic acidosis, bradycardia, multi-organ failure, rhabdomyolysis (generalised break down of skeletal muscles leading to renal failure), and death if not recognised early. Children are more prone to that syndrome.

Contraindications: circulatory shock, sedation of children for more than 24 h. Avoid high doses of propofol in the intensive care unit.

7.2.4 Etomidate

Etomidate is a strong hypnotic for anaesthesia induction, not available in all countries.

Preparation: a white lipid emulsion with 2 mg/mL for IV injection.

Indication: A good alternative for anaesthesia induction in patients with hypovolaemia (aim to treat hypovolaemia before induction), ileus, shock, cardiac disease; short GA for cardioversion of patients with tachyarrhythmia.

Effects: amnesia, hypnosis. No side effects on cardiovascular system.

Dose: 0.2–0.3 mg/kg IV in adults, but usually 1 amp =20 mg is adequate dose for adult patients. Pain and myoclonic movements during injection are possible. PONV. Reversible suppression of the adrenal gland.

Onset and duration: maximum effect within 1 min, duration 3–5 min.

Side effects: PONV, very short-lasting respiratory depression, pain on injection, jerking movements of the limbs although patient is unconscious (not seen when muscle relaxant is added); reversible depression of the cortisol and aldosterone synthesis in the adrenal glands. Therefore, the drug is not any longer used for maintenance of anaesthesia. If you really need to give repeated doses of this drug, you should add 100 mg of hydrocortisone to an adult patient to avoid problems with adrenal gland insufficiency.

Contraindications: sedation in the ICU, history of porphyria.

7.3 Opioid Analgesics

Most opioid drugs are classified as narcotic drugs and under the dangerous drugs act (DDA). Local law and dangerous drugs regulations must be strictly observed. In most countries, these drugs must be stored in a special cupboard with a lock. The key must be in a safe place, and only certain authorised persons may have access to it. Discuss that with the pharmacy keeper if your health facility is about to get such drugs for the first time. A book must be kept where every ampoule is listed with the name of the patient, the dose and date of administration, and with the name of the prescriber. A signature is also required, and the remaining stock is always to be recorded. A broken ampoule is recorded as "broken and discarded ampoule". However, all efforts should be made to avoid breaking ampoules since that may lead to suspicion of misuse. Risk for addiction is almost zero if narcotic drugs are used to treat acute pain (trauma, surgery) or chronic pain, e.g. in cancer patients. Misuse as recreational drug is of cause illegal and may rather quickly lead to addiction.

Alfentanil, sufentanil, and remifentanil are opioids which are, similar to fentanyl, used during anaesthesia. They have almost the same effects and side effects as fentanyl but different potency and duration of action. However, they are not available in many countries and not listed below.

7.3.1 Morphine

Morphine is a strong opioid (narcotic) analgesic drug. It is the oldest analgesic drug worldwide, used as chemically isolated morphine since more than 200 years while the more complex plant extract opium has been used for several thousands of years. Morphine is one of the natural alkaloids in opium, made from the fruits of a flower called opium poppy. In ancient times, opium was used for recreational use (its addictive effects were not yet known), for pain relief and to help people with insomnia. Morphine is nowadays still one of the most prescribed opioid analgesics worldwide. Effects and side effects are caused at MOP receptors (μ opioid receptors) in the central nervous system and some inner organs like the guts and the urinary tract.

Preparation: 1 mL ampoule containing 10 mg for SC, IM, or IV injection. Tablets with different doses are available.

Indication: moderate to severe pain.

Effects: anti-pain (analgesic), sedation, anti-cough (antitussive). Asking the patient regularly about the level of pain to adjust the dose to the individual requirements is vital.

Dose: Dose varies and needs to be titrated individually. Average dose is 0.1 mg/kg IV, SC, or IM; huge variation depending on level of pain, combination with other analgesics/anaesthetics and individual variability of drug response. As part of balanced anaesthesia: adults 10 mg in the beginning of major surgery if no fentanyl is used, or 3–5 mg IV at the end of major surgery followed by increments when required, or 10 mg SC or IM at the end of major surgery when severe postoperative pain is anticipated. Often, morphine needs to be repeated TDS or QDS for up to 3 days and sometimes even longer. Some patients, e.g. after severe injury, need morphine every 4 h and may need higher dose than 10 mg morphine to get sufficient pain relief. Close observation of SpO_2 and respiratory rate is necessary in these patients.

Onset and duration: Onset of effect after 5–10 min, full effect after approximately 20 min. Duration of effect 3–6 h.

Side effects: respiratory depression, nausea, vomiting, pruritus without rash, small, constricted pupils, chest wall rigidity with difficulty breathing, histamine release and bronchospasm, urinary retention, constipation, biliary tract spasm, dreams, and hallucinations. Observation in a recovery unit or HDU is recommended after morphine. Pulse oximetry and counting respiratory rate regularly is very helpful. Patients who receive repeated doses of morphine or huge doses should receive oxygen.

Contraindications: gall bladder colic, choledocholithiasis, paralytic ileus, severe asthma with respiratory insufficiency, patients with respiratory depression unless on ventilator.

7.3.2 Fentanyl

Preparation: most commonly in ampoules with 2 mL at 0.05 mg/mL.

Indication: intra-operative analgesia in artificially ventilated patients.

Effects: around 100 times stronger analgesic than morphine, fentanyl produces analgesia and some sedation but not hypnosis and no amnesia so that fentanyl should never be the sole anaesthetic agent.

Dose: 1–2 μg/kg or 0.05–0.1 mg IV in adults. Higher or more than once repeated doses may be used if the patient is intubated, controlled ventilated, and delayed extubation with postoperative care in a fully equipped HDU is planned.

Onset and duration: onset around 3 minutes, max effect after 5 min, duration of action 30–60 minutes. Duration after higher doses and after repeated doses lasts longer since the drug accumulates in the body.

Side effects: respiratory depression, especially after high or repeated doses can be marked and long-lasting. Nausea and vomiting are common. No effects on cardiovascular system.

Contraindications: fentanyl must not be used if no oxygen is available or if respiratory arrest is not manageable. Postoperative observation including pulse oximetry and counting respiratory rate regularly is mandatory.

7.3.3 Pethidine

Pethidine (also called meperidine) is a synthetic opioid (narcotic) drug under DDA.

Preparation: ampoules with 1 or 2 mL of 50 mg/mL for SC, IM, or IV injection.

Indication: treatment of moderate to severe pain, even for gall bladder and kidney colic, prevents shivering and may decrease fever. In the rare situation where no LA agent is available for intrathecal use, pethidine 1 mg/kg may be used for spinal anaesthesia instead.

Effects: analgesia and sedation via opioid receptors; even local anaesthetic effects.

Dose: 50–100 mg for adults or 1 mg/kg; TDS or QDS.

Onset and duration: 10–20 min; duration dependent on dose and level of pain 2–6 h.

Side effects: nausea and vomiting, respiratory depression if overdosed, constipation if used for several days. If pethidine is used to treat labour pain, the neonate may show respiratory depression. Therefore, it must only be used during the first stage of labour. In hypovolaemic patients, it may cause hypotension. No gall spasm. Pethidine has an active metabolite, normeperidine which may accumulate in renal failure. That metabolite may cause reversible neurotoxic effects like agitation, hallucination (rare), and very rare, seizures, particularly in small infants after repeated doses.

Contraindications: hypotension, impaired consciousness unless patient is intubated and on ventilator.

7.3.4 Tramadol

Tramadol is currently the most commonly prescribed opioid analgesic worldwide. It is weaker than most of the other narcotic drugs, and in many countries, it is not under DDA. That means it would not need to be kept in a special locked DDA cupboard and no special bookkeeping would be required. However, it is recommended to store all anaesthesia drugs in locked cupboards because that increases safety and diminishes misuse. Local regulations must always be observed.

Preparations: 2 mL ampoules with 50 mg/mL for IM, IV injection, tablets with 50 or 100 mg, additionally slow-release tablets with up to 400 mg.

Indication: moderate to severe pain. Tramadol is rather safe during labour pain as only 1% is crossing the placenta.

Effects: analgesia, less sedation than morphine or pethidine.

Dose: 1 mg/kg or 50–100 mg for adults depending on severity of pain. In contrast to other opioids, tramadol has a maximum dose that is 600 mg/24 h for adults. Probably, higher doses would not add to effect, so that stronger opioids are needed if tramadol max dose is insufficient. For patients who don't get sufficient analgesia with 100 mg tramadol, 10 mg of morphine is a better choice or combination of tramadol with one ampoule of diclofenac. Patients with chronic renal failure should get lower daily doses, e.g. 100 mg BD as max dose.

Onset and duration: 30 min after injection and after oral administration, duration 6 h.

Side effects: less respiratory depression and constipation than the other opioids, especially compared to morphine. Fast injection is likely to cause nausea. Slow injection or short infusion over 30 min is better tolerated. Tramadol may cause seizures in patients on antidepressant drugs.

Contraindications: epileptic patients.

7.3.5 Codeine

Although codeine is also an opioid drug, it is weak and not suited for treatment of severe pain. Not classified as DDA. A proportion of codeine is metabolised to morphine by liver enzymes. The analgesic effect is quite variable due to fast or slow metabolising conditions (genetic variability) in different people.

Preparation: tablets with 30 mg or ampoules containing 60 mg in 1 mL for IM injection; not for IV administration. Dihydrocodeine is twice as potent as codeine.

Indication: mild to moderate pain, cough, acute diarrhoea.

Effects: analgesic, anti-cough, sedation, anti-diarrhoeal.

Dose: codeine 30–60 mg, dihydrocodeine 15–30 mg.

Onset and duration: onset 15–30 min, duration 4–6 h.

Side effects: respiratory depression is possible if overdosed and in fast metabolisers who are reaching high peak effect; dizziness, constipation, nausea, abdominal cramps.

Contraindications: allergy; codeine should be used with caution in children <12 years.

7.3.6 Naloxone

Naloxone is a pure opioid antagonist with no intrinsic effects. That means a patient who is receiving naloxone would not show any effects if no opioid was in the body.

Preparation: ampoules with 0.4 mg in 1 mL.

Indication: respiratory depression caused by opioid overdose.

Effects: antagonises all effects of opioids.

Dose: dilute 1 ampoule with 9 mL NS to make 0.04 mg/mL, titrate to effect with 0.04 mg increments. In an emergency with no availability to ventilate a patient, a higher dose may be given, around 0.1–0.2 mg; only in very rare situations, the whole ampoule is needed.

Onset and duration: onset 1–2 min, duration around 20–40 min which may be shorter than the effects to be antagonised. Observation of the patients in a HDU on pulse oximeter and counting respiratory rate is mandatory. Repeated doses may be needed.

Side effects: hypertension, tachycardia, arrhythmia, sweating, severe pain.

Contraindications: acute myocardial ischaemia, known allergy (hypersensitivity) (extremely rare).

7.3.7 Pentazocine

Like codeine or tramadol, pentazocine is one of the weaker opioids and usually not under DDA. The drug is not available in a number of countries but used a lot in other countries.

Preparation: ampoules with 1 mL at 30 mg/mL for SC and IM injection (not for IV injection), tablets for oral intake.

Indication: treatment of moderate to severe pain.

Effects: while all other opioids listed in this chapter are mainly acting at the MOP receptors (μ opioid receptors), pentazocine is an agonist at KOP (κ or kappa opioid receptors) and σ or sigma receptors and acting as antagonist at MOP receptors. Therefore, it has a ceiling effect and should not be used in much higher dose than 0.5 mg/kg since that would add to side effects without causing better analgesia.

Dose: 30 mg IM or 50–100 mg orally in adults.

Onset and duration: 15–30 min after injection, 1–3 h after oral administration, duration 3–4 h.

Side effects: less respiratory depression, nausea and constipation than equivalent doses of morphine; dry mouth, sweating; hallucinations and nightmares are not uncommon especially if higher doses are administered.

Contraindications: allergy (very rare); addiction to any opioid drug.

7.3.8 Buprenorphine

Buprenorphine is a very strong opioid drug with long duration of action and mixed agonist and antagonistic effects at opioid receptors. It cannot be reversed with naloxone; instead it can antagonise effects of morphine, although not reliably, and should not be combined with other opioids. If respiratory depression does occur, oxygen and ventilation support may be needed for prolonged hours.

Preparation: ampoules with 0.6 mg in 2 mL at 0.3 mg/mL for IM and IV injection; tablets for sublingual administration with 0.2 and 0.4 mg.

Indication: severe pain.

Effects: same as morphine; analgesia, sedation, anti-cough, miosis.

Dose: 0.3–0.6 mg IM or IV; 0.2–0.4 mg sublingually for adults >50 kg; 0.15 mg IM or 0.1 mg sublingually for children >30 kg.

Onset and duration: 10–20 min; duration 6–8 h.

Side effects: respiratory depression especially if combined with other sedative drugs; nausea, vomiting; drowsiness, dysphoria; anaphylactoid reactions.

Contraindications: known allergy.

7.4 NSAIDs and Other Non-opioid Analgesics

7.4.1 Diclofenac

Diclofenac is a nonsteroidal anti-inflammatory drug (NSAID, analgesic drug which is mainly acting at peripheral COX-1 and COX-2 receptors). NSAIDs produce analgesia and show anti-inflammatory and antipyretic (anti-fever) effects.

Preparation: tablets with 25, 50 or 75 mg; 3 mL ampoules with 75 mg at 25 mg/mL for IM injection; some preparations are also for IV infusion (put 1 ampoule in a small amount of NS) or slow IV injection.

Indication: mild to moderate pain, fever; in combination with opioid analgesic even for severe pain.

Effects: analgesia, decreases fever, suppresses inflammation.

Dose: 1–2 mg/kg TDS for max 2 days in acute pain, thereafter 0.5–1 mg/kg TDS.

Onset and duration: 15-30 min, lasting 6–8 h.

Side effects: IM injection may be very painful and should be omitted in children unless they are anaesthetised. Inject diclofenac before waking the patients at the end of surgery. Later after surgery, patients should receive oral drugs instead of painful injection. The function of platelets is inhibited reversibly; however, this effect is usually mild and no contraindication for postoperative pain relief after most types of surgery (do not use it if bleeding during operation unusually severe).

Contraindications: asthma, kidney insufficiency, elderly patients who are on ACE blockers, acute severe bleeding, head injury with TBI, gastric ulcer.

7.4.2 Ketorolac

Ketorolac belongs to the NSAID.

Preparation: ampoules with 30 mg per 1 mL, tablets with 10 mg.

Indication: short-term treatment of moderate to severe pain.

Effects: analgesic and anti-inflammatory.

Dose: adults 15–60 mg IV, the max dose for treatment of acute pain is 120 mg per day 1, 15–30 mg TDS from day 2 or 10 mg QDS orally no longer than few days; children 0.5 mg/kg.

Onset and duration: 30 min, 4–6 h.

Side effects: gastritis, impaired platelet aggregation, thrombotic events if used for prolonged time in high dose.

Contraindications: allergy, NSAID provoked asthma, kidney disease, peptic ulcer, myocardial infarction, pre- and postpartum bleeding, any major bleeding, head injury, craniotomy, intracranial bleeding.

7.4.3 Ibuprofen

Ibuprofen belongs to the NSAID.

Preparation: tablets with 200, 400, or 600 mg, suspension for oral intake, no injectable preparation.

Indication: mild to moderate pain, migraine, fever.

Effects: analgesic, anti-fever and anti-inflammatory.

Dose: adults 400 mg TDS or QDS, the max dose for treatment of acute pain is 800 mg TDS no longer than few days; 10 mg/kg children.

Onset and duration: 15–30 min, 4–6 h.

Side effects: gastritis, high dose may have effects on platelet aggregation, thrombotic events if used for prolonged time in high dose.

Contraindications: allergy, NSAID provoked asthma, renal failure, peptic ulcer, myocardial infarction, major bleeding.

7.4.4 Paracetamol

Paracetamol is a weak analgesic and antipyretic drug which is not NSAID due to its lacking anti-inflammatory effect.

Preparation: tablets with 250 or 500 mg, suspension, suppositories, IV infusion with 100 mL containing 500 or 1000 mg.

Indication: mild to moderate pain and fever.

Effects: anti-pain, anti-fever.

Dose: 15 mg/kg QDS, adults >50 kg BW 500–1000 mg QDS.

Onset and duration: 10–20 min, 4–6 h.

Side effects: usually no side effects unless overdosed. A toxic dose of >100 mg/kg may lead to nausea and vomiting, abdominal pain, sweating, shock, and finally liver failure.

Contraindications: severe liver disease, liver failure.

7.4.5 Metamizole

Metamizole (dipyrone, noramidopyrine, Novalgin®) is a strong non-opioid analgesic with less effect on platelet function than diclofenac or ketorolac. Is has no anti-inflammatory effects. It is not available in all countries. In combination with opioids like morphine it is producing a supra-additive effect with excellent analgesia but no increased risk for respiratory depression.

Preparation: ampoules with 500 mg/mL; usually 2 mL ampoules; tablets with 500 mg.

Indication: moderate to severe pain, fever; also suitable for treatment of cancer pain.

Effects: anti-pain, anti-fever.

Dose: 0.5–1 g slowly IV > 10 min, or orally in adults; 10–20 mg/kg in children.

Onset and duration: 10–20 min; 4–6 h.

Side effects: hypotension (avoid rapid IV injection), nausea, gastritis, dizziness, vertigo; rare: haemolytic anaemia, thrombocytopenia, leucopenia, anaphylactic shock.

Contraindications: children <3 months or 5 kg; pregnancy and breast-feeding mothers; dehydration, hypotension, severe liver/kidney impairment, allergy to NSAID, bone marrow disease with severe leucopenia or anaemia.

7.5 Sedatives

Some of the drugs causing sedation may lead to addiction and should only be used for limited time and due to clear indications. Indications can be anxiety before surgery, sedation during procedures like gastroscopy, or combination with anaesthetic drugs as a part of balanced anaesthesia, as well as acute agitation or acute psychosis. Other sedative drugs have also excellent antiemetic effects, often at lower doses than the sedative effect, and can be used for that purpose as well. They are not producing analgesia but may increase the pain threshold and enhance the effect of analgesics. Clonidine is a drug with many different effects and not fitting in just one of the classes in this chapter, however, it is listed here. It has sedative and antihypertensive effects, diminishes the stress response to surgery, is useful as part of balanced anaesthesia since it decreases the requirements of the anaesthetics, and it has analgesic and antiemetic properties.

7.5.1 Diazepam

Diazepam, Midazolam, and Lorazepam are belonging to the benzodiazepines, drugs acting on the $GABA_A$, the most widespread inhibitory receptors in the CNS. Children need higher doses per kg than adults.

Preparation: 2 mL-ampoules with 5 mg/mL for IV injection. Tablets with 5 or 10 mg.

Indication: Nice as premedication or a few minutes before start of anaesthesia, even for sedation during regional anaesthesia. It produces sedation, in combination with fentanyl or ketamine hypnosis; no analgesic effects; common drug for treatment of seizures; no effects on circulation. Only single dose since the drug would accumulate (exception: treatment of tetanus where long-lasting effects are required).

Effects: anxiolysis, amnesia, sedation, may induce sleep, antiepileptic (= anticonvulsive), slight muscle relaxation.

Dose: Average dose is 5–10 mg IV in adults, 2.5–5 mg in children.

Onset and duration: onset within 3–5 min after IV injection, 15–30 min after oral intake. Duration depends on the dose and is at least 1 h, can be much longer, especially after repeated doses.

Side effects: Pain on injection. Inject slowly and have a fast-running infusion going. The combination of diazepam with opioids like morphine, fentanyl or pethidine may cause profound respiratory depression (have pulse oximeter attached and observe respiration).

Contraindications: caesarean section before the baby is delivered, because it may cause a "flabby baby" which is not breathing and has little muscle tone.

7.5.2 Midazolam

Preparation: ampoules with 5 mg in 5 mL, or with 15 mg in 3 mL; in some countries even tablets and oral suspension.

Indication: sedation for premedication or procedures or in the ICU; combination with ketamine for short GA.

Effects: Amnesia, anxiolysis, sedation both short term and in intensive care, anticonvulsive; that is the same effects and side effects as diazepam, but shorter acting and stronger.

Dose: 1–5 mg IV per adult or more if required (titrate to desired effect); around 0.1 mg/kg IV for children; 5 mg for grand mal epilepsy; around 0.1 mg/kg for premedication orally, 0.3 mg/kg orally for children.

Onset and duration: 3–5 min after IV injection, 5–10 min after IM, and 10–20 min after oral administration. Duration 1–2 h.

Side effects: in combination with opioids, respiratory depression possible.

Contraindications: same as for diazepam.

7.5.3 Lorazepam

Preparation: ampoules with 1 or 2 mg; tablets with 2 mg.

Indication: premedication, sedation (e.g. agitated patients in the recovery area), treating epileptic seizures.

Effects: same as for diazepam and midazolam.

Dose: 1–2 mg in adults for sedation, max dose 4 mg in status epilepticus, children 0.05 mg/kg.

Onset and duration: 10–20 min, several hours.

Side effects: same as for diazepam and midazolam.

Contraindications: same as for diazepam.

7.5.4 Chlorpromazine

Chlorpromazine is a neuroleptic agent producing sedation, anti-psychotic and antiemetic effects; even antihistamine, but nowadays rarely used to treat allergic reactions.

Preparation: ampoules with 50 mg in 1 mL (50 mg/mL) or in 2 mL (25 mg/mL) for IV or IM injection.

Indication: sedation, premedication, prevention and treatment of PONV, acute psychosis, combination with anaesthetics for balanced anaesthesia.

Effects: sedation, sleep inducing, antiemetic, reduces MAC of inhalational anaesthetics.

Dose: 25–50 mg.

Onset and duration: onset 10–20 min after IV, 4–6 h sedation; up to 12 h antiemetic effect.

Side effects: mild hypotension, hypothermia (keep patient warm); rare: malignant neuroleptic syndrome.

Contraindications: hypersensitivity to chlorpromazine or promethazine.

7.5.5 Promethazine

Promethazine is a neuroleptic and antihistamine agent of same class as chlorpromazine. Since it has many different effects and only mild side effects it is a useful drug for many purposes and is listed here and under antiemetic drugs.

Preparation: ampoules with 50 mg in 1 mL (50 mg/mL) or in 2 mL (25 mg/mL) for IV or IM injection.

Indication: premedication, sedation, balanced anaesthesia, treatment of allergy, motion sickness, PONV, upper airway tract infections.

Effects: sedation, sleep induction, antiemetic, antihistamine (antiallergic), bronchodilatation, reduces secretions in the airways, anticough.

Dose: 25–50 mg.

Onset and duration: 10–20 min; 6–8 h, antiemetic effect up to 12 h.

Side effects: drowsiness, dizziness, nightmares (uncommon if combined with diazepam or midazolam).

Contraindications: hypersensitivity to chlorpromazine or promethazine.

7.5.6 Clonidine

Clonidine acts at α_2-receptors of the sympathetic nervous system in the brain and in pain modulating pathways in the spinal cord.

Preparation: ampoules with 0.15 mg in 1 mL for dilution with 9 mL NS to make 0.015 mg/mL (=15 μg/mL); tablets.

Indication: inhibiting stress response to surgical stimulus; as part of balanced anaesthesia; treatment of acute hypertension; analgesic during or after surgery; prophylaxis and treatment of PONV; shivering after anaesthesia and surgery; agitation during recovery from anaesthesia.

Effects: reducing the requirements for inhalation anaesthetics by up to 50%; antihypertensive; antiemetic; analgesic; anti-shivering; sedation. After initial increase of BP, clonidine causes some hypotension or normalising high BP.

Dose: 1–2 μg/kg that is 4–10 mL of the dilution with 0.015 mg/mL; divide the dose in small increments of 15–30 μg every few minutes to avoid short-lasting hypertension.

Onset and duration: 3–5 min, 3–8 h duration.

Side effects: dry mouth, drowsiness, bradycardia.

Contraindications: hypersensitivity; cautions in patients with heart block, bradycardia, hypotension.

7.6 Muscle Relaxants and Reversal Agents

NMBA (neuromuscular blocking agents or muscle relaxants MR) are acting at the neuromuscular junction that is the place where the motor nerve is ending in the muscle fibre. There are two types: short-acting, depolarising (succinylcholine) and longer acting, non-depolarising muscle relaxants (all other). They act only at the peripheral nerve endings where they block the neuromuscular junction and thus paralyse skeletal muscles. They are not producing any effects on the brain. Make always sure that the patient is unconscious before giving muscle relaxant and that you are able to ventilate as soon as the diaphragm is paralysed.

Remember, MR are not providing analgesia or hypnosis and must not be used instead of anaesthetics or to treat inadequate anaesthesia.

See Sect. 15.9 for "prolonged effects of MR".

See Sect. 15.7 for MH.

Nerve stimulator for monitoring effects of MR, TOF Train of four—test for residual muscle paralysis is recommended since the duration of effect is varying a lot between patients. Residual block is potentially dangerous postoperatively if patients are unable to keep airways free of secretions and produce effective cough. Airway muscles may remain weak even though a nerve stimulator might show full recovery. Different muscle groups in the body are showing different sensitivity for MR. The airway muscles are more sensitive than muscles of the abdominal wall or the limbs.

NMBA are decreasing the respiratory response to hypoxia (mediated by chemoreceptors in the carotid bodies). Long-acting MR like pancuronium must not be used if oxygen is not continuously available during surgery and postoperatively. Patients who received these agents should be put on oxygen for several hours after extubation.

7.6.1 Suxamethonium

Suxamethonium is a short acting muscle relaxant and the only MR with depolarising mechanism of action at the receptors of the neuromuscular junction. This means, the drug causes muscles to fasciculate shortly before achieving a profound but short-lasting relaxation. Since suxamethonium may cause severe bradycardia, it should always be combined with atropine.

Preparation: ampoules with 20 or 50 mg/mL, usually 100 mg per ampoule, for IV or IM injection (IM only if venous access is missing and emergency situation or inhalational induction before venous access is established).

Indication: to facilitate endotracheal intubation or surgery where muscle relaxation is required; to break severe laryngospasm (but not effective in bronchospasm), sometimes even indicated to facilitate insertion of LM.

Effects: short lasting muscle relaxation for intubation and surgery.

Dose: adults 1 mg/kg, children 1.5–2 mg/kg, increments during surgery <0.5 mg/kg or 25 mg in adults, excellent effect, e.g. for opening or closing the abdomen. It is not recommended to use more than around 300 mg in adult patients as total dose.

Onset and duration: 30–60 s, 3–5 min. Duration depends on the level of the enzyme plasma cholinesterase and may be slightly prolonged in some patients, especially in pregnant mothers and in very sick patients, but is still shorter than with all other MR. In the unlikely event that more than 500 mg have been used, a long-lasting neuromuscular block can occur which cannot be reversed until it subsides after a few hours. Some patients have a genetic disorder with decreased plasma cholinesterase activity. In those patients, duration of effect is prolonged to 10 min or, more seldom, to several hours (very rare but important to recognise; see Sect. 15.9 for details).

Side effects: bradycardia, arrhythmia, mild to moderate muscle pain postoperatively, anaphylactic reaction (especially after repeated exposure), MH (rare). Masseter muscle rigidity occurs seldom but would mean that laryngoscopy for intubation impossible; insertion of LMA in some of these cases possible (→ give propofol; a non-depolarising MR like pancuronium is likely not to be helpful). Intraocular pressure and intracerebral pressure may rise shortly but this is no reason not to use the drug and is usually not significant if suxa is combined with a hypnotic agent. Elevation of serum potassium may cause cardiac arrest, see contraindications.

Contraindications: Inability to ventilate the patient and to secure the airway until the effect has worn off. Known or suspected allergy/hypersensitivity. Risk for or history of malignant hyperthermia. Increased risk for dangerous hyperkalaemia in patients with neurologic disease, paraplegia, patients after burns, patients after crush trauma (massive trauma with destroyed muscle tissue), patients with progressive muscle disease, and bed-ridden patients >5 days.

7.6.2 Pancuronium

Pancuronium is a long-acting muscle relaxant drug with slow onset of action. It may be the only available muscle relaxant making rapid sequence induction difficult (see Chap. 6).

Preparation: ampoules with 4 mg in 2 mL for IV injection.

Indication: muscle relaxation during surgery which requires muscles relaxed, especially abdominal surgery with duration of operation of more than 1 h.

Effects: Non-depolarising muscle relaxant.

Dose: 0.05–0.1 mg/kg; usually only single dose since the drug may accumulate and duration of effect may be prolonged.

Onset and duration: onset after 3 min, long and unpredictable duration of 45–90 min, longer effect in the muscles of the throat; prolonged action if urine output low and in patients with impaired kidney function, in patients of old age or at impaired general condition. Only slight residual effect after more than 45 min is reversible with atropine and neostigmine.

Side effects: slightly increased heart rate; longer lasting weakness of the muscles in the throat and inability to effectively cough may cause pulmonary aspiration of secretions and lead to pneumonia postoperatively.

Contraindications: Inability to ventilate the patient and to secure the airway until the effect has worn off.

7.6.3 Vecuronium

Vecuronium is the only muscle relaxant which does not need storage in a fridge but remains stable at ambient temperature since it is presented as a powder for solution before use. Unfortunately, it is not always available in many countries.

Preparation: vials with a powder containing 10 mg for solution and dilution with finally 10 mL to make 1 mg/mL.

Indication: Non-depolarising muscle relaxant.

Effects: muscle relaxation during surgery which requires muscles relaxed.

Dose: 0.05–0.1 mg/kg, increments 0.03 mg/kg.

Onset and duration: 1.5–2 min, duration of surgical relaxation 30–40 min, weakness of the pharyngeal muscles last longer, around 60 min or more.

Side effects: usually none; very rare allergic reaction.

Contraindications: Inability to ventilate the patient and to secure the airway until the effect has worn off.

7.6.4 Atracurium

Preparation: ampoules with 2.5 or 5 mL at 10 mg/mL.

Indication: Non-depolarising muscle relaxant. 0.5 mg/kg. Onset after 2 min. Duration of action 30–45 min. Elimination is predictable and independent of liver and kidney function but prolonged by hypothermia.

Effects: muscle relaxation during surgery which requires muscles relaxed.

Dose: 0.5 mg/kg, increments 0.2 mg/kg.

Onset and duration: 1.5–3 min, duration of surgical relaxation around 30 min, weakness of the pharyngeal muscles lasts around 60 min and sometimes longer.

Side effects: flush, redness of the skin, rash, bronchospasm, wheezing due to histamine liberation (but usually harmless and no anaphylactoid reaction); can be prevented or treated with promethazine. Increased effect if gentamicin or magnesium are administered.

Contraindications: Inability to ventilate the patient and to secure the airway until the effect has worn off.

7.6.5 Rocuronium

Rocuronium is a non-depolarising muscle relaxant with fast onset and long duration.

Preparation: ampoules with 5 mL containing 50 mg at 10 mg/mL.

Indication: long-lasting MR during surgery. Rocuronium may be used for intubation in patients with contraindication for suxamethonium. Due to its longer lasting effect, it may only be used if you are sure to be able to establish an artificial airway; or if huge amounts of the reversal drug sugammadex are at hands. Remember that most patients can be intubated safely without muscle relaxant if a sufficient dose of propofol (2–4 mg/kg) plus analgesic (e.g. ketamine) is used.

Effects: muscle relaxation for intubation and during surgery.

Dose: 0.6 mg/kg, increments 0.2 mg/kg.

Onset and duration: 90 seconds, duration dependent on the dose 30–60 min or longer. Effect on respiratory muscles and upper airway muscles may last much longer. Elimination is prolonged in renal or liver failure.

Side effects: usually no direct side effects but beware of residual block, see above. Anaphylactoid reaction: only symptom may be sudden hypotension with non-measurable BP requiring small dose of adrenaline to resolve.

Contraindications: Inability to ventilate the patient and to secure the airway until the effect has worn off; known or suspected hypersensitivity.

7.6.6 Reversal Agents for MR (NMBA)

7.6.6.1 Neostigmine

Neostigmine is the most common reversal agent for muscle-relaxant drugs.

Preparation: 2.5 mg/mL ampoules for IV injection. Tablets with 15 mg.

Indication: IV: reversal of non-depolarising muscle relaxants (all MR with the exception of suxamethonium which cannot be reversed) 30 min or more after injection of the relaxant. The drug is also used for treatment of certain types of intoxication and some snake bites. Details are beyond the scope of this book. Tablets are used in the treatment of myasthenia gravis, a chronic autoimmune disease with progressive muscle weakness.

Effects: It does only reverse a light residual effect. A full dose of relaxant cannot be antagonised with neostigmine. Reversal may be incomplete, and the patient may still be unable to keep a patent airway, especially after more than one dose of MR. The use of a peripheral nerve stimulator to assess recovery of neuromuscular function is very useful. See also Sect. 15.9 for more details.

Dose: 2.5 mg IV for adults, 0.05 mg/kg (with atropine 0.02 mg/kg) for children.

Onset and duration: 2–5 min, max effect after 10 min, duration around 1 h.

Side effects: Can cause bradycardia, nausea, abdominal cramps, bronchospasm, and secretions in the airways. Combination with atropine 0.5 mg is decreasing the side effects. Neostigmine may cause muscle weakness if given to patients who did not get a non-depolarising MR.

Contraindications: neuromuscular block caused by suxamethonium, mechanical obstruction of bowels or urinary tract, allergy towards bromide or neostigmine.

7.6.6.2 Pyridostigmine

Preparation: ampoules with 2 mL containing 5 mg/mL. tablets with 60 mg.

Indication: the same as for neostigmine. It is mainly used for treatment of myasthenia gravis.

Effects: the same as for neostigmine.

Dose: 10 mg IV in adults for reversal of MR after more than 30 min.

Onset and duration: 5–10 min after IV injection, duration 2–3 h.

Side effects: the same as for neostigmine.

Contraindications: the same as for neostigmine.

7.6.6.3 Sugammadex

Although at present not available in many countries and expensive, it is to be mentioned in this book because of excellent effects as a unique and complete reversal drug for rocuronium and pancuronium (but not for atracurium) without side effects. Hopefully, it will be more affordable and available in the future.

Preparation: vials with 200 mg in 2 mL for IV injection.

Indication: reversal of neuromuscular block exclusively of rocuronium and pancuronium.

Effects: irreversible antagonism of neuromuscular blocking effects of rocuronium or pancuronium by encapsulating the drug molecules in the body.

Dose: for reversal of residual effects 200 mg in adults, several times higher doses for reversal of full muscle relaxation.

Onset and duration: onset 1–2 min; duration is permanent.

Side effects: extremely rare cardiac failure due to extreme bradycardia, usually no side effects.

Contraindications: allergy; neuromuscular block with other agents than rocuronium or pancuronium.

7.7 Local Anaesthetics

Local anaesthetics are blocking nerve impulses in a discrete region of the body where feeling of pain, touch, temperature, and motor reaction are blocked for a time period after which these functions are recovering automatically.

For local anaesthetic toxicity see Sect. 15.8. See Chap. 10 for spinal anaesthesia.

LA may be combined with vasoconstrictor, usually adrenaline 0.005 mg/mL (5 μg/mL), to decrease toxicity and increase duration of effect due to decreased rate of tissue absorption. Don't use adrenaline for LA in areas at risk for ischaemia due to vasoconstriction like the fingers, toes, or the penis.

7.7.1 Lidocaine

Lidocaine is the most commonly available LA agent. It can be mixed with adrenaline to extend duration of effect or to produce vasoconstriction during surgery thus minimising bleeding. Add 0.5 mL of adrenaline 1 mg/mL to 100 mL of local anaesthetic (or 0.2 mL = 0.2 mg for 40 mL of LA) to make 5 μg/mL adrenaline. Higher concentrations of adrenaline are likely to cause dangerous hypertension and tachycardia and should be avoided.

Preparation: 10 mg/mL (1%) and 20 mg/mL (2%) with and without adrenaline for local infiltration and regional block; 50 mg/mL (5%) lidocaine with dextrose for spinal anaesthesia.

Indication: local or infiltration anaesthesia, regional block; IV: treatment of ventricular arrhythmia; prevention of laryngeal reflexes on intubation.

Effects: local or regional anaesthesia that is numbness in the target region of effect. Lidocaine IV is even acting on nerve fibres in the heart, thereby stabilising ectopic ventricular rhythms. Lidocaine IV prevents from laryngospasm during intubation.

Dose: dependent on the type of block; max dose 7 mg/kg with and 4 mg/kg without adrenaline.

Onset and duration: 2–5 min; duration 30–90 min, with adrenaline up to 2 h.

Side effects: short-lasting hypotension due to vasodilatation; hypertension (sometimes extreme), and tachycardia if combined with adrenaline. Local nerve toxicity, very rare cauda equina syndrome after spinal anaesthesia (pain in buttocks and legs, motor dysfunction, numbness, incontinence; more frequently TNS = transient neurological symptoms, usually pain, which resolves within a few days and responds to ordinary analgetics).

Contraindications: allergy (extremely rare).

7.7.2 Bupivacaine

Preparation: 2.5 mg/mL or 5 mg/mL with and without adrenaline in vials or ampoules with different volumes.

Indication: local or infiltration anaesthesia, regional block, spinal or epidural anaesthesia.

Effects: local or regional block during surgery, for postoperative pain relief or for labour pain.

Dose: dependent on the type of block; max dose 2 mg/kg with and without adrenaline; for continuous blockade not more than 0.5 mg/kg/h. For average adult, max dose means approximately 30 mL of bupivacaine 5 mg/mL or 60 mL of 2.5 mg/mL. Remember that some plexus anaesthesia methods may require 40 mL volume, and that 2.5 mg/mL bupivacaine is not strong enough for that regional block. Mix lidocaine and bupivacaine in such cases to avoid overdose of bupivacaine.

Onset and duration: onset 5–10 min; duration 2–4 h without, 4–8 h with adrenaline; for spinal 1.5–2.5 h.

Side effects: local tissue toxicity, especially nerve toxicity as with lidocaine but more seldom; systemic toxicity see Chap. 15. Bupivacaine shows the highest risk for cardiac toxicity of all local anaesthetics. Be very careful not to use more than the maximum dose of 2 mg/kg. For children, dilute bupivacaine to avoid toxic dose.

Contraindications: drug allergy (very rare).

7.8 Cardiovascular Drugs for Increasing Heart Rate and Treating Hypotension During Anaesthesia and Critical Care

7.8.1 Adrenaline (Epinephrine)

Adrenaline, in some countries called epinephrine, is a natural neurotransmitter produced in the adrenal glands. It is extremely short-lived with a half-life of only 3 min due to metabolic breakdown. Adrenaline is the strongest agent acting on the sympathetic nervous system. It is also produced as drug, is normally available worldwide and should not be missing in any operating theatre, maternity, ICU, HDU, or emergency department.

Preparation: 1 mg/mL (sometimes labelled 1:1000) in ampoules for IV injection after further dilution, or IM undiluted (treatment of anaphylaxis), even via nebuliser for post-extubation croup or other types of severe bronchospasm. In some countries, 1 mg per 10 mL = 0.1 mg/mL in ampoules is ready for resuscitation.

Indication: circulatory shock, cardiac arrest, anaphylactoid reaction, hypotension during spinal anaesthesia or GA, severe bronchospasm.

Effects: on the heart: increased contractility, increased heart rate, stroke volume and cardiac output; on circulation: vasoconstriction; increased blood pressure; on bronchi: bronchodilation; on pupil size: dilatation; visual accommodation: impaired; glucose and fat metabolism in the liver: gluconeogenesis with increased blood glucose; platelet aggregation; prolonged action of local anaesthetic when mixed at 0.005 mg/mL (0.5 mg per 100 mL) with LA.

Dose: 0.005 mg – 1 mg dependent on the indication and situation. A dilution as into an infusion is only stable for max 24 h, thereafter effect of adrenaline is declining or absent.

Onset and duration: 0.5–1 min after IV bolus, duration only 3 min. Due to the short duration of action, it is often administered with infusion or syringe pump.

Side effects: hypertension, tachycardia, arrhythmia, urinary retention, increased sweating.

Contraindications: as additive for LA of digits, toes, penis (risk for ischaemia).

7.8.2 Atropine

Atropine is a parasympatholytic, anticholinergic agent, antagonising effects of the vagal nerve and other parts of the parasympathetic nervous system, in higher doses also causing central nervous effects.

Preparation: most common in ampoules with 0.5 mg/mL, some preparations are 1 mg/mL or 0.6 mg/mL.

Indication: prevention and treatment of bradycardia, prevention of salivation/reducing secretion in the pharynx, blocking reflexes of the larynx, treating nausea during caesarean section.

Effects: faster heart rate, decreased salivation and secretion, prevents reflex bradycardia and asystole, reducing risk of laryngospasm, bronchodilator, antiemetic.

Dose: usually 0.5 mg in adults IV, 0.01–0.02 mg/kg in children IV or IM.

Onset and duration: onset of effect within 1 min, duration 30–60 min.

Side effects: tachycardia, dry mouth, dilated pupils, stops sweating, increasing body temperature especially in children. Overdose may cause sedation, hallucinations, agitation.

Contraindications: thyrotoxicosis, closed angle glaucoma.

7.8.3 Ephedrine

Ephedrine is a synthetic sympathomimetic agent for treatment of acute hypotension which is mainly acting on heart rate and systemic vascular resistance.

Preparation: ampoules with 30 mg/mL or 50 mg/mL.

Indication: low blood pressure during general and regional anaesthesia.

Effects: vasoconstriction, increased heart rate and cardiac output, bronchodilation.

Dose: 1 mL is diluted to 10 mL. Increments of 3–5 mg IV.

Onset and duration: onset within 1 min, duration around 20–30 min. Effective only after short-term administration due to tolerance (so-called tachyphylaxia) after repeated doses.

Side effects: hypertension, tachycardia, arrhythmia especially when given during halothane anaesthesia.

Contraindications: closed angle glaucoma, thyroid storm,

7.8.4 Noradrenaline (Norepinephrine)

Noradrenaline is not available in all countries. It is the strongest vasopressor and first choice in patients with septic shock who may otherwise receive adrenaline infusion.

Preparation: 1 mg/mL (1:1000) in ampoules for dilution for continuous infusion via syringe pump, e.g. 1 mg + 49 mL saline or 2 mg + 98 mL to make 20 µg/mL.

Indication: patients with cardiac failure, septic shock, severe hypotension during anaesthesia.

Effects: the drug is a potent vasopressor and produces vasoconstriction; on the heart: increased contractility; no change or decrease of heart rate.

Dose: 0.03–0.15 mg/kg/min approximately; the dose is titrated to effect.

Onset and duration: 0.5–1 min after IV bolus, duration only 3 min. Due to the short duration of action is administered with infusion or with syringe pump.

Side effects: hypertension, bradycardia, diminished organ perfusion if vasoconstriction is marked.

Contraindications: if indicated, none; but make sure that sufficient fluids are administered. Due to very strong effect, noradrenaline should exclusively be administered via infusion pump to control exact dosing.

7.8.5 Dopamine

Dopamine is another inotropic agent which can be used as second--line drug to treat low cardiac output if adrenaline or noradrenaline are unavailable.

Presentation: ampoules with 200 mg in 5 mL (40 mg/mL) for dilution, e.g. 200 mg with 500 mL → 5–50 drops/min; or 100 mg = 2.5 mL in 50 mL with syringe pump → 3–30 mL/h titrated to desired effect.

Indication: second-line drug instead of adrenaline to treat low cardiac output, hypotension, bradycardia perioperatively (if not responding to adequate IV fluids, ephedrine, decreasing doses of anaesthesia drugs) and in intensive care patients with sepsis instead of noradrenaline.

Effects: sympathomimetic (increased heart rate and stroke volume → increased CO); increased kidney blood flow with increased diuresis; in higher dose vasoconstriction and elevating BP.

Dose: 2–10 µg/kg/min, septic shock up to 20 µg/kg/min (but noradrenaline or adrenaline more effective).

Onset and duration: onset within 5 min; duration 10 min, therefore as continuous infusion only.

Side effects: nausea, vomiting, tachycardia, arrhythmia, hypertension; accidental paravenous administration causes tissue necrosis.

Contraindications: Increased intraocular pressure.

7.8.6 Phenylephrine

Phenylephrine is a sympathomimetic agent which is producing peripheral vasoconstriction.

Preparation: ampoules with 10 mg in 1 mL for IV or IM injection or infusion after dilution, e.g. 10 mg into 100 mL or 500 mL NS to make 0.1 mg/mL or 0.02 mg/mL, resp.

Indication: treating hypotension during general or spinal anaesthesia.

Effects: vasopressor; no effects at the heart.

Dose: single bolus IV: 0.05–0.1 mg; infusion with 0.01–0.1 mg/min.

Onset and duration: within 1 min after IV bolus, duration 5–10 min; IM 15 min onset, 1 h duration.

Side effects: reflex bradycardia; dizziness, extensive hypertension in patients with toxic goitre; arrhythmia in patients on tricyclic antidepressants or quinine; extravascular injection may cause tissue necrosis.

Contraindications: hypersensitivity, hyperthyroidism.

7.9 Diuretics and Antihypertensive Drugs During Anaesthesia and Critical Care

7.9.1 Furosemide

Furosemide is a strong loop diuretic (acting on the ascending loop of Henle in the kidney) with additional antihypertensive effects.

Preparation: ampoules with 2 mL containing 10 mg/mL, even ampoules with 250 or 500 mg for IV injection and infusion; tablets.

Indication: IV for treatment of hypertensive crisis, lung oedema caused by heart failure, other states of fluid overload, during surgery of the prostate; tablets for treatment of hypertension or chronic renal failure.

Effects: after IV injection immediate pulmonary vasodilatation causing relief of dyspnoea already before diuresis; decreasing preload to the heart; decreasing arterial blood pressure; rapid and powerful diuretic effect.

Dose: 10–20 mg slowly IV; higher dose only as continuous infusion in ICU.

Onset and duration: 5 min; 2 h after IV bolus.

Side effects: hypotension, hypovolaemia, hypokalaemia.

Contraindications: anuria caused by dehydration or hypovolaemic shock.

7.9.2 Glyceryl Trinitrate

Glyceryl trinitrate (GTN) or nitroglycerin is used for the treatment of acute hypertensive crisis and angina pectoris in emergency department/HDU/ICU. It is also useful for treatment of severe hypertension in patients for emergency surgery in whom BP is not decreasing sufficiently by general or spinal anaesthesia.

Presentation: 5 mL vials/ampoules at 1 or 5 mg/mL for dilution and IV infusion; spray and tablets for sublingual administration; transdermal patches.

Indication: acute severe hypertension, angina pectoris.

Effects: vasodilatation, mainly of veins, increased coronary blood flow, bronchodilatation.

Dose: GTN must be diluted to make 0.1 mg/mL and given via syringe pump continuously with 1–10 mg/h IV (titrate to effect).

Onset and duration: onset within 3 min; duration <20 min after stopping infusion; don't stop infusion abruptly but stepwise to avoid rebound hypertension.

Side effects: hypotension, tachycardia, headache, flush, congestion of veins in the head → increased intracranial pressure, increased duration of neuromuscular block by pancuronium.

Contraindications: intracranial bleeding, brain injury.

7.9.3 Hydralazine

Hydralazine is a direct vasodilator at arterioles.

Preparation: 20 mg ampoules at 10 mg/mL or 20 mg/mL, 25 mg tablets.

Indication: acute and chronic hypertension; hypertensive crisis, preeclampsia.

Effects: vasodilatation.

Dose: 10–20 mg IV, repeat if required; infusion at 0.5–10 mg/h (severe preeclampsia).

Onset and duration: 5–20 min after IV bolus, 2–6 h duration.

Side effects: hypotension, tachycardia, headache, sweating, flushing, nausea, nasal congestion.

Contraindications: mitral valve disease, coronary heart disease, hypersensitivity.

7.9.4 Labetalol

Labetalol is a combined α and β blocker in the sympathetic nervous system with more pronounced effect at β blockers.

Preparation: ampoules with 20 mL at 5 mg/mL; tablets.

Indication: treatment of hypertension; acute hypertension, preeclampsia.

Effects: reduces systemic vascular resistance, BP, and heart rate while maintaining cerebral and coronary perfusion.

Dose: 20–100 mg IV, titrate to effect.

Onset and duration: onset 2–5 min, duration up to 4 h.

Side effects: bronchospasm, difficulty breathing, urinary retention, hyperglycaemia, headache, rashes.

Contraindications: severe asthma, bradycardia, heart failure, severe liver disease, Raynaud's syndrome.

7.9.5 Nifedipine

Nifedipine is a commonly used calcium channel blocker for treatment of acute and chronic hypertension.

Preparation: capsules with 5–10 mg for sublingual administration; tablets with 10–60 mg, no injectable preparation.

Indication: hypertension, angina pectoris.

Effects: vasodilation causing decreased BP, increased coronary blood flow, and cardiac output.

Dose: 5–20 mg.

Onset and duration: 5–10 min after sublingual administration.

Side effects: flush, tachycardia.

Contraindications: hypotension, severe aortic stenosis, unstable angina, myocardial infarction, heart failure, liver disease, Raynaud's syndrome.

7.9.6 Mannitol

Mannitol is an osmotic diuretic which is mainly used in emergencies to reduce fluid volume in the skull and brain and thereby decreasing intracranial pressure (ICP).

Preparation: infusion bottles with 150 mg/mL mannitol at 100 or 500 mL.

Indication: rescue therapy in situation with raised intracranial pressure before surgery.

Effects: diuretic; moves volume from intracellular to extracellular space from where it is removed by diuresis; when used for raised ICP, the amount of diuresis should be replaced with RL or NS to avoid hypotension; RL or NS would not cross the blood–brain barrier so that net effect is still intracranial volume decrease.

Dose: 0.25–1 g/kg IV (max 2 g/kg) as fast infusion bolus over few minutes; for average adult 100–400 mL. Monitor urine output and calculate fluid balance of the patient.

Onset and duration: 15–30 min; 6 h.

Side effects: in higher or repeated doses intracranial pressure may rise – rebound effect, especially if blood brain barrier is not working, and mannitol would enter the brain thereby causing the intracranial fluid volume to expand instead of decreasing.

Contraindications: fluid overload, dehydration, heart failure, lung oedema, anuria, pathologic blood brain barrier (if known), active intracranial bleeding unless during surgery.

7.10 Antiemetic Drugs

PONV is a quite common side effect of anaesthesia and surgery. The vomiting centre in the brain stem, together with the chemoreceptor trigger zone (CTZ) on the floor of the fourth ventricle in the brain, is coordinating vomiting via the vomiting reflex. Antiemetic drugs act mainly on receptors of the CTZ, but also in the efferent organs of the gastrointestinal tract. As the CTZ has different types of receptors, some patients need a combination of drugs to get relief for PONV. If one antiemetic proves ineffective, it wouldn't help to add more of the same drug but combination with a drug with different mechanism of action is recommended.

7.10.1 Ondansetrone

Ondansetrone is used for prevention and treatment of PONV and nausea during chemotherapy.

Preparation: ampoules with 4 mg at 2 mg/mL for IV injection, tablets with 4 or 8 mg.

Indication: nausea and vomiting.

Effects: acting at serotonin receptors in the vomiting centre in the brain and in the intestine.

Dose: 4–8 mg every 6 h; children >2 years 0.1 mg/kg.

Onset and duration: onset 30 min; duration 6–8 h.

Side effects: usually no side effects; bradycardia after fast IV injection is possible.

Contraindications: hypersensitivity.

7.10.2 Metoclopramide

Metoclopramide is acting at dopaminergic receptors in the gastrointestinal tract and in the vomiting centre.

Preparation: 2 mL ampoules with 5 mg/mL for IM and IV injection; tablets with 10 mg.

Indication: nausea and vomiting; impaired motility of the stomach.

Effects: increases gastrointestinal motility; antiemetic.

Dose: 10–20 mg slowly IV or IM or orally.

Onset and duration: 1–5 min after IV injection; 1–2 h duration, but should not be administered more than 8-hourly.

Side effects: sedation, drowsiness, dizziness, movement disorders, rare: malignant neuroleptic syndrome.

Contraindications: bowel obstruction, perforated gastric ulcer.

7.10.3 Droperidol

Preparation: ampoules with 2.5 mg/mL for IV or IM injection.

Indication: nausea and vomiting after anaesthesia and during pain therapy with opioids; sedation of agitated patients; migraine.

Effects: potent antiemetic at very low doses, increases analgesic effect of opioids, sedative and antipsychotic at higher doses.

Dose: 0.625–2.5 mg; usually, 0.625–1.25 mg is sufficient as antiemetic in adults; higher doses are sometimes administered for sedation where droperidol should not be the first-line drug.

Onset and duration: 10–30 min for antiemetic effect which may last for up to 12 h.

Side effects: jerking, twisting movements, stiffness (extrapyramidal symptoms); dose-dependent QT prolongation in the ECG is unlikely at low doses for antiemetic purpose while more common if used at high doses (> 10 mg) for antipsychotic indications.

Contraindications: hypersensitivity.

7.10.4 Promethazine

For sedative effects see Sect. 7.4.

Preparation: ampoules with 25 or 50 mg/mL for IM or IV injection.

Indication: prevention and treatment of PONV.

Effects: antiemetic, sedative.

Dose: 12.5–25 mg.

Onset and duration: 10–20 min; antiemetic effect up to 12 h.

Side effects: usually no or mild side effects after antiemetic doses; dry mouth.

Contraindications: hypersensitivity.

7.11 Antibiotic Prophylaxis

Antibiotic prophylaxis is widely performed to decrease surgical site infections. Not all types of operations require prophylactic antibiotics while antibiotics are mandatory in other operations, e.g. with implant of foreign body (ORIF for fractures; ventriculoperitoneal shunt implant), laparotomy in patients with peritonitis or bowel perforation, and many other types of surgery. It is always the surgeon who is prescribing antibiotics but often, anaesthesia personnel is administering it and should remind the surgeon in case he/she is forgetting about it. Timing is key; the antibiotic should be administered within 60 min before start of surgery and is less effective when given later. The entire dose of the antibiotic must be completed before incision, especially before tourniquet inflation. During preoperative evaluation ask the patient about any drug allergies, e.g. towards penicillines. There are many different antibiotics used worldwide; only a few of them are listed below.

7.11.1 Cloxacillin/Flucloxacillin

Cloxacillin and flucloxacillin are quite similar narrow-spectrum penicillines which are effective against gram-positive bacteria including staphylococcus.

Preparation: vials with 250/500/1000/2000 mg.

Indication: prevention and treatment of surgical site infection, treatment of infections like pneumonia, osteomyelitis, cellulitis, infected burns.

Effects: bactericidal antibiotic.

Dose: 30–50 mg/kg; adults 2 g IV for prophylaxis; 1–2 g TDS for treatment.

Onset and duration: 30 min; 3 h.

Side effects: allergic reactions with rashes and itching, usually no other side effects when used short-term, but may cause nausea, diarrhoea.

Contraindications: penicillin/beta-lactam allergy, combination with gentamicin.

7.11.2 Ampicillin/Amoxicillin

Ampicillin and amoxicillin are rather similar broad spectrum penicillines.

Preparation: vials with 250/500/1000 mg.

Indication: antibiotic prophylaxis, e.g. for caesarean section, treatment of many different types of infections; treatment of infections and sepsis with suspected sensitive bacteria.

Effects: bactericidal with wide spectrum, less effective for staphylococcus.

Dose: 30–50 mg/kg; adults 1 g.

Onset and duration: 30 min; 4 h.

Side effects: allergic reactions with rashes and itching, usually no other side effects when used short-term, but may cause nausea, diarrhoea.

Contraindications: penicillin/beta-lactam allergy, combination with gentamicin.

7.11.3 Clindamycin

Preparation: ampoules with 150 mg/mL for dilution and IV infusion.

Indication: antibiotic prophylaxis in patients with penicillin/betalactam allergy.

Effects: bacteriostatic, in high doses bactericidal.

Dose: 10 mg/kg, adults 600 mg slowly IV.

Onset and duration: 30–60 min; 6 h.

Side effects: nausea, vomiting, abdominal cramps, diarrhoea, colitis.

Contraindications: allergy, history of colitis.

7.11.4 Gentamicin

Gentamicin is very effective but not first-line drug because of rare but serious side effects.

Preparation: ampoules with 40 mg/mL for IM or IV administration.

Indication: prophylaxis and treatment of infections, e.g. compound fractures; effective against many gram-negative and gram-positive bacteria including staphylococcus.

Effects: bactericidal.

Dose: 3–5 mg/kg slowly (> 3 min) IV, better with infusion over 30–60 min; adjusted dose for obese patients (give same dose as for normal body weight).

Onset and duration: onset within 1 h, duration 8–12 h,

Side effects: muscle weakness, potentiation of muscle relaxants, esp. pancuronium; dose-dependent renal impairment, often reversible; rare but devastating ototoxicity of the balance organ in the inner ear so that even a single dose may cause irreversible loss of balance (difficulty walking, high risk of falls).

Contraindications: dehydration, renal insufficiency, combination with furosemide, pregnancy, myasthenia gravis; use with caution in patients at old age; gentamicin is inactivated by penicillines and cephalosporines.

7.11.5 Ceftriaxone

Preparation: vials with 1 g powder for dilution shortly before injection.

Indication: surgical prophylaxis, treatment of infections like abdominal infections, pelvic inflammatory disease, infections of bones.

Effects: bactericide with broad spectrum.

Dose: 100 mg/kg, for prophylaxis adults 1 g, for treatment adults 0.5–2 g OD slowly IV.

Onset and duration: 30 min; 12–24 h.

Side effects: diarrhoea, rashes, elevated liver levels, anaemia, leucopenia.

Contraindications: beta-lactam allergy, neonates with jaundice, premature neonates.

7.11.6 Cefuroxime

Preparation: vials with 0.75 g or 1.5 g powder for dilution before injection/infusion.

Indication: surgical prophylaxis, treatment of infections like pneumonia, urinary tract infections, meningitis, bone infections, sepsis.

Effects: bactericide with broad spectrum.

Dose: adults 1.5 g for prophylaxis; 750–1500 mg TDS for treatment of different infections.

Onset and duration: 30 min; 3–6 h.

Side effects: nausea, diarrhoea, rashes, itching, seldom serious side effects like disturbance of liver function or haematological side effects.

Contraindications: beta-lactam allergy.

7.11.7 Metronidazole

Preparation: 500 mg in 100 mL.

Indication: infection caused by anaerobe pathogens, e.g. colorectal surgery, pelvic inflammatory disease, dental abscess.

Effects: bactericidal against anaerobes and protozoa like amoeba.

Dose: 15 mg/kg; adults 500 mg TDS or 1500 mg single dose as infusion over 1 h.

Onset and duration: 30 min; 6–8 h.

Side effects: usually no side effects; nausea are possible.

Contraindications: allergy.

7.12 Hormones: Corticoids, Insulin, Oxytocin

Hydrocortisone and dexamethasone are two corticoid drugs which are frequently used perioperatviely. Hydrocortisone is a synthetic preparation of the natural hormone cortisol which is produced in the adrenal glands with a peak concentration early in the morning. It has many effects and is regulating metabolism of proteins, lipids, and glucose. Deficiency is causing generalised vasodilatation with hypotension; weakness, fatigue, tiredness, weight loss, hypoglycaemia, pain, apathia, depression, chronic inflammation, and poor immune reaction. Under conditions of stress, trauma, acute severe disease, or circulatory shock, increased cortisol production and release are essential for survival.

7.12.1 Hydrocortisone

Preparation: vials with 100 mg powder for dilution before injection; tablets.

Indication: allergy, severe asthma or status asthmaticus, post-extubation croup (airway obstruction after intubation or intubating attempts), during ENT surgery to prevent oedema in the airways.

Effects: anti-allergic, anti-inflammatory, anti-asthmatic.

Dose: 1–5 mg/kg; adults 100–500 mg IV.

Onset and duration: within 2 h; 6–8 h.

Side effects: hyperglycaemia, immunosuppressive (in several chronic diseases, immunosuppression is the intended effect), sleep disorder, psychosis, fluid retention, peptic ulcer, and osteoporosis (not after short-term administration), Cushing syndrome, cataract after prolonged administration with high doses.

Contraindications: severe hypertension, cataract, heart failure, gastric ulcer.

7.12.2 Dexamethasone

Preparation: ampoules with 4 mg/mL for IV injection, tablets.

Indication: same as for hydrocortisone and antenatal use in preterm pregnancy to induce lung maturation in the infant; PONV prophylaxis, brain oedema, pain, allergy, bacterial meningitis.

Effects: similar to hydrocortisone but much stronger; decreases brain oedema, antiemetic, prevents hearing loss in patients with meningitis, immunosuppression after organ transplantation.

Dose: adults 4–8 mg IV; severe acute asthma single dose of 12 mg IV.

Onset and duration: 1–2 h, duration 36–72 h.

Side effects: same as with hydrocortisone.

Contraindications: allergy towards dexamethasone; same contraindications as with hydrocortisone.

7.12.3 Insulin

Insulin is a hormone which is normally produced in the pancreas. It is essential for regulating glucose metabolism. With insulin deficiency, a patient will be suffering from diabetes mellitus. Many pharmaceutical presentations of insulin are available which are similar to human insulin or modified as long-acting, slow-release insulins for treatment of diabetes.

Preparation: vials containing 100 IU/mL.

Indication: treatment of diabetes mellitus and other causes of hyperglycaemia; treatment of hyperkalaemia (usually in ICU and together with glucose infusion to avoid hypoglycaemia as side effect).

Effects: glucose and potassium transport from plasma into cells (from extracellular fluid to intracellular fluid), decreasing blood glucose and K^+ in plasma, stimulation of carbohydrate metabolism, lipid and protein synthesis.

Dose: 4–40 IU SC, IV or with infusion.

Onset and duration: within 1 h; 3–7 h; long-acting insulin: onset within 4 h, duration 18–36 h.

Side effects: hypoglycaemia, hypokalaemia (= low potassium); blood glucose must be monitored regularly during therapy with insulin.

Contraindications: hypoglycaemia.

7.12.4 Oxytocin

Oxytocin is a hormone which is produced by the posterior pituitary gland. It is contracting the uterus during and after labour. It is also produced as drug for the same purpose.

Preparation: ampoules with 5 or 10 IU (that is 8.4 or 16.7 μg, resp.) per mL for IV or IM injection or infusion; store in a fridge is recommended; at room temperature stable for approximately 1 month, thereafter the effect may decline.

Indication: uterine atony, promote or induce labour, PPH.

Effects: uterine contraction.

Dose: 5 IU slowly IV after delivery of the newborn; repeat once if required (slowly over several minutes; dilute the drug!); if more oxytocin is needed, use infusion with 30 IU at 10 IU/h.

Onset and duration: 1–5 min; 1–2 h.

Side effects: hypotension caused by vasodilatation; dangerous when IV bolus given in actively bleeding, hypovolaemic patients who should get it injected very slowly over several minutes; even cardiac arrest when injected too quickly; flushing; decreased diuresis; overdose may cause uterine rupture.

Contraindications: known hypersensitivity; increased risk for uterine rupture.

7.13 Bronchorelaxation

Drugs for bronchodilatation are used in the treatment of asthma and during acute bronchospasm perioperatively. Patients with severe asthma should also receive corticosteroids like dexamethasone or hydrocortisone. Although not a first-line drug for treatment of bronchospasm, it is good to remember that ephedrine is a potent bronchodilator and often at hands for the AP. For longer lasting effect, 1 ampoule of ephedrine may be injected IM.

7.13.1 Salbutamol

Preparation: ampoules with 0.5 mg/1 mL for SC injection, 2.5 mg/2.5 mL nebuliser; aerosol, tablets.

Indication: first-line treatment of asthma, COPD, to prolong preterm pregnancy by inhibiting preterm labour; special indication: treating acute hyperkalaemia.

Effects: acting on beta-adrenergic receptors of the sympathetic nervous system; bronchodilatation, increasing heart rate, uterine relaxation.

Dose: 0.5 mg SC/IM every 4 h; 2–4 mg orally 6–8 hourly.

Onset and duration: 5–15 min; 4 h.

Side effects: tachycardia, shift of potassium ions from extracellular (plasma) to intracellular, tremor, sweating, sleeping disorder, anxiety, potentiates long-acting muscle relaxants.

Contraindications: severe, uncontrolled hypertension; hypokalaemia; pre-eclampsia, eclampsia, uterine haemorrhage.

7.13.2 Aminophylline

Preparation: ampoules with 10 mL at 25 mg/mL; tablets.

Indication: second-line treatment for severe bronchospasm alone or in combination with salbutamol or other beta-adrenergic, COPD, sometimes used for treatment of heart failure.

Effects: bronchodilatation and improved contractility of diaphragm; improved lung function; increases heart rate and cardiac output and decreases systemic vascular resistance; increased renal blood flow and acts as mild diuretic.

Dose: initially 5 mg/kg or 1 ampoule 250 mg for normal size adults slowly IV over >10 min; in life-threatening bronchospasm a second ampoule may be given with infusion over 1 h, but check heart rate, have ECG attached and stop infusion when tachycardia/arrhythmia occurs; maintenance: 125 mg every 4–6 hours or 0.5 mg/kg/h infusion for maintenance in ICU/HDU; total daily dose in adults around 750 mg (max 900 mg); overdose is likely to produce severe arrhythmia.

Onset and duration: 15 min; 4–6 h.

Side effects: headache, tremor, nausea, gastric pain, allergy, sleeping disorder, tachyarrhythmia can often be avoided by slow injection over several min, hypokalaemia, ventricular fibrillation, convulsions if overdosed.

Contraindications: tachycardia >130/min, cardiomyopathy, aortic stenosis, myocardial infarction; concomitant use of halothane increases risk for arrhythmia.

7.14 Pharmacological Treatment of Severe Bleeding

7.14.1 Tranexamic Acid (TXA)

Tranexamic acid is an antifibrinolytic agent which prevents blood clots from being dissolved, however, only in the early phase after onset of bleeding. Additionally, it has anti-inflammatory actions. It is sometimes called cyclokapron.

Preparation: ampoules with 0.5 g or 1 g TXA at 100 mg/mL for IV injection after dilution.

Indication: acute, major bleeding >1 l in adults (15–20 mL/kg in children) as early as possible and within the first 3 h after onset of the bleeding; all cases of PPH within 3 h after childbirth; trauma: within 3 h after the accident.

Effects: TXA decreases perioperative blood loss and helps stop bleeding in PPH or after trauma; reduces mortality caused by bleeding.

Dose: 20 mg/kg for children or 1 g for adults diluted for slow IV injection over 10 min. The dose may be repeated once only, recommended 30 min after initial dose if bleeding not stopped; in children, only half dose may be repeated.

Onset and duration: 5–15 min; duration of action 3 h.

Side effects: hypotension if injected fast (dangerous in patients with severe bleeding), pain, vomiting, seizures, impaired colour vision, anaphylaxis, thromboembolism.

Contraindication: > 3 h after start of bleed, intracranial bleeding without head trauma, allergy.

7.14.2 Aminocaproic Acid

Epsilon-Amino-N-caproic acid, EACA, is a pro-coagulant drug with similar mechanism of action as TXA and is used for the same indications.

Preparation: 20 mL vials with 5 g at 250 mg/mL IV; tablets with 1 g; oral solution.

Indication: excessive acute bleeding.

Effects: decreases blood loss and helps stop the bleeding due to more efficient blood coagulation (inhibits the breakdown of fibrinogen and fibrin clots).

Dose: adults: 4–5 g IV with infusion over 1 h followed by 1 g/h over 8 h or until the bleeding is stopped; children 100–200 mg/kg slowly IV followed by 100 mg/kg after 6 h.

Onset and duration: onset around 1 h; duration 3–4 h.

Side effects: increased risk for thrombosis and embolism.

Contraindications: DIC (disseminated intravascular coagulation).

7.14.3 FFP

Fresh frozen plasma (FFP) is prepared during blood donation when the whole blood is separated into erythrocyte concentrate (PRBC or packed red blood cells) and plasma which is frozen within 6 h after donation. Disadvantage: It takes 30 min or more to thaw and warm FFP before it can be transfused. While coagulation factors remain active for less than 24 h in whole blood and are absent in PRBCs, they are >50% active in FFP. Massive haemorrhage is complicated by loss of coagulation factors and platelets which may increase the amount of blood loss. Therefore, if bleeding exceeds around 2–3 l or 50% of total blood volume, FFP should be added to the transfusion of PRBCs. Fresh whole blood is even better at preserving coagulation than FFP because of full activity of coagulation factors and platelets are still functioning in warm blood of "walking donors" which should not be cooled before urgent transfusion while FFP does not contain active platelets.

Preparation: plastic bags containing 200–250 mL; FFP should be AB0 compatible.

Indication: massive bleeding, coagulation deficiency.

Effects: volume expander, supporting normal blood coagulation.

Dose: initially 10 mL/kg; up to half the estimated volume of blood loss.

Onset and duration: immediate; effect of coagulation factor 7 only 6 h, other factors and volume effect 12–24 h.

Side effects: fluid overload if given in too large amounts, allergic reaction, haemolysis, transfusion-related acute lung injury, transfusion-related infection.

Contraindications: blood group incompatibility.

Further Reading

Australian and New Zealand College of Anaesthetists (2020) Guideline for the safe management and use of medications in anaesthesia. bit.ly/3bFD5Ex

Farhan H, Moreno-Duarte I, McLean D, Eikermann M (2014) Residual paralysis: does it influence outcome after ambulatory surgery? Curr Anesthesiol Rep 4(4):290–302

National Department of Health, South Africa (2019) Essential drugs programme hospital level (Adults) standard treatment guidelines and essential medicines list, 5th edn. National Department of Health, South Africa, Kimberley

Peck TE, Hill SA (2021) Pharmacology for Anaesthesia and intensive care, 5th edn. Cambridge University Press, Cambridge

Scarth E, Smith S (2016) Drugs in anaesthesia and intensive care, 5th edn. Oxford University Press, Oxford

WHO (2021) World Health Organization model List of essential medicines—22nd List. World Health Organization, Geneva 2021 (WHO/MHP/HPS/EML/2021.02). Licence: CC BY-NC-SA 3.0 IGO

8 General Anaesthesia for Major Operations

Abstract

General anaesthesia for major surgery consists of amnesia, analgesia, unconsciousness, and immobility. These effects can be achieved with a single inhalational anaesthetic, with a combination of IV anaesthetics, or as balanced anaesthesia, a combination of IV anaesthetics with inhalational agents +/− muscle relaxants.

Inhalational anaesthetics are delivered via calibrated vaporisers. With each single breath a small amount of anaesthetic is inhaled. In the lungs it is taken up into the blood, from where it is taken up by the brain and also by all other tissues. Induction of anaesthesia takes more time than with IV anaesthetics. The minimal alveolar concentration (MAC) at which 50% of all patients would not move during skin incision is agent specific, greater at young age and is a measure for dosage. With pure inhalational anaesthesia, 1.2–1.5 MAC is needed for surgical anaesthesia, which is approximately equal to 1–1.5% halothane, or 1.5–2.2% of isoflurane, or 2.5–3.5% of sevoflurane.

During balanced anaesthesia, the dose of inhalational agents can be reduced significantly, thus minimising side effects.

Overdose of inhalational agents is dangerous and may lead to cardiac failure.

Total intravenous anaesthesia (TIVA) can be achieved with a combination of hypnotic, analgesic, and if required, a muscle relaxant drug. Propofol and fentanyl or ketamine; or ketamine and diazepam or midazolam are common combinations. The latter can be used for anaesthesia with spontaneous breathing, while the combinations with propofol or fentanyl require intubation or laryngeal mask airway, and manual or mechanical ventilation of the patient.

Keywords

Balanced anaesthesia for major surgery · General principles of inhaled anaesthetics · Halothane anaesthesia in resource-limited settings · Ketamine for anaesthesia maintenance · Neuromuscular blocking agents (muscle relaxants) in resource-limited settings · TIVA (total intravenous anaesthesia) in resource-limited settings

General anaesthesia for major surgery consists of four components: amnesia (not remembering anything), analgesia (not feeling pain), hypnosis (sleeping, being unconscious), muscle relaxation (immobility, not moving). These effects can be achieved with a single inhalational anaesthetic agent in sufficient dose; however, as this would lead to significant side effects on circulation, the

D. Kietzmann, *Anaesthesia in Remote Hospitals*, Sustainable Development Goals Series,
https://doi.org/10.1007/978-3-031-46610-6_8

combination of different drugs is a better option and is called balanced anaesthesia. Elective major surgery with site of operation below the umbilicus can often be performed as spinal anaesthesia and even upper abdominal surgery can be performed with spinal if the spread of local anaesthetic in the subarachnoid space is high enough. If general anaesthesia is planned, a combination of inhalational anaesthetics and IV anaesthetics or narcotics will be preferred. Muscle relaxants may also be needed depending on the type of surgery. Ketamine as the sole anaesthetic is rather safe but does not produce deep anaesthesia with muscle relaxation as required for abdominal surgery and other operations with long duration.

8.1 General Principles of Inhalation Anaesthesia

During inhalational anaesthesia, a vaporised anaesthetic like halothane, isoflurane, or sevoflurane is added to the inhaled air / oxygen mixture and would cross through the alveolocapillary membrane together with O_2. The speed of uptake in the lungs is different for different volatile anaesthetics so that anaesthesia induction and recovery can be faster or more slowly (halothane slowest, sevoflurane fastest of the three mentioned above). Increased ventilation would always increase speed of induction since the amount of anaesthetic which reaches the alveoli would increase with increased ventilation. The goal of delivering inhaled anaesthetics is to produce anaesthesia by establishing a specific concentration in the central nervous system. This is achieved by establishing the desired concentration in the lungs that ultimately equilibrates with the brain.

Volatile anaesthetics are applied by inhalation. During inspiration, they reach the alveoli, the parts of the lungs where any gas exchange takes place and where inhaled anaesthetics are taken up into the blood. From the blood, the anaesthetic is taken up by the brain and by the tissues (the vessel-rich organs as liver, kidney, heart, lungs, the muscle group, and the fat group). The amount of uptake is dependent on the solubility of the drug in each tissue. For example, high lipid solubility means extensive uptake by the brain and fatty tissues. High blood solubility means that it will take longer for the agent to reach equilibrium with the brain, because it will first be taken up extensively by the blood.

With each single breath, only a small amount of anaesthetic is entering the lungs so that it takes much more time to get an effect than with IV induction where the whole dose is injected over around 30 s and reaches the brain within a minute. Since the uptake of the volatile anaesthetic into the brain takes a while, it is more comfortable, faster, and safer for the patient to induce anaesthesia with an intravenous anaesthetic. However, induction by inhalation is also possible, especially with halothane or sevoflurane which have a sweetish, non-irritant smell. That takes about 10–20 min until a sufficient level of anaesthesia is achieved for endotracheal intubation and surgery if no intravenous drugs are added.

The level of anaesthesia is related to the principle of MAC—minimum alveolar concentration of the anaesthetic. For details of the MAC concept, see Sect. 8.2. During steady state, that is after more than 1 h of inhalational anaesthesia when the concentration of anaesthetic in the alveoli is in equilibrium with the concentration in the blood and the one in the brain, the concentration in the lungs reflects the effect concentration in the brain. With sophisticated modern anaesthesia machines that concentration can be measured together with capnography for exhaled CO_2. It is a useful measure since the required concentration for desired effect is relatively constant between patients, showing little variability. With isoflurane inhalational induction is difficult and not recommended. If isoflurane is the only inhalational agent and IV access before induction is not possible, e.g. in small children, ketamine may be given IM (5 mg /kg) followed by isoflurane induction 3 min later.

The speed of uptake is dependent on cardiac output, alveolar ventilation, concentration of anaesthetic in the inspired gas mixture, and on its blood and lipid solubility. Table 8.1 gives the physicochemical properties and the potency of inhalational anaesthetics. Uptake is faster if high

Table 8.1 Properties of inhaled anaesthetics. MAC (minimal alveolar concentration) is given for 40-year-old adults and is a measure of the potency of the agent. Note that halothane and isoflurane have nearly the same boiling point. That means a halothane vaporiser can be used for isoflurane and vice versa since calibration is the same. Of course, the agents must never be mixed, and the vaporiser must be labelled for the agent used

	Halothane	Isoflurane	Sevoflurane	Desflurane	N_2O
Vol% minimal alveolar concentration (MAC)	0.75	1.16	2.0	6.0	105
Blood/gas partition coefficient	2.5	1.4	0.68	0.42	0.46
Oil/gas partition coefficient (lipid solubility)	224	98	47	18.7	1.4
Boiling point °C	50	49	58.5	23.5	- 88.5

FGF (fresh gas flow) of 4–6 L/min is used initially. 5–10 min after induction FGF should be reduced to around 2 L/min to save anaesthetic agent, and the concentration at the vaporiser must be reduced to avoid overdose. A lower FGF than 2 L/min may be applied only if a fully equipped anaesthesia machine is used with monitoring of the concentrations of oxygen and anaesthetic, and if continuous capnography is used.

For maintenance of anaesthesia in circulatory stable adults around 1–1.5% halothane, or 1.5–2% of isoflurane or 2.5–3.5% of sevoflurane are needed at the vaporiser for most types of surgery. Before skin incision and especially painful surgical stimulation like opening of the peritoneum and pulling at inner organs, 0.5 mg/kg ketamine or 50 μg fentanyl can be administered to get a balanced quality of anaesthesia. During operations which last more than 2 h, the concentration of the anaesthestic can often be reduced by approximately one-third from the second hour. 20 min before end of surgery, the concentration at the vaporiser can be reduced further, and during closure of the fascia 0.5 MAC (approximately 0.4% halothane, 0.6% isoflurane, or 1.0% sevoflurane) is often sufficient. During skin sutures, the anaesthetic may be switched off. Signs for light anaesthesia would be movement, coughing, pushing, tears, high blood pressure, or heart rate. Deep anaesthesia causes respiratory depression and finally apnoea, muscle relaxation, and low BP.

Effects of inhalational anaesthetics when used as the sole anaesthetic agent:

- Stage 1: analgesia, amnesia, normal pupil size and reflexes, normal spontaneous respiration.
- Stage 2: Excitement; irregular respiration, large pupils with light reflex, no eyelash reflex, increased laryngeal reflexes with risk for laryngospasm.
- Stage 3.1: Surgical anaesthesia with regular respiration and large tidal volumes, small pupils, no eyelid reflex but corneal reflex remaining.
- Stage 3.2: as 3.1 but corneal reflex depressed and abdominal muscles relaxed.
- Stage 4: overdose of anaesthetic; respiratory depression, pupils enlarged, risk for cardiac failure.

Note that the pupil size cannot be used to assess depth of inhalational anaesthesia if opioids are given since opioids reduce pupil size.

8.2 Inhalational Anaesthetic Drugs

Minimal alveolar concentration (MAC): Inhalational anaesthetics are producing amnesia, analgesia, sleep (unconsciousness), and immobility (muscle relaxation) in a dose dependent way. Therefore, general anaesthesia can be performed with a single inhalational agent. The potency of inhalational anaesthetics is dependent on their lipid solubility. It is measured as so-called MAC that is "minimal alveolar concentration". MAC is defined as the minimal alveolar concentration (concentration in the lungs) at which half of the patients would not move during skin incision. MAC is dependent on age and is highest in young children. For surgical anaesthesia, 1.2–1.5 MAC are usually required or combination with IV agents, than a lower MAC would be sufficient.

Each inhalational anaesthetic agent has a specific MAC which determines its potency.

Halothane: The MAC for halothane is 1 Vol% in children, 0.75% in adults and around 0.6 % in elderly patients.

Isoflurane: 1 MAC in children is around 1.6%, in adults 1.2%, in the elderly 0.9%.

Sevoflurane: Sevoflurane with a MAC of approximately 2.8% for 1-year-old infants, 2.5% for schoolchildren, 2.0 Vol.% for adults and 1.4% in the elderly is about 2–3 times less potent than halothane that means 2–3 times more anaesthestic agent is needed for the same effects (much more expensive!).

***Nitrous oxide*:** N_2O is the weakest agent theoretically needing 105% to reach 1 MAC. Of course, as the patient needs at least 21% oxygen, the theoretical max concentration for nitrous oxide is 100–21=79%, but that equals only 0,7 MAC. Even an 80-year-old patient needs still 80% N_2O for 1 MAC of anaesthetic not leaving space for sufficient oxygen. That means it is not possible to perform anaesthesia with N_2O as the sole anaesthetic drug. Usually, 60–70% N_2O with 30–40% of oxygen are combined with another anaesthetic. Nitrous oxide is a good analgesic and amnesia-causing agent at these concentrations.

***The effects of anaesthetics are additive*:** For balanced anaesthesia, two or more drugs are combined to achieve better effects while side effects will be minimised. When two anaesthetics are combined their resp. MAC are simply added. For example, 0.5 MAC Sevoflurane (1 vol %) + 0.5 MAC N_2O (52.5 vol %) results in 1 MAC total anaesthetic effect, almost the same quality of anaesthesia as with sevoflurane 2% without nitrous oxide. Combination with a strong IV analgesic like ketamine, pethidine, morphine, or fentanyl would also reduce MAC significantly.

"Alveolar concentration" means the concentration in the lungs of the patient. This concentration is not the same as that one at the vaporiser, but usually it will be somewhat lower, especially during the beginning of anaesthesia. After achieving a steady state of equilibrium with the tissues (usually not before several hours of anaesthesia), the concentration in the lung, that is the alveolar concentration, will match with the concentration in the inspired gas mixture. With highly equipped anaesthesia machines, it is possible to measure the expired concentrations of all gases, namely oxygen, nitrogen, carbon dioxide (CO_2), and of any inhalational anaesthetic. The end-expiratory concentrations approximate the alveolar concentrations. This is a useful tool, however, to provide safe anaesthesia, it is not mandatory to be able to measure the real concentrations in the patient's lungs, provided we always assess and adapt the required dose of anaesthetic by clinical signs such as blood pressure, pulse rate, or any reactions of the patient like moving, fast and deep breathing, tears in the eyes.

8.2.1 Halothane

Halothane is a halogenated hydrocarbon, bromo-chloro-trifluoro-ethane. Halothane is neither flammable nor explosive in clinical conditions. It is by far the cheapest volatile anaesthetic (diethylether not considered which is even cheaper but hardly available nowadays). The MAC is 0.75% in adults and 1% in children (reduced to approximately 0.3–0.5% in combination with opioids, ketamine, or nitrous oxide). That means halothane is a very potent anaesthetic. The concentrations used in anaesthesia vary from 0.3 to 3.0%. The agent must be used with a calibrated vaporiser to avoid overdosage. Even slight to moderate overdosage would result in cardiorespiratory depression and finally circulatory collapse. Most vaporisers are calibrated up to 5% but *more than 3% must not be used and even 3% may only be used for few minutes.* Keep your hand at the vaporiser lever to make sure you wouldn't forget to reduce concentration. Blood pressure should be measured at least every 5 min and monitored carefully. The concentration must be reduced if blood pressure falls. Halothane should always be applied with extra oxygen (at least 35% oxygen). Even in surgical doses it may depress the cardiovascular system (decreased cardiac output and blood pressure), especially in small infants and the elderly. Many patients need to be artificially ventilated during surgery, because it causes respiratory depression dose-dependently. Patients usually need oxygen during recovery from halothane anaesthesia as well. They must never be sent to the ward immediately but be observed with pulse oximeter for a minimum of 30 min after extubation. Some patients will need oxygen in the ward for 24 hours, especially after abdominal surgery.

Halothane is a potent anaesthetic but a week analgesic. It will not result in postoperative analgesia after regaining consciousness. It can produce some muscle relaxation, especially in higher doses, but usually not always enough for abdominal surgery, where some repeated doses of suxamethonium or a single dose of a long lasting muscle relaxant might be needed additionally.

80% of the halothane are eliminated by expiration, 20% are metabolised in the liver.

Side effects of halothane: *Direct, dose dependent depression of the myocardium* (marked in patients under acute blood and fluid losses, in patients with heart disease and in infants <6 months). Halothane sensitises the heart to *arrhythmias,* especially when patients have low potassium and when adrenaline is administered with local anaesthetic (surgical infiltration with adrenaline should be with caution or avoided) or intravenously or is produced by the adrenal glands in response to surgical stress, when anaesthesia is not deep enough. Cardiac arrest due to ventricular fibrillation is the most severe possible side effect and requires immediate resuscitation. ECG monitoring is highly recommended. Dose-dependent *respiratory depression* requires artificial ventilation during surgical anaesthesia. *Bronchodilation* is marked and especially favourable in patients with bronchial asthma. Nausea and vomiting after anaesthesia may occur, but it is less frequent than with nitrous oxide and can be treated with promethazine, ondansetrone, droperidol, or other antiemetic. *Relaxation of the uterine muscle* may lead to extensive bleeding, which means halothane is not the agent of choice for caesarean section. However, it may be administered in low doses up to 0.7% (max 1.0% for very short period) at the vaporiser during C/S in combination with repeated doses of ketamine or other analgesic.

Liver damage may occur especially after repeated anaesthesia with halothane. Usually it is mild, but sometimes life-threatening, and even fatal liver failure may be caused by one of the metabolites. *Malignant hyperthermia* is extremely seldom (less than 1 in 10,000) but a complication with high mortality that is triggered by halothane or any other volatile anaesthetic and by suxamethonium. A patient who survived malignant hyperthermia must never again receive halothane or suxamethonium or any other volatile anaesthetic because that would trigger malignant hyperthermia again with high risk for cardiac arrest. Instead, the patient should receive i.v. anaesthetics as ketamine, thiopentone, propofol, fentanyl, pethidine, or spinal anaesthesia.

Contraindication: Heart failure, cardiocirculatory shock, uncorrected dehydration, history of or increased risk for MH, severe liver disease.

8.2.2 Isoflurane

Isoflurane is a non-flammable halogenated methyl ethyl ether with a pungent ethereal odour. It is not well suitable for inhalational induction. Its great advantage is that it causes minimal cardiac depression and no liver damage. Isoflurane causes marked vasodilatation with decreased BP, partly compensated by increase in heart rate. It does not trigger cardiac arrhythmia. It causes marked muscle relaxation so that a NMBA often is not required. Isoflurane is therefore safer than halothane, but it is also more expensive. Malignant hyperthermia is rare but can occur as with all inhalational agents. Its MAC is around 1.2% in adults, in combination with N_2O, fentanyl or ketamine 0.6%. Recovery is moderately faster than with halothane.

In contrast to halothane, isoflurane is suitable for neurosurgery, especially craniotomy, even in patients with elevated intracranial pressure, where it may be administered up to a max concentration of 1.2 MAC.

For maintenance of anaesthesia, isoflurane is quite ideal for all patients with only exception of patients in shock and patients with susceptibility for MH. It is significantly cheaper than sevoflurane.

8.2.3 Sevoflurane

Sevoflurane is a fluorinated isopropyl ether. Non-pungency and rapid increases in alveolar anaesthetic concentration make sevoflurane an excellent choice for smooth and rapid inhalational induction. Dose-dependent respiratory depression occurs. Muscle relaxant effect as with isoflurane. Sevoflurane only mildly depresses myocardial contractility but causes some vasodilatation. Arterial blood pressure declines slightly less than with halothane. Because sevoflurane causes little, if any, rise in heart rate, cardiac output is not maintained as well as with isoflurane but better than with halothane. Like halothane, sevoflurane is a potent bronchodilator which makes it suitable for patients with asthma. A few percent are metabolised in the liver. However, severe liver damage does not occur. Malignant hyperthermia is rare but can occur as with all inhalational agents. Unfortunately, it is rather expensive, and the MAC is high (around 2%) that means more anaesthetic agent is needed per hour of anaesthesia compared to isoflurane or halothane.

Like isoflurane, sevoflurane is also suitable for neurosurgery. Doses <1.2 MAC can safely be used even in patients with increased ICP. Concentrations above 1 MAC produce dose-dependent vasodilatation in the brain.

Emergence from sevoflurane anaesthesia is faster than from the other volatile agents. Children may undergo a phase of restlessness and delirium more frequently than with the other agents. Small doses of propofol (0.5 mg/kg) or an opioid at the end of surgery can prevent that effect.

8.2.4 Other Inhalational Agents

8.2.4.1 Nitrous Oxide

Since nitrous oxide is expensive and it is used more and more seldom worldwide. Nitrous oxide is compressed and stored in cylinders at a pressure of 50 bar when it is partly liquid, partly gas. It is difficult to assess how much N_2O remains in the cylinder, because the pressure is only that of the vapour. The amount of liquid can only be assessed by weighing the cylinder. *When the pressure begins to fall below 50 bar, the cylinder is nearly empty* (compared to a cylinder with oxygen which is half full when pressure is half).

N_2O is a weak anaesthetic which needs to be combined with other anaesthetic drugs. 60–70% N_2O are equal to only 0.57–0.67 MAC. It has good analgesic properties, produces amnesia and sedation, but no relaxation.

With the use of N_2O, it is possible to administer a dangerously hypoxic gas mixture in case the oxygen source is failing while N_2O is continued. Most anaesthesia machines have therefore an oxygen failure alarm and stop automatically N_2O when oxygen is not delivered at least 25%. If anaesthetists are using N_2O they must check if such an oxygen failure prevention is installed and working. Otherwise, N_2O should not be used to avoid the risk of ventilating a patient with 100% N_2O without oxygen which would cause death within minutes.

The safest way to administer N_2O is with the monitoring of SpO_2, FiO_2, and capnography which enables using low FGF < 3 L/min. If no oxygen sensor is available, the fresh gas flow must not be below 3 L/min (1 L O_2 plus 2 l/min of N_2O). If soda lime and/or SpO_2 unavailable, the FGF must be 6 L/min (2 L of O_2 plus 4 L/min of N_2O).

Side effects: Side effects include PONV (post-operative nausea and vomiting) to be likely. N_2O is more soluble than nitrogen in the blood. That leads to excessive diffusion of N_2O into closed gas spaces. N_2O may increase the volume of gas containing spaces in the body, e.g. the bowels, the middle ear, or the volume of pneumothorax or pneumoperitoneum. It is contraindicated for surgery of the middle ear, the retina, brain surgery, and for operation of bowel obstruction as well as for laparoscopic surgery. It has cardiac depressant effects that are often counteracted by sympathoadrenal stimulation. Exposure for more than 6 h can lead to bone marrow depression with agranulocytosis and anaemia, sometimes irreversible and should therefore be avoided.

It is not smelling anything and not irritating airways so that inhalational induction is easy. Analgesic effect is already within 3 min. Painful wound cleaning and dressing can be performed with 60% nitrous oxide in oxygen. The patient would not become unconscious but be in a state of amnesia and analgesia. 50% N_2O with oxygen (in some countries available in a fixed mixture called Entonox® within one cylinder) can be used for analgesia during labour pain under childbirth.

Its main indication is the combined use with volatile agents to reduce their doses and thereby the side effects on the cardio-respiratory system and to achieve faster recovery after the end of operation.

8.2.4.2 Desflurane

Desflurane is several times more expensive than sevoflurane and of all inhalational anaesthetics the one with the worst impact on climate. It is unavailable in many countries and was recently banned in some countries because of its greenhouse effects. For MAC and other properties, see Table 8.1. Uptake is fast so that adequate anaesthesia for surgery is achieved quickly and recovery is also fast. Desflurane is not suitable for craniotomy and contraindicated in patients with increased ICP.

8.2.4.3 Diethyl Ether

Ether was the first volatile anaesthetic agent which was used for GA since 1846 until recent years in several countries. Meanwhile it is seldom used because of difficult availability. On the other side, it can easily be manufactured locally and could still be an alternative for GA in very remote places and provided the AP is familiar with it. MAC is 2% for adults, however due to slow uptake, the concentration at the vaporiser is usually 5–15%. The *advantages of ether*: it is very cheap, does produce excellent intraoperative and even postoperative analgesia, sufficient muscle relaxation when used in higher concentration, provides cardiovascular stability due to vasoconstriction and increased heart rate (advantageous in patients with hypovolaemia), causes respiratory depression only when overdosed, and bronchodilation is also a positive side effect. Ether anaesthesia can be performed with room air and without adding oxygen in most patients. *Disadvantages*: slow uptake during inhalational induction which is unpleasant and takes longer time than with halothane; risk for laryngospasm and increased airway secretions (atropine premedication is mandatory), and often PONV. The main reason why it is hardly used nowadays is that it is easily flammable and explosive. Therefore, ether is relatively safe only in simple operation rooms without oxygen (oxygen is increasing risk for fire), without electricity, and especially without the use of electric devices like diathermy. A long tube should be used connected to the expiratory limb and scavenge the ether through a hole towards the outside of the building, since ether would accumulate on the floor and easily catch fire or explode. Filling the vaporiser should be with caution, and spillage of ether must be avoided. The same is true if industrial grade ether is to be used, since it is delivered in large containers unsuitable for theatre. Decanting into smaller bottles must be performed very carefully and with the help of a funnel, if available, in a place without any flammable or electric device, and spilling be avoided.

In health facilities where a functioning source for oxygen is present, ether should not be used; however, in settings where (unfortunately) oxygen is not available, ether may be an alternative additional to ketamine anaesthesia or in case ketamine is O/S. In better equipped operation theatres, ether should not be used because of these risks. Additionally, no modern anaesthesia machine, including those which are specially designed for low resource and remote settings, is equipped with an ether vaporiser. Instead, ether is used with a calibrated draw-over vaporiser, the EMO (Epstein Macintosh Oxford vaporiser), connected to a non-rebreathing system for spontaneous and manual ventilation which is open for room air.

8.3 Total Intravenous Anaesthesia TIVA

With IV anaesthetics, induction is fast while inhalational induction takes at least 10 min. After a single dose of an IV anaesthetic, the onset of effect is within 1 min due to rapid distribution into the brain. Redistribution into other organs is also rapid, so that the concentration in the brain decreases within few minutes. Duration of hypnotic effect after single dose of IV anaesthetic is 5–10 min for all of them (thiopentone, propofol, ketamine, etomidate). However, if used for maintenance with infusion via syringe pumps or after repeated bolus doses, the duration of effect is prolonged, and that extent is different for the different drugs due to their volume of distribution and their metabolism. Thiopentone would accumulate so markedly that maintenance of anaesthesia is almost impossible with that drug while propofol and ketamine are well suited for maintenance. Etomidate must not be used for maintenance since it depresses the adrenal glands so that physiological cortisol synthesis is blocked.

The major difference between inhalation anaesthesia and TIVA is that with a single volatile agent all components of anaesthesia are provided while several drugs must be combined for TIVA to achieve amnesia, analgesia, hypnosis (sleep), muscle relaxation, and alleviate sympathoadrenal stress response to surgical stimuli. Whether the AP chooses one or the other method, or balanced anaesthesia which is the combination of inhalational and intravenous anaesthesia, is depending on availability of drugs and devices for dosing (vaporisers) and continuous administration (syringe pumps) and on the personal preferences of the anaesthetist. Both methods are good and universally applicable.

Propofol is suitable for induction and maintenance of TIVA but must be combined with a strong analgesic as ketamine or fentanyl (50–100 μg/h depending on the type of surgery). Ketamine is safer than fentanyl as it does not produce respiratory depression. Many patients can be intubated with propofol in slightly higher dose plus analgesic without using a muscle relaxant, e.g. if suxamethonium is O/S or contraindicated. For maintenance, 10 mg/kg/h for 10 min followed by 8 mg/kg/h for another 10 min followed by 4–6 mg/kg/h is usually adequate dosing. Blood pressure decreases more with propofol than with any other anaesthetic agent and must not be used in patients who are hypovolaemic (dehydrated or bleeding).

Ketamine for maintenance TIVA: For adults, 100–300 mg/h are needed depending on body weight and size, the type of operation, and the general condition of the patient. Ketamine should be combined with a hypnotic agent, alternatively with propofol via syringe pump or with a single dose of midazolam, diazepam, promethazine, or chlorpromazine at the beginning of anaesthesia.

8.4 Balanced Anaesthesia

Most frequently, anaesthesia is induced with IV analgesic and hypnotic drugs, e.g. fentanyl or ketamine and thiopentone or propofol. Additionally, atropine and diazepam can be used as premedication or just before induction. Muscle relaxant is used if the patient is intubated. Balanced anaesthesia is anaesthesia where the desired effects (amnesia, analgesia, hypnosis, muscle relaxation) are achieved with a combination of different drugs. The balanced technique has long been used by anaesthetists to achieve good quality of anaesthesia with lower doses of multiple drugs, thereby limiting the risk of side effects from each agent.

Maintenance can be achieved with inhalational anaesthetic (isoflurane, sevoflurane, or halothane) alone or in combination with 60–70% N_2O. The requirements for volatile agents are reduced if additional doses of fentanyl or ketamine are injected. Inspiratory concentrations for maintenance at the vaporiser: Sevo: 1.5–3.5%, iso 0.8–2.0%, halo 0.5–1.5% if combined with N_2O and/or analgesics. The higher doses are only temporarily used to get anaesthesia deeper. They would lead to cardiac depression if administered for prolonged time.

How to estimate dose during GA is very much dependent on the experience of the AP. Different phases of the operation are causing different levels of pain and sympathetic stimulation. Anaesthesia depth must continuously be adapted to the needs of surgery. Patients show a great interindividual variability in drug response. Additionally, drug dose requirements are also dependent on the patient's general condition. A patient with decreased level of consciousness before anaesthesia needs lower doses than a fully alert person.

Analgesics during balanced anaesthesia: ketamine 25–50 mg or fentanyl 50–100 μg before surgical stimuli as skin incision, opening of peritoneum, inserting wound retractors, or at regular intervals of 15–30 min. Fentanyl is accumulating if injected several times. For maintenance, 50 μg per hour are rather safe, while with higher doses prolonged assisted ventilation after the end of surgery may be required due to long-lasting respiratory depression. The effects of fentanyl can be reversed by naloxone. However, that should only be performed in emergency with respiratory depression and no means of assisting ventilation available (e.g. in the peripheral ward). It is much better to ventilate patients as long as they are not breathing sufficiently. Naloxone is reversing effects of opioids abruptly, so that patients may suddenly suffer from severe pain and high blood pressure due to the stress.

Instead of using fentanyl, intraoperative analgesia can also be achieved with a single dose of a long-acting analgesic like morphine 10 mg or pethidine 100 mg or other opioid drugs before skin incision. Only one opioid/narcotic agent should be used to avoid severe and long-lasting respiratory depression.

Muscle-relaxant drugs are required to facilitate endotracheal intubation. Without muscle relaxant, anaesthesia must be very deep to enable intubation or insertion of laryngeal mask airway. During abdominal surgery, relaxation of the muscles is often requested by the surgeon. Either deep anaesthesia, provided, ventilation is controlled and BP not too low, or additional doses of suxamethonium 25–50 mg IV can be administered, which will produce 3–5 min of excellent relaxation, e.g. if the patient is pushing. Non-depolarising muscle relaxants like pancuronium should be used with caution, and in smaller health facilities or operation theatres without recovery room, they should not be used at all, since their effects may last unpredictably long. Patients might be awake and breathing at the end of surgery and be extubated, but the muscles in the throat would still be weak, putting patients at risk for aspiration of secretions and respiratory insufficiency with hypoxia. The risk is even higher if oxygen cannot be administered uninterruptedly from the end of surgery until several hours post surgery. Pancuronium can lead to avoidable deaths in the early postoperative phase. Therefore, it may be safer to use incremental doses of suxamethonium up to not more than a total dose of 200–300 mg. Bradycardia, a common side effect of suxamethonium, can be prevented by atropine.

After major surgery with balanced anaesthesia, patients must be observed sufficiently long by anaesthesia staff before they may be transferred to the ward. Under no circumstances patients may be transferred from operation theatre immediately after extubation. Patients who are planned for intensive care after operation can be transferred early while they are continuously ventilated and monitored on the way to the ICU.

Further Reading

Bokoch MP, Su P-YP (2023) Intravenous anesthesia. In: Pardo MC Jr (ed) Miller's basics of anesthesia, 8th edn. Elsevier, Philadelphia, pp 107–124

Chang CY, Goldstein E, Agarwal N, Swan KG (2015) Ether in the developing world: rethinking an abandoned agent. BMC Anesthesiol 15:149–153

Herbert L, Tige R (2020) General and urological surgery. In: Craven R, Edgcombe H, Gupta B (eds) Global anaesthesia, 1st edn. Oxford University Press, Oxford, pp 229–238

Kirkbride D (2019) The practical conduct of anaesthesia: Induction of anaesthesia. Maintenance of anaesthesia. In: Thompson J, Moppett I, Wiles M (eds) Smith and Aitkenhead's textbook of anaesthesia, 7th edn. Elsevier, London, pp 441–455

O'Regan M (2019) Anaesthesia in resource-poor areas. In: Thompson J, Moppett I, Wiles M (eds) Smith and Aitkenhead's textbook of anaesthesia, 7th edn. Elsevier, London, pp 850–858

Temple E, Wiles M (2019) Inhalational anaesthetic agents and medical gases. In: Thompson J, Moppett I, Wiles M (eds) Smith and Aitkenhead's textbook of anaesthesia, 7th edn. Elsevier, London, pp 49–65

9 Short General Anaesthesia for Minor Procedures

Abstract

General anaesthesia consists of amnesia, analgesia, sleep, and immobility. However, for minor procedures including incision and drainage of abscesses, repositioning of fractures, or wound debridement, and other procedures lasting less than around 30 min, deep hypnosis and muscle relaxation are often not required. This chapter contains dose recommendations for short anaesthesia without endotracheal intubation and without anaesthesia machine for infants, children, and adults. Pulse oximeter and self-inflating bag are mandatory minimum equipment. Oxygen, BP cuff, and suction device may be needed as well.

For very short procedures a combination of ketamine, diazepam (or midazolam), and atropine is often a good choice and may be drawn together into a single syringe. Most patients will keep a patent airway and breathe, cough, and swallow sufficiently. Average doses: atropine 0.01 mg/kg, diazepam 0.1 mg/kg (midazolam 0.05 mg/kg), ketamine 1–2 mg/kg. Incremental doses of ketamine 1 mg/kg are required every 5–10 min. Children without IV access may receive atropine 0.02 mg/kg and ketamine 5 mg/kg IM, onset within 5 min, duration 20–30 min.

Side effects include tachycardia, hypertension, increased salivation and secretions in the airways; and during recovery hallucinations, excitation, and confusion are common.

For patients at old age or with known hypertension, BP monitoring is mandatory. If systolic blood pressure is 180 mmHg or higher, the dose of ketamine is reduced to 0.5–1 mg/kg combined with low dose thiopentone 1–2 mg/kg or propofol 0.5–1 mg/kg. Mask ventilation is usually required shortly; oxygen and suction device must be immediately available.

Keywords

Drugs for short general anaesthesia · General anaesthesia for minor procedures · Ketamine for short procedures · Ketamine IM for minor surgery · Short general anaesthesia in resource-limited settings

The state of complete anaesthesia normally consists of analgesia, amnesia, sleep, and immobility. For short procedures, usually, muscle relaxation is not required, sleep does not need to be very deep, but analgesia must be sufficient, and amnesia is desired. Amnesia means the patient does not remember what happens after the onset of anaesthesia or sedative drugs.

This chapter contains dosage recommendations for short anaesthesia. Please notice that the AP is solely responsible for the correct dose and

D. Kietzmann, *Anaesthesia in Remote Hospitals*, Sustainable Development Goals Series,
https://doi.org/10.1007/978-3-031-46610-6_9

administration of drugs. Therefore, please check the correct dosage even on drug datasheets/product information and follow local guidelines. Always label the syringes carefully.

A combination of ketamine, diazepam, and atropine is often a good choice for short general anaesthesia (GA). An alternative for diazepam is midazolam (Dormicum®) which is not painful on injection and shorter acting, and onset is more quickly. Effects are the same as with diazepam. Notably, 1 mg of midazolam equals 2 mg of diazepam so that with midazolam half the dose as with diazepam may be used. For very short procedures, small amounts of propofol (20 mg for adults which may be repeated once) can be used instead of the longer-acting diazepam or midazolam. Equipment for resuscitation must be available and ready to use, especially oxygen, Ambu bag, or other types of self-inflating bellows, face mask, oropharyngeal (Guedel) airway, resuscitation drugs such as adrenaline, and suction devices. Use a pulse oximeter for monitoring; in known or suspected hypertensive patients and patients >60 years, add blood pressure monitoring. If you do not have a pulse oximeter, use a precordial stethoscope and feel the pulse frequently.

9.1 Indications

Minor surgery includes incisional drainage of abscess, painful wound debridement, repositioning of fractures, and other short, painful procedures which require anaesthesia. Short GA can also be used for procedures shorter than approximately 45 min if airway difficulties are anticipated and even face mask ventilation would prove to be difficult or impossible. Examples are burns of the head, face, or neck including release of contractures with limited mouth opening or neck movement. Ketamine for caesarean section please see under Chap. 11.

9.2 Relative Contraindications

- Congestive heart failure
- Heart disease with known or suspected valvular stenosis and ischaemic heart disease.
- Short GA can be difficult in patients with chronic alcohol or drug abuse.
- Poor general condition (half the normal doses might be adequate).
- Dilatation and curettage (patient might move; therefore, instead of diazepam give 2–3 mg/kg thiopentone or 1 mg/kg propofol in combination with ketamine; be ready to ventilate the patient shortly).
- Head injury (ketamine can increase intracranial pressure if the patient is not artificially ventilated). In ventilated patients, ketamine does not produce effect on intracranial pressure. Patients with head injuries are prone to lose their airways and to stop breathing when anaesthetised even with small doses. Consider intubation anaesthesia instead (see even Sect. 13.4).

9.3 Drugs for Short GA

Atropine 0.5 mg/mL plus diazepam 5 mg/mL plus ketamine 50 mg/mL or 100 mg/mL. Instead of diazepam, propofol 10 mg/mL or 20 mg/mL, or thiopentone 25 mg/mL may be used alternatively. Diazepam causes pain on injection. That may be reduced by mixing 0.5 mL lidocaine with 10 mg of diazepam. If midazolam is available, it can replace diazepam. It causes the same effects and does not cause pain on injection, and the dose is half that of diazepam.

9.3.1 Effects

Ketamine produces analgesia in low doses (0.5–1.0 mg/kg), and in high doses (>1.5 mg/kg), it produces so-called dissociative anaesthesia which consists of profound analgesia with only slightly impaired pharyngeal and laryngeal reflexes, no deep hypnosis, and often open eyes. Patients "hear" and "see", but the cerebral cortex is dissociated from perception so they are not responsive. Patients are usually able to swallow and cough and to keep their airway open. It does not cause respiratory depression unless diazepam is overdosed or thiopentone or propofol are used in combination with ketamine. The muscle tone is often a bit increased, and there is no relaxation.

9.3.2 Side Effects

Side effects include nightmares, hallucination, confusion, and excitation during recovery. In order to minimise these side effects, diazepam, midazolam, promethazine, haloperidol or chlorpromazine, or thiopentone (the latter exclusively by a trained anaesthetist) can be used. Even small doses of propofol (20 mg) are helpful. Other side effects: sympathetic activation with a mild increase in blood pressure and heart rate (can be severe in patients with untreated hypertension or with preeclampsia) and profuse salivation (therefore atropine is needed).

9.3.3 Doses

The recommended doses are approximations for average patients. The requirements for the individual patient may be different. Therefore, the effects and side effects always need to be carefully observed in order to adjust the dose properly.

Induction doses: adults and children >10 years: atropine 0.5 mg; diazepam 5 mg; ketamine 1–2 mg/kg.

Incremental doses: atropine and diazepam none; ketamine 0.5–1 mg/kg.

Children >1 year with IV access: atropine 0.01–0.02 mg/kg; diazepam 2.5 mg; ketamine 1.5–2.5 mg/kg.

Repeated doses: atropine and diazepam none; ketamine 1 mg/kg.

Children without IV access: atropine 0.02 mg/kg; diazepam none; ketamine 5–6 mg/kg IM as single dose, onset of effect 3–5 min; or 7–10 mg/kg ketamine mixed with sugar and water or sweet juice orally → onset of effect after 15 min but less reliable than after IM injection.

9.3.4 Short GA Without Available Anaesthesia Staff for Emergency Procedures

Adults for painful dressing/wound cleaning/repositioning of fractures even ***when no trained anaesthesia staff is available*** may receive a single IM injection of ketamine 100 mg plus pethidine 100 mg at the responsibility of the patient's physician. That combination provides excellent short-term analgesia for painful procedures followed by long-lasting analgesia. Contraindication is a head injury with an impaired level of consciousness or circulatory shock (in shock, ketamine may be used, but pethidine should be omitted because it would decrease blood pressure).

9.3.5 Duration of Effect

After ketamine IV 5–10 min, IM 20–30 min for surgery, the analgesic effect lasts longer. However, it may take much more time until the patient is fully awake and responsive. The patients should recover in calm places without being disturbed in order to avoid nightmares and excitation. When they have recovered, they may drink and eat unless surgery or general condition would make that impossible.

The onset of effect is within 1 min after IV injection, within 3–5 min after IM, and within 15 min after oral administration.

Propofol or thiopentone instead of diazepam: Remember that thiopentone and propofol may cause respiratory depression and hypotension. For short GA with spontaneous breathing, only small doses may be used, e.g. 20 mg propofol for adults irrespective of bodyweight or 1 mg/kg for children. In children, propofol is less effective than in adults, and with effective doses, they would stop breathing. Combination with diazepam or midazolam may be easier and safer in paediatric cases. Remember that opened propofol vials must not be used longer than 12 h due to the risk of infection. Thiopentone can be used in smaller doses compared with induction dose before major operations, e.g. 50–100 mg for adults or 2 mg/kg for children in combination with ketamine as alternative to diazepam.

Patients in poor general condition may be anaesthetised only in theatre with full anaesthesia equipment, not in the POP/wound treatment room, in the outpatient department, or elsewhere.

9.3.6 Short GA for Patients with Hypertension

Severe hypertension can lead to hypertensive crisis and heart failure if the usual dose of ketamine is given. In patients with BP > 180 mmHg, you will need a SIB and face mask, stethoscope, and oxygen source. Have pulse oximeter and BP cuff attached. If available, use even ECG. Measure BP around every 3 min. Put the patient on a drip and apply oxygen. Titrate the anaesthesia drugs with repeated small amounts until a sufficient effect is achieved. Combinations of small amounts of propofol (20–50 mg) or thiopentone (50–100 mg) with small amounts of ketamine (25–50 mg) are a good choice. If available, you can also use 50 μg of fentanyl (repeat, if necessary, only after more than 15 min) instead of ketamine and combine it with propofol or thiopentone. Most patients will need manual ventilation for some minutes until they are breathing sufficiently again.

9.3.7 Short GA for Patients with Respiratory Disease

Short GA in the same way as for other patients provided oxygen is available. Have oxygen ready and aim for SPO_2 > 94%. Ketamine has a relaxing, dilating effect on the bronchi which is advantageous for patients with asthma or COPD. Thiopentone is better avoided.

9.3.8 Short GA for Patients with Kidney Disease

Avoid dehydration but also over-infusion. The same drugs can be used for short GA in the same doses as for other patients. Patients with renal disease are often hypertensive. Then use short GA for hypertensive patients.

9.3.9 Short GA for Patients with Diabetes

The same anaesthetics can be used. Smaller doses may be adequate. Aim for glucose control. Give RL infusion, and add dextrose if glucose level < 6 mmol/L. The general condition of these patients may be impaired. Careful monitoring of vital signs including blood pressure and pulse oximetry is needed. Communication with the physician regarding fasting of the patient and administration of insulin is recommended. Oral antidiabetics must not be given when patients are fasting.

9.3.10 Table of Doses for Short General Anaesthesia "Short GA"

The doses in Table 9.1 are given for intravenous administration of atropine 0.5 mg/mL, diazepam 5 mg/mL, or ketamine 50 mg/mL. The drugs may be mixed in a single syringe immediately before injection.

Table 9.2 gives intramuscular administration for short GA single dose.

Do not use short GA IM for infants below 5 kg.

Table 9.3 gives doses for oral administration of ketamine mixed with sugar and little water or syrup, not applicable for infants below the age of approximately 6 months.

Table 9.1 Doses for short IV general anaesthesia

Bodyweight	Drug	Induction		Incremental dose	
(kg)		mg	mL	mg	mL
5–9	Atropine 0.5 mg/mL	0.1	0.2	0	
	Diazepam 5 mg/mL	2.5	0.5	0	
	Ketamine 50 mg/mL	10–15	0.2–0.3	5–10	0.1–0.2
10–15	Atropine 0.5 mg/mL	0.15	0.3	0	
	Diazepam 5 mg/mL	2.5	0.5	0	
	Ketamine 50 mg/mL	15–25	0.3–0.5	10–15	0.2–0.3
16–20	Atropine 0.5 mg/mL	0.2	0.4	0	
	Diazepam 5 mg/mL	5	1.0	0	
	Ketamine 50 mg/mL	25–40	0.5–0.8	15–20	0.3–0.4
21–25	Atropine 0.5 mg/mL	0.25	0.5	0	
	Diazepam 5 mg/mL	5	1.0	0	
	Ketamine 50 mg/mL	40–50	0.8–1.0	20–25	0.4–0.5
26–30	Atropine 0.5 mg/mL	0.3	0.6	0	
	Diazepam 5 mg/mL	5	1.0	0	
	Ketamine 50 mg/mL	50–60	1.0–1.2	25	0.5
31–40	Atropine 0.5 mg/mL	0.4	0.8	0	
	Diazepam 5 mg/mL	5	1.0	0	
	Ketamine 50 mg/mL	60–80	1.2–1.6	30–40	0.6–0.8
41–50	Atropine 0.5 mg/mL	0.5	1.0	0	
	Diazepam 5 mg/mL	5	1.0	0	
	Ketamine 50 mg/mL	80–100	1.2–1.6	50	1.0
51–70	Atropine 0.5 mg/mL	0.5	1.0	0	
	Diazepam 5 mg/mL	5	1.0	0	
	Ketamine 50 mg/mL	100–125	2–2.5	50–75	1.0–1.5
> 70	Atropine 0.5 mg/mL	0.5	1.0	0	
	Diazepam 5 mg/mL	7.5	1.5	0	
	Ketamine 50 mg/mL	125–150	2.5–3	75–100	1.5–2.0

Table 9.2 Intramuscular administration single dose

Bodyweight	Atropine 0.5 mg/mL		Ketamine 50 mg/mL	
(kg)	mg	mL	mg	mL
5	0.1	0.2	25	0.5
6–7	0.1	0.2	35	0.7
8–9	0.15	0.3	50	1.0
10–12	0.2	0.4	60	1.2
13–15	0.25	0.5	75	1.5
16–20	0.3	0.6	100	2
>20	0.4	0.8	125	2.5

Table 9.3 Oral administration single dose

Bodyweight	Atropine 0.5 mg/mL		Ketamine 50 mg/mL	
(kg)	mg	mL	mg	mL
8	0.1	0.2	80	1.6
9	0.2	0.4	90	1.8
10–12	0.2	0.4	100	2.0
13–15	0.25	0.5	125	2.5
16–20	0.3	0.6	150	3.0

10 Spinal Anaesthesia

Abstract

Spinal or subarachnoid anaesthesia is a regional block where intrathecal nerve structures near the spinal cord are anaesthetised. A small amount of local anaesthetic is injected between two lumbar vertebrae into the cerebrospinal fluid space, causing a fast and profound blockade of the body segments caudal to the level of the block, usually below the umbilicus or below the costal arch. It is suitable for caesarean section, other types of lower abdominal or perineal surgery, urological operations, hernia repair, and lower limb surgery. Duration of the block is dependent on the dose and type of local anaesthetic and usually lasts 1–2 h, rarely more than 3 h. Doses depend on the patient's height (decreased during late pregnancy and at old age): bupivacaine heavy 7.5–15 mg; pethidine (an opioid with additional local anaesthetic properties) 50–75 mg diluted with 1–2 mL NS. Spinal anaesthesia is cheaper than general anaesthesia and safer, provided the anaesthesia practitioner is able to recognise and treat complications. The most common side effects are bradycardia and hypotension, which are marked if the spread of the block is higher than required. Give infusions prior to and during anaesthesia. Always have atropine and a vasoconstrictor such as ephedrine ready plus resuscitation drugs such as adrenaline available.

Post-dural-puncture headache is less common if small (25–27 gauge) and blunt (pencil-point) spinal needles are used.

Contraindications include acute bleeding, infection with fever or infection of the site of injection, and bleeding disorder. Anticoagulant drugs must be paused before performing a spinal block.

Keywords

Complications of spinal anaesthesia · Local anaesthetics for spinal anaesthesia · Pethidine for spinal anaesthesia · Spinal anaesthesia for non-specialist anaesthesia providers

10.1 General Considerations and Anatomy

Spinal anaesthesia is a regional anaesthetic technique that, together with epidural and caudal anaesthesia, belongs to the central neuraxial blocks. "Central neuraxial" means that structures near the spinal cord are anaesthetised. For spinal anaesthesia, only a small amount of local anaesthetic is injected on the back between two lumbar vertebrae into the cerebrospinal fluid (subarachnoid) space The local anaesthetic will produce a fast and profound blockade of the body segments caudal to the cranial level of the block (usually legs and inguinal and lower abdominal regions are

D. Kietzmann, *Anaesthesia in Remote Hospitals*, Sustainable Development Goals Series,
https://doi.org/10.1007/978-3-031-46610-6_10

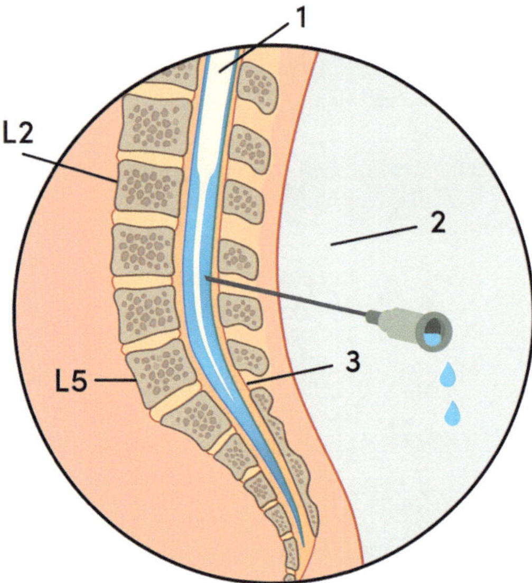

Fig. 10.1 Section of lumbar vertebrae showing the spinal needle in the correct place. 1 spinal cord, 2 spinal needle in the correct place with cerebrospinal fluid (liquor) dropping, 3 ligamentum flavum, and L2 and L5 = body of lumbar 2 and 5

anaesthetised). The nerve roots of the spinal nerves with their sensory, motor, and sympathetic fibres are anaesthetised within a few minutes. The maximum block height is different for motor block, pain reception (can be tested as a response to pinprick), and cold sensation. Anaesthesia to touch is around two segments lower than a block of cold sensation. Pinprick is in between.

Spinal anaesthesia is generally a safer alternative compared with general anaesthesia, if used correctly; however, one must be aware of anatomy (see Fig. 10.1), technique, and possible complications. Equipment and drugs for cardiopulmonary resuscitation must be available. Thorough training and supervision are necessary a couple of times until you can perform it on your own. Anaesthesia providers may perform spinal anaesthesia only when they have fully understood the possible complications, how to recognise them, and how to treat them.

10.1.1 Indications

Spinal anaesthesia is suitable for lower abdominal surgery, caesarean section, gynaecological and urological operations, inguinal hernia repair, hydrocelectomy, lower limb surgery, and perineal and anal surgery in adult patients. Spinal anaesthesia can even be performed in cooperative teenagers provided that the anaesthesia practitioner is experienced. Adjust the dose to their body size and add a light sedative, e.g. diazepam 5 mg IV or midazolam 2 mg. If you have a syringe pump and are familiar with it, sedation with approximately 2 mg/kg/h propofol is an excellent alternative after an initial bolus dose of 20 mg IV. Even adults may feel more comfortable with sedation during surgery. With spinal anaesthesia up to the level of thoracic 6, upper abdominal surgery is possible if the surgeon is familiar with operating in spinal rather than in general anaesthesia. The level of anaesthesia needs to be assessed very carefully to be sure that it works sufficiently; otherwise, a top-up with GA is required. Some patients may have difficulty breathing. Give oxygen and comfort them, and observe the movements of the diaphragm. Light sedation is often helpful in such cases. As the diaphragm is innervated by the phrenic nerve from the cervical 4 segment, it is unlikely that a patient cannot breathe sufficiently, but the intercostal muscles may be partly paralysed and coughing may be difficult. The duration of surgery is limited as the effect of the spinal is wearing off after 90–120 min in most patients. Sometimes, the effect lasts longer, but that is not predictable.

10.1.2 Contraindications

Contraindications include local infection or generalised sepsis, known bleeding disorder/patient on anticoagulants (e.g. warfarin), platelets <80,000, lack of sterile equipment, unresuscitated patient who is hypovolaemic (cannot tolerate a drop in BP), prolonged surgery (spinal lasts only 1–2–3 h), known allergy towards the local anaesthetic drug, difficult anatomy, and uncooperative patient.

10.2 Technique

Prepare the patient as for GA with usual assessment, fasting for 6 h, have rescue equipment available, check laryngoscope and tubes, know where your drugs are, and draw up some ephedrine/atropine. Insert a large bore venous cannula with running infusion. Consider preloading with 500 mL if the patient was fasting for many hours. Check vital signs and start to write the anaesthesia record. Correct positioning of the patient is very important, so request help from theatre staff, and ask the patient for cooperation ("please bend your back like an angry cat"), which makes life so much easier for everyone. Palpate the last rib and trace back to the lumbar bone from where it originates which is thoracic 12 (T12). A palpated line between the iliac crests (anterior superior iliac spine) usually crosses the body of lumbar 4 (L4) or the interspace L3/4. After disinfecting your hands, put on sterile gloves and put a sterile drape or the paper of the sterile gloves as a sterile working surface behind the patient's back. Disinfect the skin thoroughly. Povidone-iodine needs 3 min on the skin surface to be effective; chlorhexidine or methylated spirit needs 1 min. Start when comfortable with everything including asepsis and the smallest spinal needle available, e.g. 25 g. Several types of spinal needles exist; some of them are blunt with a 20 g introducer needle and others are sharp without introducer. Interspace L3/4 is often best; alternatively, L4/5 or L2/3 may be used. The subarachnoid space is often quite shallow so go slowly and you have a better chance of getting it the first time, and do not push in the whole way unless necessary (usually not). If you fail to get the spinal first attempt, it is worth checking the position of the patient and checking your anatomy again.

The spinal needle will pass through the following anatomical structures as shown in Fig. 10.1: skin, subcutaneous tissue, supraspinous ligament, interspinous ligament, ligamentum flavum, epidural space (3–5 mm thick), dura, and intrathecal space = subarachnoid space with CSF. The epidural space contains fat and blood vessels. If you obtain blood, you need to quickly insert the needle a little further before the blood clots and obstructs the tip of the cannula. If you do not get CSF, you need to remove the cannula and flush it with a little normal saline or LA before inserting it at a different interspace. Often, you can feel a "give" after being through the ligamentum flavum. Painful sensation in the patient should mean you stop inserting the needle any further which often already is in the subarachnoid space if the patient is feeling a sudden pain.

Look at one of the following or similar videos on YouTube to see the technique:

https://www.youtube.com/watch?v=SZ2TClYz4zI

https://www.youtube.com/watch?v=iUYr05be-OM

When you get CSF try to aspirate a small bit slowly, secure the immobile needle in one hand using the back as support and slowly (over 10–15 s) inject local anaesthetic. Generally, 2–3 mL 0.5% bupivacaine (that is 10–15 mg) or 2 mL 5% lidocaine (that is 100 mg) is used for most surgeries and 1.5 mL for C-sections (75 mg lidocaine) but considering the size of the patient. Small patients need less volume than tall patients. For old patients with low body weight, the dose is reduced by a quarter. Once placed, help the patient into position and tell them their legs will be heavily numb for a few hours, but this will return to normal. It is a good idea if you have time to check the level of the block and that it is working before the surgeon does!

Regular monitoring is mandatory: check the pulse oximeter continuously and BP every 2 min for the first 10 min, then every 5 min for 30 min, and thereafter every 15 min if the patient is not losing blood. It is recommended to use an ECG monitor as well. At least in high-risk patients, for caesarean section, and whenever pulse oximeter reading is poor, an ECG monitor is necessary if available. (If disposable electrodes are O/S, just use a little jelly on the skin, attach ECG, and fix it with adhesive tape.) Communicate with the patient; they often feel unwell as a first clinical sign before blood pressure or heart rate drops. Try to ensure that they are comfortable and prone to getting cold sometimes a blanket makes life more comfortable or something soft under their head if possible. Ephedrine/atropine should be used if needed. Atropine is also often effective in cases of nausea/vomiting during spinal anaesthesia.

In case the spinal is not effective, perform general anaesthesia, e.g. with ketamine or inhalational anaesthesia. Do not perform a second spinal at least 20 min after the first dose. The first spinal might become effective as well, however, unusually late, and then the total amount of LA is too much causing life-threatening high spinal anaesthesia. The patient would stop breathing and get circulatory collapse needing adrenaline infusion: 1 mg adrenaline into 500 mL infusion, let it drip, and drip rate is adjusted to response. Aim systolic BP around 100. Establish a second venous line with NS or RL 1 L full speed.

The local anaesthetic is injected into the cerebrospinal fluid in the subarachnoid space in the lumbar region through a lumbar punction below interspace L1/L2 where the spinal cord ends. That means the interspaces L2/L3, L3/L4, or L4/L5 may be used only in order to avoid damage to the spinal cord. Below L5, spinal anaesthesia is usually not possible due to anatomy. Spinal anaesthesia results in a block of spinal nerve roots by blocking nerve impulses before they reach the CNS and it decreases the excitability of the tissues by blocking Na^+ (sodium) channels which are necessary for impulse conduction. Pain and temperature fibres are the smallest and thinnest and are affected first, next touch, and lastly motor (largest and thickest nerve fibres). Therefore, motor blockade indicates sufficient anaesthesia.

10.3 Local Anaesthetic Drugs for Spinal Anaesthesia

There are two types of local anaesthetics (LA) for spinal: hyperbaric "heavy" and isobaric. ***Isobaric*** or "plain" solutions show almost the same density as cerebrospinal fluid. Their spread is not dependent on the position of the patient during the injection or afterwards but on the volume injected and the speed of injection. Usually, 0.5–1 mL more than a heavy solution is needed for the same effect. ***Hyperbaric*** means a solution denser ("heavier") than cerebrospinal fluid. This is usually achieved with a mixture of the local anaesthetic with 7.5% dextrose. These solutions allow the level of the block to be controlled by positioning the patient so that the drug flows "downhill" to the segments that need to be blocked. For example, injection with the patient in the sitting position will result in a block of the sacral nerve roots; injection with the patient in the lateral position, if the position is maintained, will produce unilateral anaesthesia on the lower side.

The spread of hyperbaric LA is influenced very much by positioning after injection: For procedures performed in the perineal, vulva, or anal regions, let patients sit 5 min after injection of lidocaine/prilocaine or 10 min after injection of heavy bupivacaine. Then let them lie down. Let them in a *head-done position first 10 min after injection of lidocaine/prilocaine* or 15 min after injection of bupivacaine, because thereafter the LA is fixed and will not spread any further. By doing that, the spread will only be in the sacral and lower lumbar segments (the so-called **saddle block**; this block requires only 1.0 mL of LA; otherwise, the concentration of LA in those segments would become too high and potentially neurotoxic).

For all other procedures, let the patients lie horizontally immediately after injection, but avoid head-down positioning because this would let the drug spread too high. If the block is too high, patients have difficulties with breathing and blood pressure drops markedly. In the horizontal position, the spread is usually up to the thoracic segment Th8 to Th4. In cases where spread to Th10–12 is sufficient (surgery of a leg), a slight head-up position is appropriate for the first 5–10 min after injection.

For surgery of the thigh (e.g. femur ORIF) in the lateral position, the patient must remain around 10 min in a supine position before turning to the side to avoid the local anaesthetic flowing downhill to that side which is not to be operated.

Too early head-down position or overdose may cause high spinal anaesthesia with life-threatening circulatory failure and respiratory insufficiency or respiratory arrest. In worst cases, patients become unconscious, stop breathing, and need immediate ventilation with oxygen, tracheal intubation, and cardiac resuscitation. Usually, in that condition, you will find the pupils to be dilated and not reacting to light. Unconscious patients do not need muscle relaxation for intubation and do not need general anaesthetic drugs. Just secure the airway and ventilate until the patient is recovering and treat the hypotension and bradycardia with adrenaline. If endotracheal intubation is difficult or unsuccessful, use a laryngeal mask instead, and if unavailable, use nasopharyngeal or oropharyngeal airway and ventilation via a face mask. Call for help from a senior anaesthetist!

10.3.1 Doses of LA for Spinal Anaesthesia

Bupivacaine 0.5% hyperbaric contains 5 mg/mL with dextrose/glucose 7.2%: 1.5–2.0 mL = 7.5–10 mg for C/S; 2.5–3 mL = 12.5–15 mg for other procedures. For saddle block, give 1 mL hyperbaric.

Bupivacaine 0.5% without dextrose ("plain"): 2–2.5 mL = 10–12.5 mg for C/S, 3–4 mL = 15–20 mg for all other procedures. Saddle block is impossible with a plain local anaesthetic.

Lidocaine 5% hyperbaric contains 50 mg per mL with dextrose/glucose 7.5%. For saddle block, 1.0 mL = 50 mg is sufficient, for caesarean section 1.5 mL = 75 mg (however, if the woman is <50 kg and < 155 cm, give only 1.2–1.3 mL). For all other procedures 2.0 mL = 100 mg, but for patients <50 kg and < 155 cm, give 1.5 mL only. Add 0.1–0.2 mL adrenaline 1% if required duration of effect >60 min.

Lidocaine 2% contains 20 mg/mL lidocaine HCl (lignocaine hydrochloride). Unfortunately, most preparations of lidocaine 2% additionally contain a preservative like methylparabene which should not be used intrathecally. Lidocaine 2% in 5 mL or 10 mL vials is usually free of preservatives (read the label carefully) and may be used for spinal. The preservative may cause several weeks-long neurological problems with pain, weakness, and numbness in the legs. It may only be used in emergencies if there are no alternatives. Give 3.0 mL = 60 mg for C/S, and 4 mL = 80 mg for all other procedures. Duration of action is usually short and may be prolonged by adding adrenaline 0.05 mg = 0.05 mL (one drop) of adrenaline 1 mg/mL.

Prilocaine 2% plain or hyperbaric: 2–3 mL = 40–60 mg; for saddle block, 1 mL hyperbaric.

In case the injection of the local anaesthetic does not produce a sufficient effect within 10 min after lidocaine or 15 min after bupivacaine injection, ***a second dose as spinal should not be given as this can lead to a life-threatening high or total spinal block.*** Sometimes there is the effect of spinal with delay or there is insufficient spread of the LA.

Instead, one should wait 20–30 min, or general anaesthesia may be performed.

10.3.2 Duration of Effect

The duration of lidocaine is approximately 40–70 min and may be extended to approximately 80–100 min by mixing lidocaine with 0.05–0.1 mL adrenaline 1 mg/mL. The duration of bupivacaine is 1.5–3 h and can be extended a little (10–30 min longer lasting effect) with 0.1 mL adrenaline. Prilocaine duration of the block is 60–80 min and can be prolonged by adding adrenaline.

With lidocaine and prilocaine, the onset is faster (2–10 min) than with bupivacaine (4–20 min). Heavy LA produces a faster onset than plain.

If surgery lasts longer than spinal anaesthesia, conversion to GA is needed in most cases. Ketamine can be used if just some minutes are to be bridged until the end of the operation.

10.3.3 Pethidine for Spinal Anaesthesia

If local anaesthetics for spinal anaesthesia are O/S, pethidine can be used instead as the drug is preservative-free in ampoules with 50 or 100 mg at 50 mg/mL, and it is hyperbaric. Pethidine is unique among opioid drugs as it is not only acting at the opioid receptors but also acting as a local anaesthetic. It is the only opioid that produces a sensory and motor block in the same way as LA do when injected intrathecally. Indications include allergy towards LA and LA out of stock. Pethidine is cheaper than bupivacaine, which is also an advantage.

For saddle block, 0.5 mg/kg is injected and the patient is sitting for 10 min and thereafter put into lithotomy position. For procedures at the legs or lower abdomen, 50–75 mg of pethidine is usually adequate. If diluted with 1–2 mL of NS, the spread would be higher (more cephalad). For caesarean section, 50–75 mg = 1–1.5 mL pethidine plus 1–2 mL NS could be injected to get a spread up to thoracic 4–6. If the woman is <155 cm, dilute 50 mg pethidine with 2 mL NS and inject only 2 mL of these 3 mL (equal to 33 mg). Women 156–165 cm may get 50 mg + 1 mL NS, and above 165 cm, 75 mg + 1 mL NS. The patient can be put in a slight head-up position if the spread gets too high in the cephalad direction, or in a supine position if the spread is required to be higher. Very tall adults may get up to 100 mg of pethidine plus 1 ml NS intrathecally for spinal anaesthesia. Duration of effect is a bit shorter than with bupivacaine, which is around 80–120 min and cannot be prolonged by adding adrenaline.

Side effects include hypotension as with local anaesthetics for spinal anaesthesia. Have ephedrine or diluted adrenaline with 0.01 mg/mL (10 μg/mL) ready or other vasoconstrictor. Pethidine for spinal anaesthesia is also likely to produce some degree of sedation.

As pethidine is an opioid, respiratory depression is possible but not common and would present early when the patient is still in theatre and vital signs are observed. However, during spinal anaesthesia with pethidine, patients must not receive any sedative drug like diazepam as that combination of drugs is likely to cause severe respiratory depression. Always have a self-inflating bag and face mask at hand when giving spinal anaesthesia.

Please note that an equipotent dose of *morphine* (e.g. 5 mg morphine instead of 50 mg of pethidine) *must not be used* for spinal anaesthesia! Morphine would not produce spinal anaesthesia but only analgesia and would be very likely to produce severe long-lasting respiratory depression when injected intrathecally because it spreads cephalad into the cerebrospinal fluid around the brain stem. Even respiratory depression with delayed onset after several hours is possible and might cause death in the ward. *Pethidine is the only opioid drug that can be used for spinal anaesthesia.*

10.4 Side Effects and Complications of Spinal Anaesthesia

10.4.1 Post Dural Puncture Headache

This is relatively common and can be quite debilitating for the patient, with cases recorded of headaches occasionally (rare) lasting up to 2 years. It is caused by leakage of cerebrospinal fluid (CSF) through a dural puncture which causes traction on the meninges, often relieved by lying down, and aggravated by standing/mobilisation, occipital mainly, sometimes neck stiffness or hearing loss. ***Treatment*** includes sufficient fluid intake, paracetamol, ibuprofen, or diclofenac, sometimes caffeine helps (coke/tea/coffee), and bed rest. However, continuous bed rest must be avoided to minimise the risk of thrombosis. If severe and no improvement with conservative measures after several days, if possible, refer the patient for a blood patch (20 mL of the patient's own blood injected into epidural space with a special needle for epidural puncture; the blood forms a seal, and in >90% cases, it gives immediate relief, but the technique requires a lot of experience and the special equipment). *Prevention* is by using small and blunt needles.

Reduce the incidence of headache by using the smallest available, e.g. 25 g or 27 g needle, preferably Whitacre (pencil point top) where possible! By preparing and getting the patient into the optimum position *before* commencing the procedure, you have a better chance of getting it the first time and avoiding multiple attempts. However, if spinal is very difficult to perform, or when spinal needles are out of stock, even the inner needle of a 20 g indwelling venous cannula or other thin and sufficiently long cannula may be used but has a higher incidence of post-puncture headache (up to 30%). **Lower backache** and ache in the buttocks are seldom but sometimes severe, usually temporary within a few days, and it is most common after lidocaine. Lidocaine with preservative methylparabene is indicated for local anaesthesia, but not for spinal anaesthesia. When used for spinal anaesthesia, it may cause long-lasting severe pain, numbness, and weakness of the legs and should therefore be avoided.

10.4.2 High Spinal

Spinal anaesthesia with a block above the level of Th4 is too high. This complication is not as common but ***potentially fatal*** and important to be recognised quickly. The patient may complain of weakness, inability to squeeze hand when asked, drowsiness, and difficulty with breathing. They may have severe hypotension. Check the height of the block immediately, and do pulse and blood pressure checks frequently. Treatment is supportive; remember A, B, and C. It may need O_2/+ intubation, ventilation, fluids, and ephedrine, atropine and phenylephrine, or adrenaline infusion. Usually wears off quite quickly, but one must be very attentive until stable. Remember to explain to the patient what is going on and that it is treatable. It is a very frightening sensation. A guideline from South Africa's Society of Anaesthesiologists on "Management of high spinal anaesthesia" is cited under "Further readings".

10.4.3 Total Spinal Anaesthesia

Total spinal is a complication when the spinal block is total which means all vertebral segments including the cervical segments and the brain are anaesthetized. The cerebrospinal fluid covers the brain and the spinal cord, and if the concentration and the spread of the drug are complete, the patient would be completely paralysed with the pupils being wide and not reacting to light. The patient would be unconscious and not breathing, and circulation would collapse to extremely low BP and heart rate around 30–35/min. Without adequate and fast treatment, the patient would die quickly from respiratory and cardiac arrest.

Call for help and perform CPR, ventilate with oxygen, and give infusion full speed plus adrenaline infusion titrated to BP > 80.

Total spinal anaesthesia is caused by a massive overdose of local anaesthetic agents. Most often, it is caused when an epidural anaesthesia (EDA) was intended, but accidentally, the local anaesthetic was injected into the subarachnoid space instead of the epidural space. For epidural anaesthesia, the LA dose is more than five times higher than for spinal. epidural anaesthesia (EDA) should normally be performed by specialist anaesthesiologists only or by physicians under the supervision of a specialist. The method is beyond the scope of this book.

The second possible cause for total spinal is by insufficiently trained anaesthesia provider who injects the contents of "one ampoule" or "one vial" instead of knowing the adequate dose. LA drugs are often provided in ampoules at 4–10, sometimes in 20 mL multi-dose vials. If you inject the whole ampoule, you are causing total spinal anaesthesia.

10.4.4 Hypotension and Bradycardia

Low blood pressure immediately after injecting the LA is common. Always get baseline BP before commencement. A volume of 500–1000 mL Ringer's or NS in healthy adults helps. Less common when injecting LA slowly over 10–15 s, titrate ephedrine to effect, 3–6 mg per time. Often the first symptom is nausea, especially in ladies for caesarean section. It is advised to treat if symptomatic or systolic BP < 90 mmHg. Regularly check BP every 2 min over the first 10 min after injection and thereafter every 5 min. Bradycardia: If the heart rate drops, atropine 0.5 mg is usually very effective. Do not wait until the pulse is very low.

10.4.5 Infection

Always use aseptic technique or no technique! Always do a thorough washing of hands, gloves, and mask and a thorough washing of the patient's back before final disinfection. Remember that the disinfectant needs at least 60 s (methylated spirit, chlorhexidine) or 3 min (povidone-iodine) to kill the germs. Therefore, do not dry the back too early. First, perform cleaning, then disinfection, and then prepare the drugs and syringes. Thereby enough time will have elapsed for the disinfectant to be effective. The triad: fever, backache, and neurological symptoms are typical for spinal abscess.

Because of the risk of infection, an open ampoule with LA must not be used for more than 1 day and be kept sterile. Multi-dose vials with a rubber may be used for several days, and the rubber should be disinfected before use. Ampoules should not be left open for longer than a few hours. They can only be used on the same day. In hospitals with low caseloads and large ampoules with LA, you can prepare sterile syringes with proper amounts of LA, e.g. 2–3 mL per syringe. After putting on the face mask, surgical hand washing, and disinfection, use sterile gloves and a sterile table with a sterile cloth, and have an assistant who gives the syringes and needle to you sterile and helps you to draw the LA while keeping sterility. The syringes can be put into a sterile kidney dish and wrapped with a sterile cloth. Label it with the date and contents. Store these sterile syringes in a fridge. You may use them for up to 2 weeks, approximately. When there is plenty of LA stocked, and the costs are not high, the remains of one ampoule should rather be discarded than stored.

10.4.6 Spinal or Epidural Haematoma

Bleeding disorders are a contraindication for spinal anaesthesia. Check if the patient is on anticoagulants and discuss with his responsible physician how long that medication is to be paused. Consider GA instead of spinal. Haematoma near to the spinal cord is a very rare complication but may lead to permanent paralysis of the legs, the urinary bladder sphincter, and the anal sphincter. Treatment is only possible at hospitals with MRI scans and neurosurgery. Even there, the paralysis may last permanently in spite of immediate operation.

Further Reading

Casey WF (2000) Spinal anaesthesia—a practical guide. Update Anesth 12:21–34

Hewson DW, Hardman J. Regional anaesthetic techniques. In: Thompson J, Moppett I, Wiles M. Smith and Aitkenhead's textbook of anaesthesia. 7th. London: Elsevier; 2019:527–557

Kee WDN (1998) Intrathecal pethidine: pharmacology and clinical applications. Anaesth Intensive Care 26(2):137–146

Macfarlane AJR, Hewson DW, Brull R (2023) Spinal, epidural, and caudal anesthesia. In: Pardo MC Jr (ed) Miller's basics of anesthesia, 8th edn. Elsevier, Philadelphia, PA, pp 289–317

van Rensburg G, van Dyk D, Bishop D, Swanevelder JL, Farina Z, Reed AR, Dyer RA (2016) The management of high spinal anaesthesia in obstetrics: suggested clinical guideline in the South African context [this is a guideline published by the south African Society of Anaesthesiologists (SASA) through the efforts and work of the obstetric Anaesthesia special interest society (OASIS), a special interest group of SASA]. South African J Anaesth Analg 22(1(Supplement 1)):S1–S5

11 Obstetric Anaesthesia

Abstract

Anaesthesia for caesarean section: the gold standard is spinal anaesthesia, e.g. with bupivacaine heavy 7.5–10 mg dependent on patient's height. Put a pillow or wedge under the right hip until the neonate is delivered to minimise the supine hypotension syndrome which is caused by the uterus compressing the aorta and v. cava. This potentially life-threatening complication can be mixed up with high or total spinal anaesthesia as symptoms may be similar (severe hypotension, unconsciousness, and hypoventilation). During spinal anaesthesia HR >60 and systolic BP >90 mmHg is required to assure sufficient foetal circulation. Always have atropine and ephedrine, phenylephrine, noradrenaline, or adrenaline (double dilution to 0.01 mg/mL) ready.

General anaesthesia includes increased risk for desaturation, pulmonary aspiration of stomach contents, and difficult airway management. Anaesthetics may cross the placenta and affect the foetus. Diazepam and opioids are contraindicated before delivery. Hypoxia or hypotension of the mother is also affecting the foetus. In resource poor setting ketamine 2 mg/kg plus small increments may be used as sole anaesthetic with spontaneous breathing followed by diazepam after delivery.

Preeclampsia: spinal anaesthesia, if possible, avoid hypertension, consider magnesium, labetalol, hydralazine, nifedipine.

Neonatal resuscitation: Keep the neonate warm and dry. Suction shortly, and if required, perform mask ventilation, but do not intubate if fully equipped intensive care is not available.

Patient with haemorrhagic shock: two venous cannulae, infusion full speed, oxygen, ephedrine, adrenaline 1 mg=1 ampoule into 500 mL NS, drip rate with target SBP >80 mmHg, consider tranexamic acid and blood transfusion.

Keywords

Anaesthesia for caesarean section in resource-limited settings · Anaesthetic management of pre- and postpartum bleeding · Anaesthetic management of ruptured ectopic pregnancy · Neonatal resuscitation in remote health facilities · Physiological changes during pregnancy · Supine hypotension syndrome in pregnancy

11.1 Physiologic Changes During Pregnancy

Alveolar ventilation is increased and the functional residual capacity of the lungs is decreased while the oxygen demand is increased. Therefore, patients are very prone to hypoxaemia during

D. Kietzmann, *Anaesthesia in Remote Hospitals*, Sustainable Development Goals Series,
https://doi.org/10.1007/978-3-031-46610-6_11

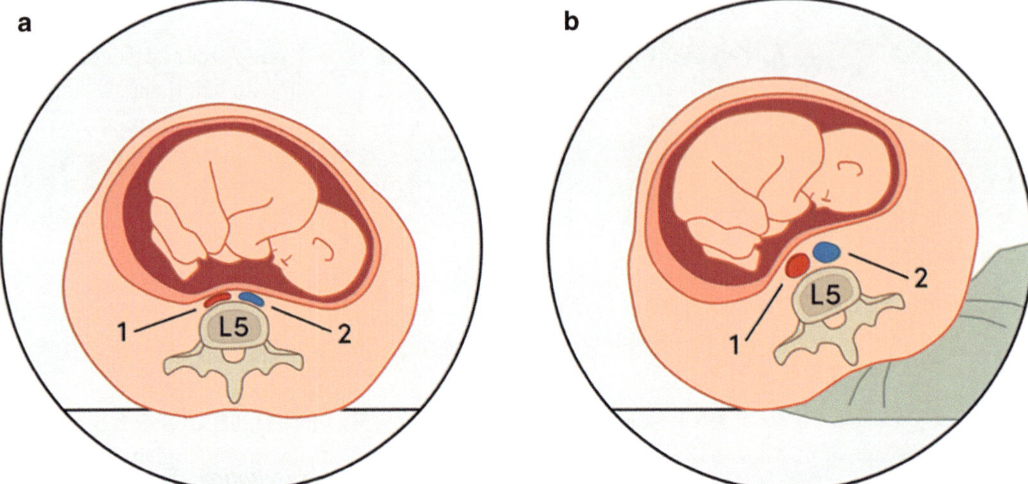

Fig. 11.1 Supine hypotension syndrome which is caused by aortocaval compression as shown in the left figure (**a**) and relief by positioning with a wedge under the right hip in the right figure (**b**)

even short periods of apnoea (e.g. during endotracheal intubation). The cardiac output is increased during pregnancy and especially during labour, and therefore the heart rate is higher and needs to be higher to ensure sufficient cardiac output. Atropine should be given if the heart rate decreases below 70/min during anaesthesia or surgery. Gastro-oesophageal reflux and gastritis are common. Gastric motility is reduced, and the stomach is displaced by the uterus, so the risk for pulmonary aspiration is increased during anaesthesia. Blood coagulability is increased with risk for thrombosis and lung embolism. Blood volume is increased, but Hb level is slightly decreased.

Aortocaval compression from occlusion of the vena cava inferior by the uterus in a supine position can cause the ***supine hypotension syndrome*** with pallor, hypotension, sweating, and nausea. It is caused by the weight of the enlarged uterus compressing the aorta and the vena cava leading to decreased venous return to the heart. In severe cases, unconsciousness and circulatory failure may occur. Therefore, a slight tilting position or left lateral position of the patient is highly recommended. This can be achieved with a tilt of the table of around 15° or with a wedge under the right hip 10–15 cm high as in Fig. 11.1. Even improvisation with a roll of a towel can be helpful.

11.2 Anaesthesia for Caesarean Section

The theatre must be warm. Switch off the air conditioning or adjust it to at least 25 °C. If the neonate becomes hypothermic, there is a great risk for severe respiratory and cardiac depression, especially in the case of asphyxia.

Always have at least one large-bore venous line equipped with an infusion at full speed. Before the induction of any kind of anaesthesia, whether regional or general, and immediately after spinal injection, the mother should be tilted 15° to her left side in order to prevent compression of the vena cava and the uterine vessels, causing the supine hypotensive syndrome (sudden decrease of venous return to the heart and very low BP) which can be life-threatening for both, mother and foetus.

Spinal anaesthesia is worldwide regarded as the first choice of anaesthetic method for elective and acute caesarean section (the latter provided that time allows). GA increases the risk for the mother as difficulty with airway management is more common during pregnancy, and the risk for pulmonary aspiration is increased. However, if the AP is not sufficiently familiar with spinal anaesthesia, GA with ketamine may be the safer choice. Efforts should be made by all health facilities where C/S is performed to have their anaesthesia staff sufficiently trained.

11.2.1 Spinal Anaesthesia

Spinal anaesthesia is preferred, e.g. with bupivacaine 7.5–10 mg (1.5–2 mL of bupivacaine 0.5%) or with lidocaine 5% in dextrose 60–75 mg (1.2–1.5 mL), or with any other suitable local anaesthetic drug. The dose is dependent on body height and on the size of the uterus. Small women need 7.5 mg, while women >160 cm may need 9 mg and > 170 cm 10 mg. Very tall women >175 cm might need 11 mg of bupivacaine. A large uterus increases abdominal pressure and leads to the spread of the LA more cephalad, while the caesarean section in case of a premature or small neonate with a small uterus may need a little higher dose (approximately 0.2 mL more) than stated above to achieve an adequate spread of anaesthesia. If anaesthesia during operation is not complete, ketamine 25–50 mg IV may be injected as a supplement and repeated if required. Immediately after giving the spinal anaesthesia, the patient must be put supine with a tilted pelvis as in Fig. 11.1 and the operation should start as soon as anaesthesia is achieved.

Onset with bupivacaine is 2–4 min, and the duration is 60–120 min; onset with lidocaine is 1–3 min, and the duration is 45–75 min. A hyperbaric anaesthetic (LA with dextrose) is heavier than cerebrospinal fluid and usually produces a better quality of anaesthesia for C/S. Isobaric or plain LA: 0.5 mL larger dose than stated above is needed, but spread of block is more unpredictable, and onset may be delayed.

Contraindications for spinal anaesthesia: Contraindications include severe hypovolaemia, haemorrhagic shock, restless patient who is not cooperative, severe eclampsia with uncontrolled seizures, HELLP (**H**aemolytic anaemia, **E**levated **L**iver enzymes, and **L**ow **P**latelets) syndrome if platelets are below 80,000, anticoagulation with insufficient time elapsed after last dose, any other bleeding disorder, and severe problems of the spine.

11.2.2 General Anaesthesia

During pregnancy, from the second trimester until 48 h after delivery, the risk for aspiration of gastric contents is increased. Therefore, the golden standard for GA is intubation anaesthesia with RSI. However, in a low-resource setting, this is not always the safest method. Consider not performing intubation anaesthesia in the following situations: If the AP is alone and is not familiar with intubation, if intubation is only seldom performed at the health facility, if the equipment is not complete or not functioning (laryngoscope), or if essential drugs are out of stock like suxamethonium or thiopental, ketamine anaesthesia with spontaneous breathing may be the safer alternative. The same applies in a situation with an anticipated not manageable difficult airway.

If available, 30 mL of sodium citrate should be given orally within 30 min before anaesthesia induction to make gastric contents less acidic and less dangerous in case of pulmonary aspiration. Before induction, oxygen should be given over several minutes.

Intubation anaesthesia with rapid sequence induction: Give atropine 0.5 mg, thiopentone 5 mg/kg (250–350) mg plus ketamine 50–75 mg (thiopental 7 mg/kg, max 500 mg, if no ketamine is added), and succinylcholine 50–75 mg; or atropine 0.5 mg, propofol 2.5 mg/kg (125–200 mg) (contraindicated in severe hypovolaemia or shock) plus ketamine 50–75 mg, and succinylcholine 50–75 mg. The addition of ketamine makes the quality of anaesthesia better by providing an excellent analgesic effect for intubation and surgery before the infant is delivered without adding to the risk. Notably, 30–45 s after injection of suxa, the trachea is intubated. Cricoid pressure can be applied (see Chap. 6). If endotracheal intubation fails after two attempts, the patient should gently be ventilated with a face mask in order to improve oxygenation. Then, a laryngeal mask airway (size 3 for 30–50 kg BW and size 4 for >50–60 kg) can be inserted, because this airway device provides better protection from aspiration than the face mask/oropharyngeal airway. After intubation, give halothane 0.5–0.8%, isoflurane 0.7–1.2%, or sevoflurane 1.6–2.0%. Volatile anaesthetics should not be given in higher concentrations than the above-mentioned 0.8–1 MAC (MAC = minimal alveolar concentration for adequate anaesthesia, specific for each volatile anaesthetic agent), because they may lead to uterine relaxation with severe bleeding. Nitrous oxide is rare, but, if available, it may be added at 50–60% concentration, and halothane/isoflurane may be reduced by 50%. Ketamine bolus doses of around 25–50 mg can also be used in combination with halothane/isoflurane. Volatile agents are contraindicated in patients with severe haemorrhage before the bleeding is controlled and the circulation is stable, after which they may be added carefully at 0.5–0.8 MAC (equal to 0.4–0.6% halothane, 0.6–0.9% isoflurane, or 1.1–1.6% of sevoflurane). All other inhalational agents may also be administered as alternative.

Ketamine anaesthesia with spontaneous breathing can be performed without endotracheal intubation, but a laryngoscope and endotracheal tube (ETT) should be ready in case of problems. Drugs for induction: atropine 0.5 mg and ketamine 100 mg (relatively contraindicated in eclampsia, see later in this chapter), after 1 min start of surgery (tell the surgeon). After delivery of the neonate give diazepam 10 mg, and give additional ketamine 50 mg increments when required.

No diazepam, no pethidine or morphine, and no fentanyl before delivery of the neonate, as they may affect the outcome of the neonate by causing respiratory depression and low muscle tone.

Until delivery of the neonate, all patients should receive 100% oxygen. ***Immediately after delivery, oxytocin*** 10 units IV are administered (5 units IV as a slowly injected bolus and 5 units into the infusion) for uterus contraction. Fast injection of oxytocin must be avoided because it may cause marked hypotension, especially in patients with major bleeding or the mother with cardiac disease. In cases of severe bleeding, additional doses of oxytocin may be given up to a maximum of 30 units with an infusion over several hours. Oxytocin potentiates the action of succinylcholine, so that muscle relaxation may last up to 20 min.

Postoperative pain therapy: At the end of the surgery, give diclofenac 50–75 mg IM unless there is ongoing bleeding or renal disease, or pethidine 50–100 mg IM or a combination of both which is more effective and provides excellent analgesia. Alternatively, morphine 5–10 mg SC or tramadol 100 mg IM or pentazocine 30 mg IV/IM/SC may be used. A short infusion of paracetamol (Perfalgan®) 1 g is recommended if available, but, usually, it is not strong enough to be the sole analgesic. Postoperative nausea and vomiting can be treated with promethazine, ondansetrone, or metoclopramide. It is better to give the analgesic before the effects of the spinal or general anaesthesia have worn off as preventive analgesia is more effective.

11.3 Complications of Anaesthesia for Caesarean Section

- Maternal mortality, if caused by anaesthesia, is most often related to hypoxaemia during airway management difficulties.
- Pulmonary aspiration of gastric contents, leading to severe pneumonia, less severe if sodium citrate was given immediately before starting anaesthesia.
- Hypotension is common, most often caused by hypovolaemia (bleeding) or high spinal anaesthesia (avoid too high doses and always have vasoactive drugs ready to inject). A guideline from South Africa's Society of Anaesthesiologists on "Management of high spinal anaesthesia" is cited under "Further readings". However, a sudden marked drop in BP, bradycardia, and unconsciousness may also be caused by the supine hypotension syndrome (aortocaval compression, see above under physiology during pregnancy). Needs immediate action and the help of a second person, if available a second anaes-

thetist. Tilt the table or move the uterus to the left side and speed up the surgery until the infant is delivered which would stop the compression immediately and help circulation to restore. Differential diagnosis: Even a lung embolism can cause severe circulatory collapse and circulatory arrest. Always have adrenaline, oxygen, and, if possible, laryngoscope and ETT available and four hands to work as a team.
- Post-dural-puncture headache.

That is a common complication with thick, reusable spinal needles. The risk is moderate (around 2–5%) with 22 g single-use needles and minimised (but still around 0.5–2%) by a single use of small needle sizes (25 g) with atraumatic tips plus orientating the needle bevel parallel with the axis of the spine. The best type of needle is that with a pencil-point tip (Whitacre or Sprotte) followed by a diamond-shaped Quincke tip. Treatment of headache: Paracetamol and ibuprofen for 3 days, let the patient be lying flat as much as possible without complete immobilisation as that would increase the risk for thrombosis. Around 3 litres of fluid intake per 24 h may be encouraged during the next 3 days. In very severe and prolonged cases, an epidural blood patch may be indicated if skills and equipment are available. That procedure may only be performed by an *experienced* anaesthetist who is skilled in epidural puncture with an epidural Tuohy needle and a special loss of resistance syringe. A second person has to take 20 mL of blood from the patient under sterile conditions which is immediately injected into the epidural space where the Tuohy needle has already been placed. Relief of the headache is usually immediate in around 75–80% of patients. The other patients might need a second blood patch a day later which has again around 75% chance of success. Differential diagnosis: The post-dural puncture headache is more severe in sitting or upright position, while other causes of headache, including severe neurological causes like subarachnoid bleeding or cerebral sinus venous thrombosis, would be worse in the supine position or unaffected by position.

11.4 Anaesthesia in Preeclampsia and Eclampsia

5–8% of all pregnant women suffer from preeclampsia. Symptoms are hypertension with or without proteinuria and peripheral oedema, less than 1% plus congestive heart failure with pulmonary oedema as a possible complication. The foetus is often showing insufficient growth. Preeclampsia begins after gestation week 20 and is considered severe if BP > 160/110. Patients may also suffer from headache, blurred vision, nausea, and dizziness. Treatment is essential, and often the pregnancy must be terminated before completed gestation. Some of these patients get eclampsia (seizures, sometimes even intracerebral bleeding) or HELLP syndrome (**H**aemolytic anaemia, **E**levated **L**iver enzymes, and **L**ow **P**latelets) including coagulation disorders and sometimes severely impaired renal function with oliguria both of which are associated with significant mortality.

The underlying problem is a generalised vasospasm which may affect all organ systems and the foetus (intrauterine growth retardation).

Eclampsia, severe preeclampsia, and HELLP are acute life-threatening for both, mother and child. Perform caesarean section as soon as possible that is as soon as the foetus is mature enough but do not wait if the life of the mother is in acute danger. A dexamethasone or betamethasone dose of 12 mg IM to the mother, if time allows, repeated once after 24 h, reduces the risk of the preterm foetus for developing respiratory distress syndrome and other complications of prematurity. In all cases with coagulation disorders (platelets <80,000) and uncontrolled cramps or seizures, general anaesthesia with rapid sequence induction and endotracheal intubation should be performed instead of spinal anaesthesia. The decision for spinal or GA is not easy as a difficult airway is also often associated with preeclampsia because of swelling due to oedema inside the pharynx. If the AP is not sufficiently trained to perform endotracheal intubation, general anaesthesia with a face mask and spontaneous/gently manually assisted ventilation may be safer. LM airway is an alternative in case of difficult intubation. In all other patients, spinal anaesthesia is the best choice, especially in those with high BP.

Prevent or control seizures: *Magnesium sulphate* 4 g ($MgSO_4$) as fast infusion is the most effective drug. Urine output should be 0.5–1.0 mL/kg/h. (that is approximately 25–70 mL/h), but do not force diuresis with huge amounts of fluids. During C/S, no fluid bolus but only 90 mL/h. (30 drops/min) of NS or RL and replacement of blood loss is given due to the high risk of pulmonary oedema with fast infusions.

Hypertension should be treated with hydralazine IV and/or labetalol, and/or nifedipine. Very severe cases need magnesium infusion of 1 g/h additionally for 24 h.

Coagulation abnormalities should be corrected if possible.

Spinal anaesthesia: If there is no increased risk for coagulation disorder that means if platelets are >80,000, then spinal anaesthesia is the method of choice (either with bupivacaine heavy 7.5–10 mg = 1.5–2 mL, 2–2.5 mL bupivacaine plain, or (if bupivacaine is unavailable) with lidocaine/dextrose 5% 60–75 mg = 1.2–1.5 mL).

Oxygen via a face mask should always be administered at least until the neonate is delivered.

If the blood pressure is still high (>180/90) at 15–20 min after injection of the spinal, hydralazine 5 mg IV is the drug of choice. Hydralazine may be repeated after 20 min if required until a max dose of 25 mg after 80 min is administered. Labetalol in 10 mg increments every 10 min is the second-line treatment of hypertension.

After delivery, oxytocin 10 units are given slowly (risk for severe hypotension), that is over 10 min. If more than 10 units are needed, they must be given with infusion at a rate of max 10 units per hour.

General anaesthesia with endotracheal intubation: Always two persons are needed. Place the mother in a left uterine displacement position (15° tilted position) to avoid occlusion of the vena cava. If blood pressure > 160/90 mmHg, give hydralazine 5 mg IV. Preoxygenation for at least 3 min (ask a second anaesthesia staff or theatre nurse or midwife to hold the face mask with 5 L/min oxygen while you are preparing the anaesthetic). Avoid atropine. Rapid sequence induction with thiopentone (5–7 mg/kg BW which means 250–500 mg) or propofol 2.5 mg/kg (125–250 mg) + succinylcholine 1 mg/kg = 50–100 mg. A smaller dose of thiopentone or propofol is associated with an increased risk for intraoperative awareness. ***Ketamine is relatively contraindicated in preeclampsia and eclampsia.*** If ketamine is the only available anaesthetic, it should be administered in small, titrating bolus doses to avoid extreme hypertension. There is also an increased risk for excessive hypertension due to intubation. According to the rapid sequence intubation (RSI) algorithm, avoid mask ventilation as long as the patient is not getting hypoxic. Immediately after intubation give 0.7% of halothane or 1.0% isoflurane or 1.6% sevoflurane. After delivery of the neonate, 10 mg of morphine, 100 mg of pethidine, or 100 µg of fentanyl IV, or 60% N_2O, is useful for analgesia in combination with halothane <0.7 Vol%, isoflurane <1%, or sevoflurane <1.6%. Even tramadol 100 mg can be used but is less effective than the other opioids. Intraoperative hypertension should be treated with hydralazine as a drug of first choice. Other antihypertensives are also possible, e.g. labetalol.

All of these patients should get two IV lines and Ringer's solution (not too fast, avoid fluid bolus). In spite of hypertension, the intravascular volume is decreased. Expected blood loss during C/S is 500–1000 mL but may be more.

Avoid hypervolaemia as there is a risk for pulmonary oedema, but give enough fluid if BP decreases too much. In very severe preeclampsia, IV volume is not well tolerated and often not necessary as BP remains high in spite of spinal anaesthesia and blood loss. Measure blood pressure every 2 min until it has normalised.

Patients with seizures: In addition to magnesium infusion, thiopentone (2–3 mg/kg) or diazepam are the drugs of choice for the treatment of seizures due to their excellent anticonvulsive effects, but avoid diazepam before the delivery of the neonate (asphyxia). After delivery, oxytocin 10 units are given slowly IV.

Magnesium sulphate is the drug of first choice for all patients with severe preeclampsia and with eclampsia. Magnesium prevents or controls seizures. Side effects are muscle weakness and potentiation of muscle relaxants. However, it has to be given in very high doses: The initial dose is 4 g in 100 mL infusion over approximately 20–30 min, followed by 1 g/h magnesium as an infusion up to 24 h after delivery of the newborn.

Magnesium is usually provided in 20 mL vials containing 50% magnesium sulphate that is 10 g in 20 mL. Each ml is equal to 0.5 g.

The initial dose is 8 mL of magnesium sulphate 50% in 100 mL DNS or 100 mL NS as an infusion with high speed. If 100 mL infusions are unavailable but only 500 mL bottles are in stock, please discard approximately 400 mL from the bottle before adding magnesium to avoid fluid overload. Thereafter, 12 mL magnesium sulphate 50% is administered with 500 mL infusion over approximately 6 h that is slowly with 25–30 drops/min. Thereafter, give 10 mL magnesium sulphate in 400 ml infusion over 5 h.

11.5 Dilatation and Curettage

Short procedures like D&C may be performed with short GA (see Chap. 9). Often, this procedure is performed in the maternity that is remote from the major operation theatre. Be sure you have all resuscitation equipment at hand including drugs, infusions, oxygen, self-inflating bag, and suction device. Use monitoring at least with pulse oximetry and BP control. Be prepared if the patient is bleeding significantly and call for help if necessary.

11.6 Pre- or Postpartum Bleeding, Major Bleeding During Caesarean Section, and Ruptured Ectopic Pregnancy

Blood loss during labour and caesarean section can be very high. In case of estimated blood loss of >1 L, give infusions at full speed, uninterrupted even while the patient is waiting on a stretcher. This is absolutely essential and must be continued until the patient is stable and the bleeding is stopped. It is very important that the midwife assesses the amount of blood loss continuously and applies abdominal pressure or uterine massage to reduce bleeding and not to wait until circulatory shock is established. Tachycardia with normal blood pressure but increased capillary refill time > 2 s usually means blood loss between 1000 and 1500 mL. *Low BP is a late sign during bleeding.* In other words: A woman who is showing tachycardia, fast breathing, *and* low blood pressure or decreased level of consciousness has often lost more than 50% of her blood volume, that is more than 1500–2000 mL, and must be treated very urgently (compare Sect. 15.2.2).

If ***tranexamic acid (TXA)*** 100 mg/ml is available, give 1 g (equivalent to one or two ampoules) slowly IV over 10 min. A second and last dose of 1 g over 10 min is given if the bleeding has not stopped 30 min after the first dose. TXA must be given early during bleeding, within 3 h after childbirth or 3 h after onset of bleeding, as the benefit is only seen after early administration.

Theoretically, around 3 L of RL or NS is needed to replace the loss of 1 L of blood, because crystalloids are distributed in the blood volume plus interstitial space, leaving only one-third of them within the circulating blood volume. However, it is not recommended to give many litres of crystalloids, because of the risk of lung and peripheral oedema and dilution coagulopathy. If available, 0.5–1 L of colloid infusions, so-called plasma expanders (e.g. HES and albumin), should be given additionally to NS/RL or similar. If bleeding exceeds around 1.5–2 L, or Hb decreases below approximately 7–8 g/dL, erythrocyte concentrates (packed red blood cells or PRBC) and fresh frozen plasma, or fresh whole blood should be transfused, as one unit of them would replace the same volume of blood.

Most important: Stop the bleeding! Immediate surgical intervention is necessary to be started *before* or while stabilising the patient. *Do not wait for surgery*. During surgery, direct aortic compression against the spine by the surgical assistant may be lifesaving until the source of bleeding is stopped. In very severe cases, bilateral ligation of the uterine artery or even hysterectomy may be required.

If ephedrine or phenylephrine is available, it is useful in cases where, in spite of volume administration, BP is <80–90 mmHg; dose for ephedrine 3–6 mg IV, phenylephrine 0.05–0.1 mg, may be repeated every 5 min. Alternatively, if those drugs are unavailable or ineffective: 1 mg = 1 mL adrenaline in 1 L of NS or 0.5 mg = 0.5 mL adrenaline in 500 mL NS, or 0.2 mg in 200 mL NS, let drip through a second venous line or via a three-way connector together with the other infusion at 20–200 drops/min. Or draw from this dilution of adrenaline into a 10-mL syringe and inject increments of 3–10 mL every 3 min until BP is stable. Measure BP every 2–3 min and aim for systolic BP of 80–100 mmHg and HR of 80–140/min. You need at least four hands to keep up with that.

Fast and systematic actions are key to preventing a mother from losing her life under such complications. Have briefings with your team and simulate such scenarios regularly. Establish a clear plan for how to act in such emergency situations. Keep regular contact with the lab and establish a plan for fast availability of blood products in emergency. If the blood bank is reporting lack of units with certain blood groups, identify walking donors and always have a plan to obtain fresh whole blood for such emergency patients.

The above-mentioned conditions are life-threatening emergency situations where the time window is small to save the patient. Call for help to form a team of at least two APs. You need four hands. Insert one to two large-bore venous cannulae and give RL/NS full speed. Give 5 L/min 100% oxygen. Check ABC = airway, breathing, and circulation (vital signs monitored with pulse oximetry, ECG, and NIBP). A pulse oximeter might not show anything in case fingers are cold and peripheral perfusion poor. Try to perform a massage of a finger to get it warmer for SPO_2 monitoring. Use ECG if available. If not available, use a precordial stethoscope. Measure blood pressure every 1–2 min. Record the vital signs on a record form every 5 min. A warm blanket helps keep the patient warm. If possible, use warm (37–43 °C) infusions. Switch off the AC and have the theatre warm. Low body temperature is not just unpleasant but increases the risk for platelet dysfunction (more bleeding) and impairs wound healing. Have two anaesthesia staff (if unavailable, one anaesthesia staff and one theatre staff or another nurse), two large bore venous cannulae, no spinal anaesthesia but light general anaesthesia with 100 mg ketamine/ketamine drip (500 mg ketamine into 500 mL infusion, drip rate 20–100 drops/min) and spontaneous breathing or intubation (intubation is highly recommended if the patient is unconscious and does not keep a patent airway or is not breathing sufficiently). If intubation is indicated but impossible to perform, use an oropharyngeal (Guedel) or nasopharyngeal airway and a face mask with oxygen. When vital signs are better that means BP is recordable and a peripheral pulse is palpable, a combination with 0.5 MAC volatile anaesthetic or diazepam or midazolam is possible to assure amnesia. Muscle relaxation is not necessary (only for intubation) and can add to the high perioperative risk for the patient, but some surgeons need to be convinced that they can perform without it. If they do insist on muscle relaxation, use only small doses (0.2–0.5 mg/kg) of suxamethonium instead of long-acting MR, and give atropine before the first dose to avoid bradycardia.

Brief summary: Call for help, administer RL or NS at full speed, provide oxygen, use plasma expander if available, Perform a cross-match and blood transfusion if Hb level is low, and use vasoconstrictor drugs if systolic BP is still <80. If surgery is indicated, this must be started without delay which is simultaneously with the resuscitation. Use ketamine for anaesthesia in patients with major bleeding. If time does not allow waiting for a cross-match, give blood that is ABO and Rh compatible or 0-Rh negative red blood cells and AB plasma which are compatible with anyone.

Postoperatively, intermediate care or prolonged stay in the postoperative recovery room is necessary. An observation room in the maternity can also be adequate for intermediate care with vital signs monitoring including pulse rate, BP, and urinary output. Carefully recorded observation chart every hour and oxygen 2–4 L/min is needed for the next 24 h. Acute kidney failure may develop as a complication after circulatory shock. Have a urinary catheter inserted and record output until a stable urinary output is established.

11.7 Neonatal Resuscitation

11.7.1 Equipment

- A resuscitation table, if possible with a radiant heater and a clock
- Warm towels and cloth
- Plastic bag or plastic wrapping for small preterm babies
- Smallest size of self-inflating bellows and face mask
- Optional small Guedel airways, LMA size 1
- Suction device, can be a bulb sucker
- Stethoscope and pulse oximeter
- Record form and a pen
- Optional: oxygen and CPAP
- Resuscitation drugs (see below), syringes, and needles
- Optional that is if a skilled person is available to use it: umbilical vein catheters
- Optional that is if a highly equipped NICU and team of paediatricians are available: laryngoscope and ETT

11.7.2 Procedure: Temperature, Airway, and Breathing

Little delayed cord clamping lets neonates earlier get normal oxygen saturation and improves initial outcome. Keep the environment as warm as possible for the neonate. Switch off the AC and have towels and a warming blanket ready. If possible, use a radiant heat source. Low body temperature would suppress respiratory drive and keep the foetal circulation remaining with cyanosis due to shunts between venous and arterial blood – therefore body temperature below 35° must be avoided, and temperature > 36° must be the goal. Moist skin means temperature drops 20 times faster than with dry skin. For very small preterm infants, food-grade plastic wrapping, if available, may be used, alternatively a clean, clear plastic bag with the face exposed plus a blanket. Before wrapping them in plastic, they should be rubbed and dried quickly as all neonates have to be. That stimulation usually lets the infant start crying. Assess APGAR score (see Table 11.1). Gently suck nostrils and mouth, preferably with a bulb sucker. Do not apply suction longer than necessary. Check the following while having the infant in a warm dry blanket: skin colour central and peripheral, regular breathing with crying or irregular breathing or no breathing, heart rate (stethoscope) above 100 or below or absent, spontaneous movements or movement under stimulation or no movement at all, reflexes, and muscle tone. Calculate the APGAR score from these findings and record them 1, 5, and 10 min after delivery according to Table 11.1. Perform mask ventilation with a self-inflating bag if respiration is absent or weak or the skin colour remains bluish after 2 min. Start with five inflation breaths which last 2–3 s with a pressure of about 20–25 cm H_2O. Reassess the infant: The inflation breaths should lead to increased heart rate and the infant should start breathing. If the infant is yet not breathing, continue ventilation at 30–40 per min with normal

Table 11.1 With the APGAR score, a newborn is assessed at 1, 5, and 10 min after cord clamping. The score of each row is added to make a sum of 0–10. It is also a means to assess the response to resuscitation

APGAR score	Score 0	Score 1	Score 2
Skin colour	Whole body blue or pale	Peripherally blue, centrally pink	Pink
Respiration	None	Irregular, weak, no crying	Regular and crying
Heart rate	None	<100/min	100/min
Muscle tone	Limp, floppy	Flexion only	Active motion
Reflexes	None	Grimace	Cry or active withdrawal

pressure that is gently. If available and the infant is not looking well, use a pulse oximeter. SpO_2 should rise from around 60% to >85% within a few minutes. Saturation does not need to become higher than 95%. Notably, 85–95% is regarded as normal for neonates and especially preterm babies. If resuscitation is needed, usually ventilation with air will do. Oxygen is often not adding benefit initially but may be needed later if the newborn is not improving or suffering from respiratory distress syndrome. Avoid using high concentrations of oxygen when not needed, especially in preterm infants as oxygen may lead to serious complications such as retinopathy with impaired ability to see. Intubation of the trachea is hardly adding any advantage but may cause serious complications. Mask ventilation is sufficient; alternatively, consider LMA size 1 if the newborn is greater than 2 kg. If the heart rate remains <60, start heart compressions.

11.7.3 Chest Compressions and Drugs

If the heart rate remains below 60/min although sufficient ventilation is performed, adrenaline may be given. Give 10 µg/kg IV every 3 min until improvement occurs or cessation of all efforts is decided. Dilute adrenaline 1 mg/mL with 9 mL NS to make 0.1 mg/mL = 100 µg/mL. Give 0.1–0.3 mL of that dilution or 1–3 mL of double dilution (1 mL of 0.1 mg/mL +9 mL NS = 0.01 mg/mL). Perform chest compressions around 100/min using only your thumbs over the sternum with your fingers supporting the back of the infant while ventilation is continued. If the infant does not respond to adrenaline within 10 min, consider sodium bicarbonate 1–2 mmol/kg IV. The sodium bicarbonate should be 4.2%, not more concentrated, and it should be given slowly, over 30 min. However, sodium bicarbonate is optional as the use of it is nowadays controversial. If no improvement is seen, consider one bolus of 2.5 mL/kg dextrose 10% or, if only 5% dextrose is available, inject 5 mL/kg of dextrose 5%. Even a fluid bolus of 30 ml of RL or NS slowly IV can be helpful (small premature newborns 20 mL). Try to obtain a blood sugar measurement and aim for normal values.

The APGAR score should be >6 at 1 min after birth, and 7–10 at 5 resp. Ten minutes If the score is below 7, it means resuscitation is needed, and below 3 means severe birth asphyxia. A score < 3 at 10 min means a poor outcome is likely.

While many anaesthetists like to intubate a neonate who is not breathing, it is not recommended in a remote place where no option exists for putting premature infants on a ventilator in a fully equipped neonatal intensive care unit with the specialist paediatrician. Most newborns can easily be ventilated via a face mask, sometimes facilitated by a small oropharyngeal airway. If ventilation is necessary for longer than 10 min, I recommend using a laryngeal mask size 1 provided that the infant's weight is more than approximately 2 kg. Very small infants should be mask ventilated with the smallest available mask for no longer than 30–45 min while making sure to keep them warm (overhead radiator, or warming lamp and warm ambient temperature and dry clothes). The stomach may be suctioned to avoid distension by air from ventilation. Use the smallest available self-inflating bellows and avoid overinflating the infant's lungs. Small tidal volumes are best (around 7 ml/kg). LM airway is easy to insert, and when the infant is starting to breathe himself, it does not add to respiratory resistance while it is difficult to breathe through a small ETT. Intubation of neonates is not easy, and the tube may dislocate so that only one lung or the oesophagus is inflated. A laryngeal mask would hardly be in the wrong position and is a simpler and easier-to-use device. Even if the infant is successfully intubated, what is the plan thereafter if you are in a remote hospital? When do you want to extubate the patient and how should he/she be ventilated? In all settings where referral to a fully equipped neonatal intensive care unit is unrealistic, attempts for artificial ventilation should be limited below 1 h maximum while making sure that a normal body temperature is achieved.

Resuscitation should be stopped if no signs of life can be observed after 10 min. If the mother wishes, she should be given the dead body to hold it. If APGAR remains below 3 for more than 20 min, cessation of resuscitation may be considered. Make the decision in the team, not alone. If resuscitation is successful, the newborn needs further observation. Use a pulse oximeter and assess the breathing regularly. Some of these infants may need CPAP. Measure blood glucose and keep it normal. If possible, start breastfeeding within the first hour. The infant should be in skin contact with the mother as soon as possible. Babies who cannot suck may need nasogastric feeding or IV dextrose.

Bubble CPAP devices for infants are quite common in many hospitals. They are very useful and can be lifesaving for neonates with difficulty breathing or RDS (respiratory distress syndrome). They can even be homemade with materials that are available at any health facility around the world, provided that you have a functioning oxygen source.

A useful training video on "the demonstration of bubble CPAP for the low resource environment" is freely available at https://www.youtube.com/watch?v=rjmdNspYoy4.

Further Reading

American Society of Anesthesiologists Task Force on Obstetric Anesthesia (2016) Practice guidelines for obstetric anesthesia: an updated report by the American Society of Anesthesiologists Task Force on Obstetric Anesthesia and the Society for Obstetric Anesthesia and perinatology. Anesthesiology 124:270–300

Clyburn P, Collis R, Harries S (2010) Obstetric anaesthesia for developing countries. Oxford, Oxford University Press

Collis R, Harries S, Theron A (2020) Obstetric anaesthesia, 2nd edn. Oxford University Press, Oxford

Samikura H, Inada E (2019) General anaesthesia for elective caesarean section in resource-limited settings. Update in anaesthesia WFSA. J World Fed Soc Anaesth 39:14. https://doi.org/10.1029/WFSA-D-18-00032

van Rensburg G, van Dyk D, Bishop D, Swanevelder JL, Farina Z, Reed AR, Dyer RA (2016) The management of high spinal anaesthesia in obstetrics: suggested clinical guideline in the south African context [this is a guideline published by the south African Society of Anaesthesiologists (SASA) through the efforts and work of the obstetric Anaesthesia special interest society (OASIS), a special interest group of SASA]. South Afr Anaesth Analg 22(1(Supplement 1)):S1–S5

12 Anaesthesia for Major Abdominal Surgery

Abstract

This chapter is about anaesthesia for elective and emergency abdominal surgery and for laparoscopic procedures. Laparotomy is among the commonest types of major surgery. Patients present often late as emergency with peritonitis, bowel obstruction, intestinal perforation, acute appendicitis, obstructed inguinal hernia, perforated peptic ulcer, or other diagnoses.

Preoperative assessment of vital signs, heart and lung sounds, and some lab checks are mandatory. Consider urine catheter, nasogastric tube, preoperative IV fluids such as Ringer's Lactate with goal SBP >90 mmHg and urine output 0.5 ml/kg.

Anaesthesia should be performed by a team of at least two anaesthesia providers. Elective lower abdominal surgery can be performed with spinal anaesthesia, e.g. with 12.5–15 mg bupivacaine heavy. Emergency operations are performed with general anaesthesia, preferably with rapid sequence induction and endotracheal intubation followed by balanced anaesthesia with a volatile anaesthetic like halothane/isoflurane and a strong analgesic like ketamine/fentanyl plus muscle relaxant like suxamethonium (succinylcholine)/atracurium/pancuronium. Emergency drugs, such as ephedrine, atropine, and adrenaline, must be prepared. Oxygen and suction device are mandatory if available. If anaesthesia cannot be performed with intubation, or if oxygen or functioning suction machine is not available, consider transfer to a better equipped health facility. Longer acting muscle relaxants like atracurium or pancuronium should be used with caution. Always reverse effects at the end of surgery with neostigmine or similar and consider delayed extubation, because patients after major abdominal surgery are prone to respiratory problems and aspiration.

Keywords

Anaesthesia for abdominal surgery · Abdominal surgery and muscle relaxation · Intubation without neuromuscular blocking agent · Anaesthesia for emergency laparotomy · Anaesthesia for laparoscopic surgery in resource-limited settings

12.1 General Considerations

Laparotomies are among the most common types of surgery. Elective patients may present with a history of gall bladder stones, colon cancer, enlarged spleen for splenectomy, or for gynaecological procedures such as abdominal hysterectomy or removal of ovarian cyst, only to mention some. Emergency laparotomy is often performed due to acute appendicitis, obstructed inguinal

D. Kietzmann, *Anaesthesia in Remote Hospitals*, Sustainable Development Goals Series,
https://doi.org/10.1007/978-3-031-46610-6_12

hernia, peritonitis, intestinal perforation, bowel obstruction, perforated gastric ulcer, obstructive jaundice, or abdominal trauma (see Chap. 13).

Even with patients accessing the hospital without delay, more than 50% of complications after major emergency abdominal surgery are common and the mortality rate is high even in high-resource hospitals. Late presentation with impaired general condition is not rare and associated with a higher rate of complications, e.g. impaired haemodynamics and acute kidney failure caused by dehydration, respiratory failure, or pneumonia postoperatively, sepsis, and very high mortality. Sometimes the diagnosis is not clear before surgery, especially if an ultrasound or CT scan is unavailable.

Preoperative examination, at least briefly, must be performed even in emergency cases. Take BP, pulse rate, and SpO_2. Listen to the heart and lungs and check capillary refill time (CRT) which should be <2 s. Assess nutritional state, check for signs of dehydration, and ask the patient when he/she could eat and drink last time without vomiting. Look for signs of anaemia or jaundice. Ask for chronic disease and medication, drug allergies, and problems related to previous operations with anaesthesia. Check airway anatomy. Inform the patient about the planned anaesthesia and get consent.

Consider nasogastric tube (NGT) and gastric decompression in patients with distended abdomen or a history of repeated vomiting. A urine catheter should be placed before starting surgery unless the patient is in good general condition for elective surgery, and the expected duration of operation is <1.5 h. How is the urine looking? Concentrated or diluted, yellowish or brownish? Prolonged CRT is a predictor for cardiac failure after anaesthesia induction. Have ephedrine and adrenaline or other inotropic drugs ready.

Preoperative IV Fluids Establish venous access; give IV fluids and carefully record the amount and time of infusion. Severe dehydration over several days must not be compensated too fast because of the risk for lung oedema, swollen tissues, and peripheral oedema. Around 1–2 l handwarm NS or RL can be infused quickly in adults with dehydration, followed by around 100–200 ml/h plus replacement of new losses. The goal is a systolic blood pressure >90 mmHg and urine output >0.5 ml/kg/h. *All sick patients scheduled for laparotomy need a urinary catheter inserted and urine output recorded.* The ward must record infusions administered and provide anaesthetist with information about fluid balance. How many litres of infusion was given? Did the patient pass urine and how much? Was there vomiting, diarrhoea, excessive sweating, or any other loss of fluids?

Goal-Directed IV Fluid Therapy in the Operation Theatre and Postoperatively Intravenous fluids are used to restore and replace fluid loss during major surgery. Uncontrolled fluid administration which is exceeding the losses by far is not uncommon and does more harm than good. Too much fluid produces oedema, tissue inflammation, impaired wound healing, and impaired lung function with lung oedema or pneumonia and promotes anastomosis leakage. Too restrictive fluid administration may cause diminished cardiac output with poor organ blood flow and poor wound healing and increases the risk for kidney failure markedly.

During laparotomy, around 200 ml/h is needed to replace losses from evaporation plus infusions to replace losses from bleeding or fluids drained from the abdomen.

Postoperatively, 2–3 l fluid intake per day in adults without high fever is often adequate. A zero balance should be aimed for, which means the amount of fluid intake by infusion or, if allowed by the surgeon, by mouth or NGT should be the same as the output by urine, losses from drainage tubes, NGT, or sweating. Ideally, the patient's body weight would be measured daily to see if the balance is zero, negative, or positive. Standard haemodynamic parameters such as BP, pulse rate, and even central venous pressure do not reflect the volume state of a patient. If weighing scales for bed-ridden patients are unavailable, use a measuring tape and record lower leg circumference and waist circumference daily. Mark the site at which the measurement is taken.

12.1.1 Body Temperature

During abdominal surgery, patients' temperature can drop markedly, especially in OR with AC. Body temperature regulation is not working during anaesthesia. Increase room temperature above 22°C, use warm infusions, and cover all parts of the body which are not exposed for surgery with cloth/blankets. Body temperature can decrease to 33–34°C (91–93°F) if no measures are taken to keep patients warm. It is very unpleasant for the patients to suffer from shivering during recovery. Tachycardia and raised oxygen consumption due to shivering can be dangerous in patients with cardiac disease. Hypothermia also increases the risk of infection and bleeding due to impaired function of the immune system and platelet dysfunction.

12.1.2 Spinal Anaesthesia

Spinal anaesthesia is the first choice for elective lower abdominal surgery. Consider spinal anaesthesia for abdominal surgery always if oxygen, essential drugs for GA, or essential equipment are unavailable, or if mains electricity is unstable. However, spinal anaesthesia is only safe for patients who are not dehydrated, have no fever, are not bleeding, and are showing a fair general condition. For spinal anaesthesia, use the same monitoring as for general anaesthesia that is BP, pulse oximetry, and, if available, ECG, and have drugs and equipment at hand for conversion to GA if necessary.

For upper abdominal surgery, a spinal block needs to be higher than for lower abdominal surgery. Before giving the spinal, have atropine, ephedrine, and adrenaline ready and preload with 500 ml RL or NS. One to two pillows under the head and neck help avoid spreading above the level of thoracic 4 (Th4). A sensory block up to Th4 is optimal (for patients <160 cm 2.5 ml bupivacaine heavy, for patients >160 cm, 3 ml bupivacaine heavy, and for patients >180 cm, 3.5 ml bupivacaine heavy). Old patients require 0.5 ml lower doses. If bupivacaine heavy is unavailable, consider bupivacaine plain (0.5 ml more than with heavy LA that is 3–4 ml dependent on patient height and age) or give 75–100 mg pethidine (diluted with 2 ml NS in tall patients). Check the spread of the block and BP every 2 min and tilt the patient with head up if the block is spreading too high. See Chap. 10 for details. The surgeon should be experienced and perform the operation rather quickly. A delay between the onset of the spinal anaesthesia and starting operation is to be avoided due to the limited duration of action of spinal anaesthesia. If the spinal is wearing off before the end of surgery and the peritoneum is already closed, add small doses of ketamine plus a sedative drug such as diazepam, midazolam, or chlorpromazine. If the spinal is wearing off in the middle of the operation, ask the surgeon to pause shortly until intubation anaesthesia is established. Continue with GA.

12.1.3 Balanced Anaesthesia

GA for abdominal/gynaecological surgery is best performed as balanced anaesthesia which is a combination of IV hypnotics, analgesics, and muscle relaxant agents with inhalation anaesthetics. For details, see Chap. 8. The advantage of balanced anaesthesia is minimised side effects by reducing the doses for each component of anaesthesia while optimising the desired effects. Be careful not to overdose long-acting MR or opioids and consider delayed extubation if the patient is not fully awake and has recovered to full muscle strength after the end of surgery. For intraoperative analgesia, ketamine bolus doses of 25–50 mg for adults can be administered several times plus a maximum of one single dose of an opioid if early extubation is planned and the patient is not scheduled for transfer to the intensive care unit. As a rule of thumb, only a single dose of longer-acting muscle relaxant or, even safer, only one to several doses of suxamethonium without long-acting MR should be administered. At the end of the surgery, longer-acting

MR such as atracurium or pancuronium should always be antagonised with atropine (or glycopyrrolate) and neostigmine. Postoperative analgesia should be initiated in theatre to avoid patients experiencing severe pain when fully awake.

12.1.4 How to Perform Anaesthesia for Abdominal Surgery if Muscle Relaxants Are Out of Stock

Make all efforts always to have a stock of suxamethonium and, in referral hospitals, additionally, a stock of a longer-acting non-depolarising muscle relaxant plus reversal agents. However, as the unavailability of essential drugs is a common problem, you need a plan B. Please find several versions of such a "plan B" here: All the methods described below require an experienced and skilled AP. Consider referral of the patient if anaesthesia is likely not to be performed in a safe way. In acute cases consider placing an NGT preoperatively (awake) and aim for suction to get an empty stomach before anaesthesia and surgery.

12.1.5 Intravenous Induction and Intubation Without Neuromuscular Blocking Agent

Use a timer (clock, watch, or mobile phone). Induction drugs: Ketamine has no muscle relaxant properties, while thiopentone and propofol provide some relaxation. A higher dose of propofol of 2.5–4 mg/kg would enable intubation without any neuromuscular blocking agent.

Propofol provides good intubation conditions due to sufficient muscle relaxing effect via its central nervous action. Preoxygenate for 3 min and give a sedative drug like 2.5–5 mg diazepam or 2 mg midazolam plus an analgesic like 50 mg ketamine or 0.05–0.1 mg fentanyl. Then inject propofol 2–4 mg/kg dependent on the age of the patient (the younger the patient, the higher the dose of propofol up to the maximum of 4 mg/kg). Perform gentle mask ventilation; use a Guedel tube if necessary; 90 s after propofol injection, you will find good conditions for endotracheal intubation. Measure BP shortly after intubation. Propofol can cause hypotension, especially in the elderly.

If propofol is unavailable, use thiopentone 5–7 mg/kg, and after 60 s, you may intubate.

If both propofol and thiopentone are unavailable, a combination of 5–10 mg diazepam (which has some muscle relaxing effect), 50 mg chlorpromazine, and 50–100 mg pethidine can be given while the patient is preoxygenated. With these three drugs, the muscle tone is significantly reduced. After around 5 min, 2 mg/kg ketamine is injected. One to two min later, the patient can be intubated. For maintenance of anaesthesia, either a ketamine drip or inhalational anaesthesia with 0.7–1 MAC can be used. After that combination of IV sedative drugs, requirements for maintenance doses of anaesthetics during surgery will be significantly reduced. If pethidine is unavailable, a single dose of morphine, tramadol, or another opioid drug can be used. If no opioid drugs are available, subsequent doses of ketamine 25–50 mg IV will be needed during surgery if maintenance of GA is with an inhalational anaesthetic. Emergence and recovery may be prolonged, but conditions for surgery will be appropriate.

12.1.6 Inhalational Induction and Intubation Without Neuromuscular Blocking Agent

Another method is inhalational induction. If the patient is afraid to inhale a volatile anaesthetic, premedication with diazepam or midazolam should be performed. Apply halothane or sevoflurane (but not isoflurane) via a tight-fitting face mask and increase the concentration at the vaporiser every three breaths until 2.5% for halothane or 6% for sevoflurane is achieved. Give atropine 0.5 mg IV (or 0.01 mg/kg). Let the patient breathe spontaneously until unconsciousness is achieved and the pupils are getting smaller. Halothane needs around 15–20 min until anaesthesia is deep enough for endotracheal intubation. Sevoflurane needs approximately 5–10 min. Always check the pupils. They get enlarged when patients lose consciousness, and they get small again when anaesthesia is deep enough. Never intubate in light inhalational anaesthesia as that might cause a laryngospasm which is difficult to break if you do not have muscle relaxant drugs like suxamethonium. Lidocaine is usually available. Notably, 1 mg/kg of lidocaine IV may also help prevent laryngospasm on intubation. Intubation conditions are better if you add a strong analgesic like 50 mg ketamine or 0.05 mg fentanyl.

12.1.7 Intubation Without Succinylcholine but with a Non-depolarising Muscle Relaxant

This method is only appropriate for experienced anaesthetists who are sure to be able to ventilate the patient via a secured airway. Long-acting MR instead of suxamethonium may be used for intubation if suxamethonium is O/S or contraindicated *and* the AP is experienced to handle even difficult airways safely. Intubation can be facilitated with 4 mg pancuronium (or 0.05–0.1 mg/kg), or with 35 mg (0.5 mg/kg) atracurium or 40 mg (0.6 mg/kg) rocuronium or any other MR that is available. Time to onset is a bit longer than with suxamethonium, around 2 min. Deep anaesthesia would enable intubation earlier than light anaesthesia where a higher dose of MR is required. At the end of surgery, give reversal drugs for MR, e.g. atropine 0.5 mg and neostigmine 2.5 mg unless more than 120 min has elapsed since administration of MR and the patient has obviously regained normal muscle strength (can open the eyes and lift the head). If in doubt, better perform reversal!

12.1.8 Postoperative Care

Patients after major abdominal surgery, especially after upper abdominal surgery, are prone to suffer from respiratory problems and may get pneumonia. This is partly due to pain-related superficial breathing, but also muscles have been cut and make sufficient excursions of breathing and coughing difficult. Oxygen via nasal prongs or mask may be required for a prolonged time of >24 h or until the patient is active and moving. Good pain treatment and encouragement to early mobilisation and sitting in bed rather than lying flat are vital. Exercise should be encouraged. A good tool is letting the patient blow into a home-made PEP (positive expiratory pressure) device consisting of an endotracheal tube size 8 with a powder-free disposable glove attached with adhesive tape, the "blow glove".

12.2 Elective Laparotomy

Typical operations are abdominal hysterectomy, ovarian cyst removal, and open cholecystectomy for removal of gall bladder stones, hemicolectomy, sigma or rectum resection for treatment of colon cancer, splenectomy, nephrectomy, and pancreas cyst removal.

Gynaecological laparotomy can often be performed with spinal anaesthesia. However, that is dependent on the anticipated duration of surgery, so some of these patients are operated on with intubation anaesthesia.

Ketamine anaesthesia with spontaneous breathing is not favourable for major laparotomy as surgery is difficult without some muscle relaxation, and breathing may be difficult during an operation inside the abdomen. Both spinal and intubation anaesthesia with inhalational anaesthetics provide a better quality of anaesthesia and better conditions for surgery. A slightly ramped position before intubation and extubation, if possible, would help the diaphragm into a better position and increase functional lung capacity.

The IV access must be well-secured and well-functioning. Attach full monitoring: BP cuff, pulse oximeter (or precordial stethoscope), and ECG if available, and after intubation, use capnography if available. ECG is used with jelly or moist cotton wool as improvised electrodes if disposable electrodes are O/S. Electricity must be stable (generator working) and the oxygen source must be sufficient. IV antibiotics are given before anaesthesia induction according to the surgeon's prescription. Induction is performed followed by endotracheal intubation. Have an assistant and have all the equipment for difficult airways at hand. Ventilation should be assisted or controlled as spontaneous breathing is likely to be insufficient (or impossible if muscle relaxants are used) in anaesthetised patients for laparotomy. If available, use a PEEP of 5 cm H_2O which helps prevent atelectasis.

Good intraoperative analgesia with ketamine intermittently and preventive postoperative analgesia with opioid and non-opioid combined before the patient wakes up are recommended. Muscle relaxation can be performed with 1 mg/kg of suxamethonium for intubation plus 0.5 mg/kg suxamethonium before skin incision, before inserting retractors, and before closing the peritoneum plus when required. The total dose of suxamethonium should not be more than 200–300 mg in adults. Atropine 0.5 mg would reverse bradycardia which can be a side effect of suxamethonium. This approach is usually safer than to use pancuronium or atracurium. Deep anaesthesia is required during the opening and closing of the peritoneum and inserting retractors or flushing of the abdominal cavity with warm saline. During suturing bowels, e.g. for creating anastomosis, anaesthesia can be lighter. The AP should observe the surgical field constantly and adapt anaesthesia accordingly.

Fluid requirements are dependent on the preoperative volume state of the patient. As a rule of thumb in adults, a total amount of around 2 l of RL during a 1–2 h laparotomy is needed plus replacement of blood loss.

Postoperatively, all patients must be observed for a while before being sent to the peripheral ward. Make sure that the patient is oxygenating well even, for short periods, without adding oxygen, and that no residual paralysis is present. Vital signs should be stable before transferring the patient.

12.3 Emergency Laparotomy

12.3.1 Patients with Acute Abdomen: Presentation and Pathophysiology

While the causes of acute abdomen are many, the patients have quite similar pathophysiology and clinical symptoms in common: sudden onset of abdominal pain often associated with nausea, vomiting, bloody stools or no stools, and sick appearance. Pain may be deep, dull, and poorly localised as caused by inflammation or ischaemia, colic pain caused by smooth muscle contraction, or both. Retroperitoneal causes of acute abdomen are often leading to sudden, severe back pain (e.g. pancreatitis or rupture of aortic aneurysm). The abdomen may be distended, and bowel sounds may be absent. A blood sample often shows elevated white blood cell count, patients may have fever, and urinary output may be decreased with risk for acute kidney failure. If history is prolonged over several days, patients get increasingly sick, dehydrated, and, finally, shocked from dehydration or sepsis. Abdominal X-ray may show multiple air-fluid levels in patients with ileus. Free air in the abdominal cavity indicates perforation of the stomach or the small or large intestine. Ileus can be caused by mechanical obstruction or by bowel paralysis. Syncope and shock associated with sudden onset of abdominal pain or back pain are typical for ruptured ectopic pregnancy or aortic aneurysm. While open cholecystectomy is most often elective, explorative laparotomy for obstructive jaundice is an emergency even if the case is planned as the patient is acutely sick. Treat with antibiotics and IV fluids prior to surgery if the patient is febrile. Patients should be circulatory stable and produce urine before surgery; otherwise, perioperative mortality would be very high. Stabilisation should not need more than a few hours as delayed surgery for acute abdominal problems also increases mortality. The patient who is bleeding needs to be operated on as soon as possible without waiting for stabilisation. The risk for hypoxia during anaesthesia induction is always increased in patients for emergence laparotomy.

12.3.2 Common Causes for Acute Abdomen Requiring Urgent Operation

- Bowel obstruction, e.g. caused by volvulus or cancer
- Obstructed inguinal hernia
- Acute appendicitis
- Intestinal perforation
- Acute cholecystolithiasis
- Peritonitis
- Abdominal/retroperitoneal abscess
- Perforated or bleeding gastric ulcer
- Ruptured ectopic pregnancy
- Ovarian torsion
- Ruptured abdominal aortic aneurysm
- Vascular embolism with consecutive bowel ischaemia and gangrene

12.3.3 Management

Patient preparation for emergency laparotomy: Tachycardia or low blood pressure would suggest hypovolaemia due to dehydration, sepsis, or bleeding. If bleeding is suspected, the patient must be taken to the theatre immediately and the bleeding must be stopped while resuscitation, and further diagnostic with lab tests and so on are performed simultaneously. Dehydration or sepsis is treated immediately with rapid fluid resuscitation and broad-spectrum antibiotics (if peritonitis or sepsis is suspected).

In both groups of patients, lab tests should be performed early for Hb, complete blood count and crossmatch, and blood glucose (if available plus arterial blood gas analysis, serum creatinine, serum electrolytes, and bilirubin). If no immediate improvement (systolic BP >80–90 mmHg), vasoconstrictors are administered continuously (e.g. adrenaline, noradrenaline, or phenylephrine infusion). For details, see Sect. 15.2.2.

Try to keep the patient warm as hypothermia worsens blood coagulation and wound healing and increases the risk of wound infection and pneumonia. Use warmed infusions and have towels or blankets around the patient's arms and legs unless the patient has fever.

Pain must be treated, and opioid analgesics are often required together with the administration of oxygen and close monitoring of vital signs in a high-dependency ward/area if possible.

Decompression of the stomach with a nasogastric tube and insertion of a Foley catheter for monitoring urine output should also be performed early. Simultaneously with stabilising the patient, examinations for differential diagnosis are completed with, e.g. abdominal ultrasound, X-ray, or CT scan.

A surgeon should be involved early, and as soon as the diagnosis is made with an indication for surgery, aim for a timely emergency operation. Two APs are mandatory to perform safe anaesthesia for these patients. If the health facility has only one trained AP, a second person who is trained on the job must be available as an assistant.

General anaesthesia for emergency laparotomy is performed with RSI followed by balanced anaesthesia with or without muscle relaxation (see Sects. 6.8 and 12.1). Use all monitoring that is available and measure BP at least every 2–3 min. If available, perform ventilation with a PEEP of 5 cmH_2O. The risk for hypotension after anaesthesia induction is high. Propofol or thiopentone must only be used in reduced doses (thiopentone 2–3 mg/kg and propofol 1 mg/kg) and should be combined with ketamine 1–1.5 mg/kg. Alternatively, ketamine can be used as the sole induction agent at 2 mg/kg plus diazepam 10 mg plus muscle relaxant. Have ephedrine or another vasoconstrictor drug ready. Patients with pre-existing chronic disease or old age and patients with late presentation (several days after onset of the acute abdomen) are at high risk of not surviving anaesthesia and the postoperative period. As they might not tolerate anaesthetic agents in ordinary doses, several anaesthetics should be combined in low doses and carefully titrated to effect while monitoring vital signs tightly. Instead of inhalational anaesthetic, a combination of ketamine +/– fentanyl and IV sedatives such as midazolam, diazepam, or promethazine would maintain cardiovascular stability better. Suxamethonium is usually safer than a longer-acting MR. At the end of the surgery, inject a long-acting analgesic such as morphine 5 mg IM, pethidine 50 mg IM, pentazocine 30 mg IM, or tramadol 50 mg IM and an antiemetic agent such as dexamethasone, ondansetrone, or promethazine. Add a second dose of analgesic when the patient is fully awake and experiencing moderate to severe pain. Ask the surgeon if NGT should be removed before extubation or kept for one or more postoperative days. Suction the pharynx and the NGT before extubation.

Consider delayed extubation for all patients with impaired general condition, late presentation, or prolonged duration of surgery (more than 1.5 h). Even after the reversal of long-acting MR, patients are often too weak to breathe sufficiently and maintain a patent airway. The risk for pulmonary aspiration of secretions is high even with NGT in place. Ideally, postoperative care is performed in the ICU or HDU with CPAP/PEEP and assisted ventilation if breathing is insufficient. Alternatively, if ICU or HDU with a device for delivering CPAP is unavailable, keep the patient in the theatre or improvised place for intermediate care in the ward, remaining intubated and connected to oxygen via a (homemade) T-piece until he/she is fully awake, responsive to commands and breathing, swallowing, and coughing sufficiently. A T-piece can easily be made of 20 cm of corrugated tubing with a hole cut in the middle which is exactly the size of the connector of an ETT size 7–8. Broken respirator tubes can be used as material for such T-pieces. An ordinary tube that is connected to oxygen is inserted at one end of the T-piece around 5 cm and fixed with adhesive tape. A volume of 2–4 l/min of oxygen is often required, sometimes more. The goal is SpO_2 > 93%. Do not transfer the patient to a general ward too early. Especially if the ward is far from the theatre, and no oxygen is available during transportation, the patient might become severely hypoxic and even die before reaching the ward. A health facility without an oxygen source 24/7 and staff to continuously monitor unstable patients is not suitable to operate on patients with acute abdomen.

12.4 Laparoscopy

Minimally invasive surgery (MIS) with laparoscopy has been expanding exponentially and replaced many types of open laparotomy for abdominal surgery worldwide. That process is far from being completed, and laparoscopic surgery is increasingly performed even in remote hospitals with limited anaesthesia equipment and without anaesthesiologists.

The laparoscope is a thin rod with a camera attached to visualise the abdominal and pelvic cavities. Instead of a large skin incision, small keyholes are used for surgery. Therefore, surgical stress is reduced, the wounds are much smaller, and patients are recovering from surgery faster than after open laparotomy. The abdominal muscles are left intact so that early mobilisation is facilitated. Patients feel less pain after surgery, and breathing is easier as diaphragmatic function is left intact. While the postoperative phase may be shorter and with fewer complications, operations last longer depending on the experience of the surgeon, and intraoperatively some typical and serious complications are possible.

Laparoscopy is often performed by gynaecologists: Tubal ligation, diagnostic laparoscopy, and ovarian cystectomy are the most frequent procedures. General surgeons remove the appendix or the gall bladder often via MIS. Depending on the instruments and experience of the surgeon, many other operations can also be performed with that approach.

12.4.1 Anaesthesia Specific Considerations for Laparoscopic Surgery

CO_2 is used for insufflation of the peritoneum to create a pneumoperitoneum for making structures more visible to the surgeons. Intraabdominal pressure (IAP) is increased (but must not rise >15 mmHg) and the diaphragm pushes the cephalad (towards the head). Lung volumes, especially the FRC, are decreased. CO_2 is absorbed to some extent leading to hypercapnia in the blood. Ventilation must be increased so that ET CO_2 would not rise >6.5 kPa (50 mmHg) during surgery. Patients for general surgery are often operated in head-down position which makes ventilation more difficult. Gynaecological MIS is often performed with the head-up position which makes BP difficult to maintain. A continuous vasopressor infusion may be required. Spontaneous breathing during MIS would be insufficient. *Anaesthesia is performed* as intubation anaesthesia (short gynaecological procedures even with a laryngeal mask) *with mandatory mechanical ventilation with PEEP and capnography monitoring*. For anaesthesia machine with a rebreathing circuit, make sure that the carbon dioxide absorber (soda lime) is well functioning and not expired. Respiratory rate during pneumoperitoneum needs to be 20–30% higher than usual (15–16/min in adults). ECG monitoring and automatic blood pressure recording every 2–3 min are also mandatory. Atropine is used to treat bradycardia. Antihypertensive drugs (e.g. hydralazine and labetalol) must be available as the pneumoperitoneum may lead to a significant rise in BP. Muscle paralysis is often required for longer procedures like cholecystectomy. However, pancuronium is far from ideal because urine output is often decreased and the action of pancuronium may be prolonged. Atracurium or vecuronium is safer. Reversal with neostigmine is mandatory (but may be insufficient for pancuronium), and the patient must stay intubated until full muscle recovery with the ability to swallow and to keep eyes open is achieved. Alternatively, repeated doses of suxamethonium 0.5 mg/kg can be used for muscle relaxation up to max 300 mg. Fluid requirements are less than during open laparotomy, and over-infusion should be avoided. *If any of the above-mentioned tools is not available or not functioning, or the anaesthesia provider is not trained to use them, patients must not be operated with MIS/laparoscopy.*

12.4.2 Potential Complications During Laparoscopy

- Difficulty ventilation, hypoxia, and hypercarbia
- Haemodynamic instability (hypotension or hypertension, bradycardia or tachycardia)
- Compression of abdominal organs or the aorta causing decreased venous return and cardiac failure with hypotension
- Reduced renal blood flow and diuresis, thus the prolonged effect of pancuronium
- Injury of a blood vessel with life-threatening bleeding which is more difficult to recognise and to control by the surgeon than during open laparotomy
- Injury to intraabdominal organs such as the urinary bladder or bowels
- Subcutaneous emphysema caused by extraperitoneal insufflation of CO_2; may even lead to capnomediastinum or capnothorax
- Tension pneumothorax caused by injury of mediastinum or diaphragm
- Capnopericardium or haemopericardium with cardiac tamponade causing cardiac failure
- Deep vein thrombosis and lung embolism (even caused by carbon dioxide embolism)

Consider urinary catheter and NGT to prevent injury of the urinary bladder or the stomach. Always induce pneumoperitoneum in the supine position and maintain IAP around 10–12 mmHg. Avoid extreme positioning of the patient. Prolonged head-down position is associated with brachial plexus lesions due to shoulder displacement. Parts of the lungs are not well ventilated, while other parts are not well perfused during laparoscopy, leading to ventilation–perfusion mismatch and impaired oxygenation with a risk for desaturation. Some patients may develop severe hypoxia during pneumoperitoneum, so laparoscopy must be changed to open surgery. Oxygen may even be required for some time postoperatively. Patient observation in a recovery area is mandatory.

The diaphragm is often pushed upwards (cephalad). Consequently, the carina also moves cephalad so that the endotracheal tube may be displaced into one main bronchus (usually the right one) during laparoscopy. That complication must be recognised early since only one lung would be ventilated and the other lung would get atelectasis. A sudden increase in ventilation pressure and/or decrease of SpO_2 should alert the AP to listen to both lungs and to confirm the correct position of the ETT, being ready to withdraw the tube a bit and fix it with new tape. Two anaesthesia staff are mandatory during such interventions.

The unilateral position of the ETT may be difficult to distinguish from pneumothorax. With pneumothorax, ventilation pressure would steadily increase further, and finally, cardiac collapse would occur. A tension pneumothorax is a very rare but serious complication that must be recognised and immediately treated with needle decompression (see Sect. 15.4). Address the risk for pneumothorax in the time-out briefing before the start of surgery and be prepared to treat it.

Communication with the surgeon is vital. If cardiac instability occurs, rule out that the intraabdominal pressure is >15 mmHg, or vascular injury has happened. As the surgeon would not always see bleeding from an injured blood vessel, he must be informed by the anaesthetist if the patient shows any problems with circulation or ventilation/oxygenation. Check Hb if bleeding cannot be ruled out.

Any severe intraoperative complication with high inspiratory pressure, hypoxia, severe hypercarbia, or cardiac collapse should be treated with deflation of the pneumoperitoneum, and dependent on symptoms, with open laparotomy instead of continued laparoscopy.

12.4.3 Postoperative Considerations

PONV is more common after MIS than after open abdominal surgery. Prophylaxis with a combination of two antiemetics is recommended and should be administered at the beginning of surgery or orally in the ward as premedication. An effective combination is dexamethasone 4–8 mg plus ondansetrone (or another serotonin antagonist) 4–8 mg. Even older drugs such as promethazine or metoclopramide can be effective.

Subcutaneous emphysema may postoperatively lead to hypercarbia in the blood due to absorption of carbon dioxide. Patients may present with somnolence, tachycardia, and hypertension. Treatment in severe cases is controlled hyperventilation. Perform blood gas analysis if available.

While abdominal pain is less than after open laparotomy, patients after laparoscopy may suffer from shoulder pain due to irritation of the diaphragm. Pain should be treated with a multimodal approach that is a combination of analgesics with different mechanisms of action. If the bleeding risk is not increased and surgery is uneventful, diclofenac or ketorolac IM and/or paracetamol IV at the end of the surgery, and after longer and more extensive procedures such as hernia repair or gall bladder operation, additionally, an opioid such as buprenorphine, morphine, pentazocine, pethidine, or tramadol should be given. Infiltration of surgical wounds with local anaesthetic is very effective and recommended as well. Use a long-acting LA like bupivacaine 2.5 mg/ml or lidocaine 1% with adrenaline 5 μg/ml. After LA, many patients would not need opioid drugs.

Further Reading

Aaen AA, Voldby AW, Storm N, Kildsig J, Hansen EG, Zimmermann-Nielsen E, Jensen KM, Tilbaek P, Mortensen A, Møller AM, Brandstrup B (2021) Goal-directed fluid therapy in emergency abdominal surgery: a randomised multicentre trial. Br J Anaesth 127(4):521–531

Beed M (2019) Anaesthesia for general, gynaecological and genitourinary surgery. In: Thompson J, Moppett I, Wiles M (eds) Smith and Aitkenhead's textbook of anaesthesia, 7th edn. Elsevier, London, pp 689–699

Herbert L, Tige R (2020) General and urological surgery. In: Craven R, Edgcombe H, Gupta B (eds) Global anaesthesia, 1st edn. Oxford University Press, Oxford, pp 229–238

Ilyas C, Jones J, Fortey S (2019) Management of the patient presenting for emergency laparotomy. BJA Educ 19(4):113–118

13 Anaesthesia for Trauma Surgery

Abstract

All health facilities receive trauma patients. Initial management of trauma patients should be performed according to advanced trauma life support guidelines (ATLS®). The goals are damage control resuscitation, obtaining primary diagnoses and establishing a plan for further/definitive treatment/transfer. On arrival a handover is performed with patient's name, age, gender, mechanism and time of trauma, injuries, complaints, vital signs, any previous treatment like tourniquet, wound treatment, and so on.

A primary survey is performed with (c) A-B-C-D-E approach.

(c)—catastrophic bleeding control (treat first what kills first) by compression of bleeding sites or tourniquet to limbs.

A—Airway: if patient is unresponsive, remove secretions, foreign bodies, jaw thrust without neck extension, consider oropharyngeal airway and whom to intubate.

B—Breathing: if the patient is not breathing sufficiently, give oxygen and ventilate with mask and self-inflating bag. Listen to breathing sounds and perform needle decompression if tension pneumothorax is suspected.

C—Circulation: CPR if patient is not breathing/has no pulse. IV line, fluids (RL, NS), aim for systolic BP >80 mmHg.

D—Disability: consciousness (assess with Glasgow coma scale); drugs for circulation (adrenaline), analgesia (ketamine, pethidine), coagulation (tranexamic acid).

E—Exposure and examine the whole body for injuries, try to keep warm with blankets. Limb-threatening fractures need to be treated early, reduce fractures with severe malposition.

Acute surgery may be performed with ketamine anaesthesia, but major abdominal surgery and head surgery should be performed with endotracheal intubation, controlled ventilation, and balanced anaesthesia. Keep vitals within range.

Keywords

Anaesthesia for abdominal trauma in resource-limited settings · Anaesthesia for craniotomy in head trauma · Anaesthesia management of burns in resource-limited settings · Damage control resuscitation in resource-limited settings · Prevention of secondary brain injury · Primary survey of trauma patients · Trauma management in resource-limited settings

13.1 Initial Management

A trauma patient should primarily be assessed by a multi-professional team of surgeon/orthopaedic surgeon (general physician if no specialist surgeon is available; clinical officer if no

D. Kietzmann, *Anaesthesia in Remote Hospitals*, Sustainable Development Goals Series,
https://doi.org/10.1007/978-3-031-46610-6_13

physician is available), anaesthetist, nurse, and nurse assistant. Other departments such as the lab and the radiology department should also be involved very early. A team leader is to be defined before starting any daytime shift or on-call pass at the health facility. The team leader is responsible for following a systematic approach according to advanced trauma life support (ATLS® foundation) guidelines for early management of severe trauma or local guidelines. ATLS® guidelines have been adopted by a steadily increasing number of countries all over the world. The student course manual on ATLS® by the American College of Surgeons is freely downloadable as a PDF (see further readings).

The team who is bringing the patient to the hospital, e.g. the ambulance driver and assistant, should inform the team in the emergency area with a short, standardised handover. Relatives who bring a patient should be asked systematically with the same type of handover.

13.1.1 Handover

- Name, age, and gender of the patient (if known)
- Mechanism of the trauma (what happened and when did it happen)
- Known or suspected injuries and complaints
- Vital signs (patient was/is conscious or unconscious, breathing difficulties, has pulse yes or no, any deteriorating or improving since initial trauma happened)
- Have any treatments been already performed, such as tourniquets or splints, and have any drugs or infusions been administered?

The initial goal is stabilising vital functions with (c)ABCDE approach, performing damage control resuscitation (DCR) while simultaneously obtaining primary diagnoses and establishing a plan for further/definitive treatment/transfer of the patient. Distinguish between single trauma and multiple injuries in different regions of the body. Life-threatening and limb-threatening conditions need to be addressed first.

13.1.2 Primary Survey (c)ABCDE

Treat first what kills first—for trauma patients, c—catastrophic bleeding control before A = airway.

c—Stop visible bleeding by compression of bleeding sites/tourniquet to limbs.

A—If the patient is unresponsive, check the airway and remove secretions and foreign bodies, apply jaw thrust but avoid neck movement unless an injury of cervical spine is excluded, and consider OPA (oropharyngeal airway) and whom to intubate.

B—Give oxygen and ventilate (mask and SIB) if the patient is not breathing; consider intubation; consider CPR. Listen to breathing sounds and heart sounds; immediate needle decompression is used if tension pneumothorax is suspected; in doubt, bilateral decompression is used before starting mechanical ventilation.

C—Establish IV line or, if impossible, IO (intraosseous) access and give fluids (NS and RL); aim for systolic blood pressure 70–90 if no head injury; if head injury >100 mmHg. If significant blood loss is assumed or obvious, consider blood transfusion (fresh whole blood if massive bleeding) without waiting for low Hb; aim for Hb >70; if no pulse and no BP, start CPR with chest compression: ventilation ratio of 30:2.

D—Disability—consciousness—GCS (Glasgow coma score, see Sect. 15.1). Drugs for circulation (adrenaline during CPR), pain relief (ketamine), coagulation (tranexamic acid, calcium); hypotension: ephedrine, adrenaline only if BP <70–80 despite sufficient fluids IV (head injury: aim for SBP >100).

E—Exposure and examine the whole body, front and back, then cover with blankets, and try to keep warm (remove bloody or wet clothes, and cover the head with a bonnet or towel). Apply splints for fractured limbs, reduce limb-threatening fractures and fractures presenting with severe malposition, and stabilise the pelvic fracture with a pelvic binder sited over the greater trochanters (e.g. homemade cloth). After initial stabilising, further examinations are made, e.g. with an X-ray, to establish all diagnoses and plan for further treatment or transfer.

The trauma team consists of more people than the anaesthesia team, which means the above-mentioned actions should be performed simultaneously, considering the order of priority in the list, following the (c)ABCDE principle. Perform training sessions where all staff members learn to act systematically according to their well-defined roles even in small hospitals.

Damage control resuscitation (DCR) is performed to stop acute life-threatening causes like massive bleeding.

For pathophysiology and treatment of haemorrhagic shock, see Sect. 15.2. Patients with major bleeding should receive 1 g of tranexamic acid if the trauma happened within the past 3 h. Notably, 1 g of calcium gluconate should be slowly administered IV after every 3 units of blood transfusion to keep coagulation working. Cardiopulmonary resuscitation is the subject of Sect. 15.3. Cardiac arrest in trauma patients is associated with a very poor prognosis. Resuscitation is rarely successful as the underlying cause of cardiac arrest in trauma is often the end stage of hypoxia or exsanguination, or severe hyperkalaemia caused by tissue damage. Nevertheless, CPR with chest compressions, ventilation, defibrillation if shockable rhythm, and adrenaline is often to be started until the situation is clear and the team leader decides to continue or to stop efforts. The usual algorithm is followed for CPR (see Sect. 15.3).

Acute life-threatening conditions of trauma patients include tension pneumothorax indicated by the absence of breath sounds on one side and hyper-resonance on the other side. As it can quickly cause cardiac arrest, a needle decompression is immediately indicated on suspicion (do not delay by sending the patient for an X-ray): use a large bore venous cannula or any longer and non-kinking large-bore needle and insert it perpendicular in the second intercostal space (ICS) midline until air is coming out. Alternatively, the fifth intercostal space (ICS) in the anterior axillary line can be used, especially in big patients where the cannula might be too short in the second interspace midline. As soon as possible, that is after a confirmed diagnosis of the thoracic trauma, a chest drain is placed and connected to an underwater seal.

While sending the patient to the X-ray department may be difficult if severely injured, some diagnoses can be made with ultrasound, if available. Intraabdominal bleeding (visible as free fluid), ruptured kidney, liver, or spleen, pneumothorax, or haematothorax (visible as pleura effusion), even rare cardiac tamponade would be visible with ultrasound.

A secondary survey is performed after initial stabilising and treating acute life-threatening conditions. The aim is to get all diagnoses. Ultrasound, X-ray, and, if available, trauma CT scan are performed as well as lab results such as full blood count, electrolytes, creatinine, b-glucose, and coagulation parameters like INR. A plan is established for which interventions/operations are to be performed within which time interval. Can all these operations be performed locally? Or is transfer the better option? Where is the patient to be observed? HDU, ICU, or improvised high dependence care in an area in the peripheral ward?

13.2 Abdominal and Thoracic Trauma

Ultrasound is a very useful tool in the emergency room for the diagnosis of intraabdominal damage and thoracic trauma, e.g. pneumothorax and haematothorax. In the rare case of traumatic cardiac tamponade (stab injury), ultrasound-guided pericardiocentesis may be performed by the surgeon with ketamine anaesthesia.

Chest trauma causes rib fractures, haematothorax, pneumothorax, flail chest, or open, sucking penetrating wounds, and lung contusion developing within 24 h may complicate the trauma and cause respiratory distress and failure. Chest trauma is very painful for several weeks. Good and regular analgesia is important and physiotherapy to encourage the patient to breathe deeply and to cough. Oxygen is often needed during prolonged periods. Severe chest trauma is difficult to survive if ICU care with artificial ventilation is not available.

13.2.1 Anaesthesia for Abdominal Trauma

Consider inserting urinary catheter and nasogastric tube (NGT) before starting surgery if time allows that the patient has relatively stable vital signs. Rupture of the spleen or kidney or big blood vessels and rupture of the liver or intestine are the commonest intraoperative findings. Treatment is early emergency laparotomy with rapid sequence intubation (RSI) and endotracheal intubation. Two large-bore venous cannulae are needed, and warmed IV fluids are ideal. Maintenance of anaesthesia is with ketamine ± diazepam (or other sedative agents), ± fentanyl, and muscle relaxation until the patient is circulatory stable and not bleeding when volatile anaesthetic may be added cautiously and not in too high a dose; begin with 0.5 MAC and increase stepwise if tolerated well. Have blood for transfusion prepared and take measures to keep the patient warm. Have ephedrine and adrenaline prepared.

If intubation anaesthesia is not possible due to a lack of resources, do not perform spinal anaesthesia in acute trauma patients with any significant blood loss as they might develop circulatory collapse. Instead, a combination of repeated ketamine bolus doses of 0.5–1 mg/kg is administered, oxygen is given, the best locally available vital signs monitoring is applied, and diazepam, pethidine, promethazine, or other opioids or sedatives can be combined with ketamine, and get anaesthesia more balanced. Give each drug in small titrating doses and avoid respiratory depression. Some patients do not tolerate even moderate doses without their vital signs deteriorating. In such a scenario, the surgeon should use local anaesthetic techniques to supplement that basic type of anaesthesia (e.g. rectus sheath block). Try to keep the patient warm. Switch off the AC or increase the room temperature to around 25°C. Cover arms, legs, and head with blankets or cloth. Observe the surgical field constantly to see if the patient is pushing, to see bleeding, and to see what the surgeon is doing so that anaesthesia can be adapted to the requirements.

13.2.2 Postoperative Care

Ideally, postoperative care of acute abdominal trauma patients and patients after surgery for bowel obstruction or perforated gastric ulcer should be with delayed extubation in an HDU or ICU for at least 24 h. If that is unavailable, the patient should be warmed and stabilised in the theatre before extubation. Extubation may be performed only if the patient is fully awake and responsive, able to cough and swallow, to keep eyes open, and to lift the head and hold it for some seconds. If the operation table can be tilted, a 30° head-up position is ideal before waking up. Even later, in the bed, a head-up position is better for lung function and decreases pain, especially if a roll is placed under the knees to relax the abdominal wall. In a warm environment, patients are doing better and might even feel less pain. Use a urinary catheter for at least 24 h. NGT remains in place for as long as the surgeon decides and must be connected to a urinary bag and suction applied from time to time to ensure that the stomach is kept empty. Give analgesics for postoperative pain treatment at the end of surgery; do not wait with analgesics until the patient is in the peripheral ward. Preemptive analgesia is much more effective than analgesia on request, and most adult patients need around 10 mg morphine or 100 mg pethidine or equivalent at the end of surgery; for small adults, doses should be adjusted. Many patients after major abdominal surgery need oxygen at least during the first night. If oxygen is unavailable, extubation should be even more delayed. For intubated patients, a T-piece needs to be connected, and an oxygen tube is connected with adhesive tape to that T-piece, which can be homemade from a piece of tubing with a hole in the middle, just big enough to fit on the ETT. However, much better than a T-piece is CPAP. If ICU ventilators with pressure support or CPAP do not exist, an Ambu bag or other type of SIB can be connected to the ETT, and for SIB, cheap CPAP valves can be obtained which are just connected between ETT and SIB. A PEEP of 5 cm H_2O is sufficient for most patients. Obese patients should get a PEEP of 7–8 cm H_2O. That measure helps to decrease the risk of postoperative pneumonia. Most patients who received halothane, ketamine, and pethidine or morphine ± promethazine or diazepam or chlorpromazine will be sufficiently sedated after surgery that the ETT is tolerated during the first night. If not, and if the patient would extubate himself, it is usually not a big problem. Oxygen via nasal prongs should then be given. All patients need careful observation, and infusions, drugs, and vital signs plus urine output/output from drains and gastric tubes must be recorded at least once per hour. That applies whether the patient is cared for in HDU, ICU, or normal ward. Patients after spleen removal need immunisation against meningococcal/pneumococcal-caused pneumonia or meningitis and penicillin prophylaxis.

Acute kidney injury (AKI), a deteriorating kidney function within 48 h after a critical incident, may complicate a patient's condition after shock or major emergency operation. To prevent complete renal failure with the eventual death of the patient (if no dialysis facility is available), potential causes for AKI should be treated and nephrotoxic drugs such as gentamicine or diclofenac avoided, if possible. The kidneys need a sufficient perfusion pressure which means sufficient systolic BP of >80–100 mmHg. Dehydration worsens kidney function. If urine output <0.5 ml/kg/h, check fluid balance and consider more IV fluids but avoid fluid overload with consecutive lung oedema. Hyperkalaemia is one of the complications of renal failure and can be alleviated temporarily with an insulin/glucose combination (10 IU insulin per 500 ml glucose 5% in NS) and salbutamol nebulisation or SC and calcium TDS. Furosemide is not given routinely as it might deteriorate kidney function but is indicated if fluid overload is suspected. Not all patients are responding to furosemide.

13.3 Fractures, ORIF, and Amputation

Fractures with severe malposition may cause nerve damage and are very painful. They should be reduced as fast as possible. Rupture of blood vessels may cause critical bleeding and ischaemia of the limb. The bleeding may stop on its own by maximal vasoconstriction; however, later the vessel will dilate and massively bleed again. A tourniquet initially, suture of the damaged vessels, or even amputation of the limb after a second survey may be indicated. Closed fractures with poor alignment are operated with open reduction and internal fixation (ORIF) during the next days. Open compound or comminuted fractures are operated with wound cleaning and external fixation, if possible, during the first 24 h and need antibiotic prophylaxis.

Spine injury is treated with immobilisation (cervical collar if available and fitting size; do not use a poorly fitting collar as that would do more harm than benefit) and aims to prevent secondary nerve injury. Logrolling is necessary for moving or turning the patient (two to three persons are needed). Spinal cord injury may be a complication of spine injury and leads to loss of sensory and/or motor function of parts of the body below the injury. Breathing can be affected as well, most likely with the level of injury in the cervical spine.

Anaesthesia is often with spinal anaesthesia for lower limbs and with GA for upper limbs. LM is usually sufficient for GA. Patients after severe trauma with massive muscle damage or with spinal cord injury or burns must not receive suxamethonium >24 h after trauma up to 2 months after trauma because of the risk for life-threatening hyperkalaemia which might cause cardiac arrest.

Blood loss depends on the location of the fracture and the type of operation. ORIF of the femur may cause significant blood loss and, dependent on Hb before surgery, blood transfusion may be needed.

Postoperative analgesia is always necessary, preferably with opioids plus paracetamol or a non-steroidal anti-inflammatory drug (NSAID) if no risk for re-bleeding and stable coagulation.

13.4 Head Injury with Traumatic Brain Injury (TBI)

Primary Brain Injury Primary injury is the damage to neural structure which is directly caused by the trauma and is irreversible. Secondary injury can partly be prevented with timely medical care but is a complication that is very common after TBI. Injury to the skull is different from other parts of the body as there is almost no extra space for bleeding or oedema. As volume in the cranium remains constant, bleeding causes increased intracranial pressure (ICP) instead, which diminishes cerebral perfusion pressure (CPP). The normal ICP is below 10 mmHg. At a normal BP of 120/80, the mean arterial pressure would be around 94 mmHg. Cerebral perfusion pressure (CPP) would then be equal to 94–10 = 84 mmHg. A CPP >60 mmHg is normal, and with a CPP >50 mmHg, the brain usually gets sufficient blood flow (exception: old patients and patients with chronic hypertension who need a somewhat higher CPP of >70 mmHg).

If the intracranial volume is increased due to bleeding, compensation mechanisms are started with increased absorption of cerebrospinal fluid; however, these mechanisms have very limited capacity. Therefore, increased intracranial volume by bleeding will gradually increase ICP. Clinically, symptoms for increased ICP include headache, sometimes combined with nausea, and decreased consciousness (deteriorating GCS score). High ICP means low CPP. Some patients get very high blood pressure as a compensatory mechanism if ICP is rising. All compensatory mechanisms are limited, and if ICP is very high, no sufficient cerebral perfusion is possible. Cerebral damage will occur and finally brain dead from hypoxic brain tissue. Patients with elevated ICP due to intracranial bleeding need urgent operation with evacuation of the haematoma. Such operations can be life-saving but must be undertaken within a short time interval to be beneficial.

13.4.1 Prevention of Secondary Brain Injury

Low blood pressure, hypoventilation, hypoxia, low Hb, fever, hypoglycaemia, and hyperglycaemia cause secondary brain injury and must be avoided. The CPP must be kept >60 mmHg, even if it cannot be monitored directly (which is only possible if invasive intraarterial blood pressure is monitored plus intracranial pressure measured with a line placed subcortically and attached to a pressure transducer system). Instead, systolic pressure is aimed for >100–120 mmHg.

Intracerebral vasoconstriction would decrease intracerebral blood volume and thereby the total intracranial volume. The intracranial blood vessel tone increases with decreasing $PaCO_2$, and that relationship is nearly linear. Hyperventilation decreases CO_2 in the blood and promotes cerebral vasoconstriction. Controlled hyperventilation is a very effective measure to decrease increased ICP in patients who are intubated and ventilated. However, the brain adapts to a changed level of CO_2 rather quickly, which is within several hours. Therefore, hyperventilation after a head injury should not be performed routinely but only in acute situations with suspected high ICP. Whenever possible, the underlying cause should be treated as quickly as possible, e.g. evacuation of intracranial haematoma. If surgery is no option, CT is unavailable, and no ICU with ventilators is nearby, then the treatment focuses on nursing with a 30° head-up position and to prevent secondary brain damage. Urine catheter and NGT should be inserted, and feeding should be commenced as soon as possible. Vital signs and fluids in and out are recorded on an observation chart every hour.

13.4.2 Anaesthesia for Burr Hole Evacuation of Epidural or Subdural Haematoma

Anaesthesia depends on the presentation of the patient and local resources. Burr hole evacuation of subdural haematoma in conscious and cooperative patients can be performed with local anaesthesia; otherwise, with short GA (only where LA is not sufficient and intubation cannot be performed due to limited resources) or safer, with intubation anaesthesia. Patients with head trauma are prone to lose a patent airway and stop breathing during GA. Avoid halothane as it increases ICP. High doses of ketamine in spontaneously breathing patients can also increase ICP and should be avoided.

Perioperatively, a head-up position of 30° decreases elevated ICP. Operation tables should be adjustable accordingly. It is better to only elevate the upper part of the body and keep the legs horizontal. If the whole table is tilted to reverse Trendelenburg's position, blood pressure might be difficult to keep above the minimal accepted level. If BP is low, it is better to keep the table flat. Apply oxygen and aim for SpO_2 >95%.

13.4.3 Anaesthesia for Craniotomy

Craniotomy can be performed in hospitals with CT scan and a surgeon who is trained to perform that type of surgery and with sufficient anaesthesia equipment and trained staff. At least two members of anaesthesia staff are needed to do everything which is necessary and to continuously observe the patient, the surgical field, the anaesthesia machine, and keep the anaesthesia record. Postoperatively, high-dependency care should be available including delayed extubation, especially for all patients with GCS <8. Ideally, the patient should be on a ventilator until he is fully responsive and spontaneous breathing is sufficient which may take several days in severe cases. Anaesthesia risk is quite high. Anaesthesia should only be performed with intubation anaesthesia and not with halothane for maintenance. Use the highest level of monitoring available as pulse oximeter, ECG, temperature probe, precordial stethoscope with a long tube to be accessible during surgery, capnography, and automatic blood pressure measurement. Blood grouping and cross-matched blood for transfusion should be ready at least at the time when surgery is started. Lab tests such as full blood count, coagulation tests, blood glucose, serum electrolytes, and creatinine should be performed before taking the patient to the theatre if time allows; otherwise, the blood samples are taken as early as possible. Urine catheter is mandatory as the patient might need quite a lot of IV fluids and mannitol with a diuretic effect. Fluid balance must be controlled since dehydration and fluid overload both cause secondary brain damage. Before anaesthesia induction, drugs to treat hypotension or low pulse rate must be ready and drawn up. Many of these patients need an infusion of adrenaline, dopamine, noradrenaline, or phenylephrine to keep BP at an acceptable level. Ephedrine bolus doses are often required additionally.

Anaesthesia induction is with thiopentone or propofol ± ketamine or fentanyl or morphine/pethidine, suxamethonium, and endotracheal intubation. Maintenance is with isoflurane or sevoflurane <1.2 MAC, not with halothane (desflurane and nitrous oxide are also contraindicated). TIVA with propofol and opioid plus infusion of vasoconstrictor ± invasive arterial blood pressure monitoring is an alternative but only for hospitals that are highly equipped including syringe pumps and with the presence of anaesthesiologists.

One dose of 10 mg morphine or 100 mg pethidine at the beginning of surgery is very nice as isoflurane or sevoflurane can be reduced to 0.8–1 MAC during surgery if combined with opioids. Isoflurane and sevoflurane do increase ICP at concentrations >1 MAC dose-dependently. *Suxamethonium* may be used to facilitate intubation although it increases ICP, but that effect is very short lasting and does not cause harm. *Ketamine* can also increase ICP, but only in connection with decreased breathing, not if patients are ventilated. Therefore, ketamine may be used, as it decreases the requirements of propofol or thiopentone and helps keep BP stable. *RSI* is needed but avoid periods of more than 1 min without ventilation. If intubation is not possible with the first attempt, the patient should gently be hyperventilated via a face mask to avoid too much increase of CO_2, and then the second attempt of intubation should be performed with additional equipment like the gum-elastic bougie. The optimal sniffing position of the patient's head is also vital. If the second attempt for intubation is unsuccessful, consider LMA and apply the difficult airway algorithm (see Sect. 6.6).

BP must be measured at least every 3 min and SBP kept between 100 and 160 mmHg.

Long ventilator tubing is connected straight, without an angle piece, from the endotracheal tube down towards the legs and very well fixed with tape on all connections as you will not see them and do not have access to the tubes when the sterile drapes are placed. The anaesthesia machine must have a disconnection alarm. The anaesthesia machine is moved to the side of the left leg of the patient. Anaesthesia team is working from that place because the surgical team is standing at the patient's head and arms. The arms should be placed with adduction in a neutral position alongside the body. Avoid pressure on the ulnar nerve. Use belts to avoid arms or legs slipping from the table.

The IV line may be difficult to access during surgery. An extension line with a three-way stopcock at the distal end is very useful if IV access is at the lower arm. After anaesthesia induction, a second IV cannula should be inserted on a foot if possible because the anaesthetist can see that cannula while the one on the hand could be lost without realising it when it is hidden by the drapes. A urinary catheter is necessary before starting surgery, and NGT should be placed together with intubation (oral gastric tube if the scull base is fractured). Keep the patient warm. Antibiotics are always needed as prophylaxis before incision.

Hypoxia must be avoided. Give oxygen at least 35–40% and aim for saturation >95%.

Capnography: Normoventilation to 4.5–5 before starting operation, and then hyperventilation with CO_2 4–4.5 until the bone is lifted and ICP relieved, provided that the surgeon would not prefer other target values. Controlled hyperventilation to 4.0 kPa (30 mmHg) makes sense for few hours until the increased ICP is normalised by craniotomy and evacuation of the haematoma. If capnography or arterial blood gas analysis is not available, ventilate with 6–7 ml/kg at a rate of 15/min (6 ml/kg for obese patients and 7 ml/kg for slim and normal weight patients). Manual ventilation: Use a clock with a second hand or the timer of a mobile phone and give one breath every 4 s.

Sufficiently deep anaesthesia prevents from high ICP. If the brain is obviously swollen when the scull bone is removed, IV thiopentone or propofol can be used to reduce intracranial pressure together with hyperventilation and with inotropic support to avoid low blood pressure. Usually, an infusion with adrenaline or noradrenaline is needed in addition to the basic IV fluid line. High ICP can also be treated with 2–3 ml/kg of mannitol infusion over 20–30 min IV. As mannitol causes diuresis, the amount that is urinated must be replaced with NS, RL, or Plasmalyte.

Postoperatively, extubation can be performed only if the patient is fully awake and responds to verbal commands. ICU or HDU care is required, at least in an improvised area in the ward with the best possible observation and care. Seizures may complicate the postoperative phase and need to be treated with antiepileptic drugs. Thromboembolic events can occur in adults after trauma. If available, drugs for the prevention of thrombosis should be used as soon as there is no risk of re-bleeding.

13.5 Burns

Burns patients are often small children or patients with poorly controlled epilepsy. They can occur with other injuries or without. Full-thickness burns may need several months of hospital care and require huge resources. They may leave a family bankrupt if the patient does not have health insurance. If the burned area is >50% of the body surface area, patients are unlikely to survive unless treatment in a fully equipped burns centre is possible. It may be wise to make a realistic plan together with the relatives and the patient about curative treatment or palliative care.

Primary Survey Try to obtain information about the time and kind of initial injury (fire, hot fluid, and chemicals) and chronic health problems, age of the patient, and estimated height and weight, and record them. Patients may be presenting late after the trauma. Exclude other injuries. The rule of nines is applied to estimate the burned surface area in % of body surface area. Superficial burns without blisters are not calculated. Burns charts are a good tool and should be available in every health facility (downloadable). For adults, the surface area is divided as follows: The head and each arm make 9%, each leg makes 18%, the front and the back of the trunk make another 18%, and the genitals make 1%. Children have larger heads and smaller limbs; special charts for children are used. If the patient is transferred later, the chart can accompany the patient. Also record the vital signs and administered drugs and infusions as well as other forms of initial treatment. Check Hb and blood group; if possible, check potassium and creatinine if the trauma happened >24 h ago.

Fluids Different formulas can be used to calculate fluid requirements. The Parkland formula is often used and means that a total amount of 4 ml × BW × % burned body area of RL is given during the first 24 h with a higher infusion rate during the first hours. The infusion rate is adjusted to urine output which must be measured hourly (Foley catheter) and should be 1–2 ml/kg/h. During the next days, protein-rich fluid is lost, and wound treatment causes blood loss. Packed red cells and FFP are often required.

Analgesia Burns are often very painful, so analgesics must be given at regular intervals. NSAIDs are combined with opioids like morphine or pethidine which often need to be administered at least every 4 h. Assess the level of pain and record it on the observation chart. Aim for tailored treatment. For wound cleaning, dressing, and other painful interventions, ketamine is very effective. Very severe pain can be treated with 10 mg morphine (or 100 mg pethidine) IV plus 10 mg morphine (or 100 mg pethidine) IM plus 100 mg ketamine IM. Children may receive 0.2 mg/kg morphine or 2 mg/kg pethidine slowly IV initially or IM and in case of very severe pain additionally 2 mg/kg ketamine IM. Antiemetic drugs (e.g. ondansetrone, promethazine, and dexamethasone) may be necessary to prevent nausea. Continuous observation with pulse oximetry and giving oxygen is mandatory.

Initial surgery in the first health facility, before referral of the patient to a higher-level health facility, includes escharotomy to limbs, neck, or chest if burns are circumferential, to prevent compartment syndrome. Debridement of necrotic tissue may lead to massive bleeding and should only be performed locally if blood for transfusion is available, and the level of the health facility allows for caring a patient with unstable vitals. If the patient is treated locally, subsequent surgical procedures will be needed with anaesthesia. A realistic plan should be made considering the availability of resources and the possibility of a favourable outcome.

Anaesthesia is performed as usual but omits suxamethonium because of the risk of deadly hyperkalaemia. Burns in the face or neck may predict a difficult airway. Make a thorough assessment before planning for intubation. Sometimes, LM is a good alternative; sometimes, only spontaneous breathing will be possible, and an artificial airway proves impossible unless advanced equipment for fiberoptic intubation or a videolaryngoscope can be used.

Nutrition is very important and should be started orally as early as possible or via NGT. A high-energy and -protein diet is needed with vitamins, minerals, and micronutrients not missing. If sufficient high-energy food is not available for the caretakers of the patient, extra therapeutic nutrition should be provided by the hospital. Plumpy' Nut is a brand that is ready to use and launched by UNICEF. It is produced in a number of countries, e.g. France, Kenya, Malawi, Burkina Faso, Ethiopia, India, USA, and Haiti, only to mention some. It can be stored for up to 2 years at ambient temperature, is suitable for all patients >6 months with acute malnutrition, and has saved thousands of lives. It is inexpensive and should be on the shelves in every hospital store and made available for the most needy patients.

Dressing of burn wounds can be performed with Vaseline (petroleum jelly) gauze in pieces of 10 × 15 cm which can be prepared locally and stocked in the central sterilisation department. It needs to be sterilised twice (autoclave) and is a good and inexpensive dressing material. Burns that are not healed within 14 days are full-thickness burns and need skin grafting as soon as possible to avoid contracture development. If burned areas are large, the head, neck, feet, hands, and joints need to be prioritised. Splints or casts are applied to prevent hands, arms, and legs from getting contractures.

Criteria for transfer of patients with burns are dependent on the health care system and the distance/accessibility of a centre for burns treatment. Transfer is highly recommended and should be performed without unnecessary delay after initial management of full-thickness burns if no definitive surgical treatment is locally available, i.e. all burns >10% body surface area, burns involving hands or face/neck/genitals, and major joints, inhalation injury, chemical burns, especially of head/neck, and circumferential burns of limbs or trunk.

Further Reading

Hodges S, Janjanin S, Kendell J, Lubis N, Nott D, Olim N (2020) Trauma. In: Craven R, Edgcombe H, Gupta B (eds) Global anaesthesia. Oxford handbooks in anaesthesia, 1st edn. Oxford University Press, Oxford, pp 197–228

Hormis A (2019) Emergency and trauma anaesthesia. In: Thompson J, Moppett I, Wiles M (eds) Smith and Aitkenhead's textbook of anaesthesia, 7th edn. Elsevier, London, pp 831–849

Lott C, Truhlar A, Alfonzo A, Barelli A, Gonzalez-Salvado V, Hinkelbein J et al (2021) European resuscitation council guidelines 2021: cardiac arrest in special circumstances. Resuscitation 161:152–219

Steurer MP, Lancman B (2023) Anesthesia for trauma. In: Pardo MC (ed) Miller's basics of anaesthesia, 8th edn. Elsevier, Philadelphia, pp 768–793

Stewart RM, Rotondo MF, Henry SM, Drago M, Merrick C, Haskin DS, Peterson N (eds) (2018) ATLS® advanced trauma life Support® student course manual, 10th edn. American College of Surgeons, Chicago

14 Paediatric Anaesthesia

Abstract

Anaesthesia in neonates and infants is more dangerous than for adults and should be performed by a team of two experienced anaesthesia providers in a theatre with anaesthesia machine, vital signs monitor, and airway equipment. If anything of these is unavailable, the patient should be transferred.

Children have a large head and body surface area with increased risk for hypothermia.

The trachea is short and the larynx relatively higher in the neck; a large epiglottis may cause difficult airway management.

The correct size of laryngoscope blade, tube, laryngeal mask, or oropharyngeal airway is vital (table provided in this chapter).

The functional residual capacity of the lung is reduced; infants are prone to hypoxia during apnoea.

Always take bodyweight before anaesthesia (exception huge injuries which make position on weighing scales impossible); draw drugs with proper dilution and correct doses (tables provided in this chapter); label syringes carefully.

Ketamine is safe for children as it is for adults; however, for major surgery it is not suitable as the sole anaesthetic. Avoid mask induction in fearful children, prefer midazolam 0.3–0.5 mg/kg orally, ketamine 2 mg/kg IV, or ketamine 5 mg/kg IM while the caretaker is present.

Burns patients may repeatedly receive ketamine anaesthesia or halothane with face mask for wound cleaning/debridement.

IV fluids must be balanced; avoid dehydration and fluid overload. Postoperative analgesia with local anaesthetic wound infiltration, diclofenac 2 mg/kg IM, tramadol 2 mg/kg IM, pethidine 2 mg/kg IM, or similar, is essential at the end of major surgery.

Keywords

Airway management in paediatric anaesthesia · Anaesthesia for paediatric burns patients · Anaesthesia for adenectomy and tonsillectomy · Anaesthesia induction with halothane · Dilution of drugs for paediatric anaesthesia · Fluid management for infants in resource-limited settings · General anaesthesia for infants in resource-limited settings · Management of paediatric head trauma · Paediatric anaesthesia for abdominal surgery · Postoperative analgesia for children · Preoperative evaluation of paediatric patients

14.1 General Considerations

During childhood, anaesthesia risk is inversely related to age. Providing safe paediatric anaesthesia can be very challenging.

A team of two anaesthesia staff is necessary for the safe practice of paediatric anaesthesia. In

D. Kietzmann, *Anaesthesia in Remote Hospitals*, Sustainable Development Goals Series,
https://doi.org/10.1007/978-3-031-46610-6_14

case there is only one anaesthesia provider available, ask a theatre nurse/scrub nurse/doctor to assist during anaesthesia induction and during recovery. You need four hands, and you must prepare everything you will need in advance.

Especially at high risk for anaesthesia, complications are premature infants as their organ systems are not yet functioning well. Up to a gestation age of 55 weeks, 90% of all preterm infants would show episodes of apnoea after general anaesthesia (GA), and this is independent of the choice of anaesthetic drugs. Even after sedation or short GA with ketamine, these small infants are prone to insufficient breathing. For example, 55 weeks of gestation would mean 25 weeks, nearly 5 months, after preterm birth at 30 weeks of gestation. In resource-limited settings, elective operations should not be performed in infants below 6 months after birth or below 6 kg bodyweight (BW). Even infants after term birth are at higher anaesthesia risk and should not be operated on if not absolutely necessary. If possible, and if the parents can afford it, it is better to operate on small infants in larger hospitals with anaesthesiologist plus trained anaesthesia nurses present and with more advanced equipment.

Otherwise, only emergency procedures may be performed, and ideally, the little patient should be continuously monitored in a neonatal unit (NICU), if available, where a pulse oximeter should be attached, and the respiratory rate should be counted and recorded hourly. An infant resuscitating self-inflating bag and oxygen must be available near the bedside. If there is no NICU or PICU, even in the ordinary ward, a room for sick infants should be set up with a nurse being continuously at the patient's bedside and monitoring it. After anaesthesia, the anaesthetist should observe the patient until fully awake, moving spontaneously, and circulatory stable, even if this creates problems with the timetable in that operation room. Otherwise, the risk of postoperative death in this group of patients can be really high.

Children are fearful when separated from their parent/caregiver, especially at the age between 6 months and 6 years. For patients >6 months of age, one caregiver should be allowed to be present in the operation theatre until the child is asleep. It is also possible to give a sufficient dose of sedative (e.g. midazolam 0.5 mg/kg or diazepam 5 mg >3 years orally, or ketamine 5 mg/kg IM) in the preparation area with parents present and then take the child to the OR provided that the child is well sedated and not crying. Ketamine IM is effective within 5 min, midazolam orally takes 15 min, and diazepam 30 min before taking the child to OR. At many hospitals worldwide, a parent/caretaker is allowed to change/get a theatre gown and to accompany the child into the OR until it is sleeping (e.g. mask induction with inhalational anaesthetic). That may be the least stressful way for the child providing there is a runner who would accompany the parent out of the OR as soon as the anaesthetist is deciding so. Both children and parents should be informed about what the anaesthetist is going to do (putting on a pulse oximeter, putting on a cannula, applying a face mask with oxygen/inhalational anaesthetic, the patient will fall asleep soon, and so on). At all hospitals, parents should be allowed to be present at the bed side in the recovery area after surgery. It is very stressful for the children if they do not see someone whom they know well when awakening after surgery. Additionally, patient safety is increased if a caregiver is continuously at the bedside. A child after surgery can suddenly start moving and very quickly fall off a stretcher and must never be left alone for even a minute during the whole period of recovery.

14.2 Physiological Characteristics and Their Implications for Anaesthesia

The anaesthetist should know the normal variables of children according to their age. Children have large heads and a greater body surface area in relation to their height compared with adults making them prone to lose temperature when

Table 14.1 Average body weight, size, respiratory rate (RR), heart rate (HR), systolic blood pressure (SBP), and diastolic blood pressure (DBP) in healthy, not anaesthetised children, depending on age

Age (years)	BW (kg)	Height (cm)	RR/min	HR/min	SBP (mmHg)	DBP (mmHg)
Neonate	2.5–4	46–56	40–60	90–200	50–90	25–60
6/12	7–8	61–75	30–40	80–180	60–100	50–70
1	10–11	78–83	20–30	80–160	80–105	50–65
2	12–14	84–94	18–30	80–130	85–105	50–70
4	15–18	102–108	18–28	80–120	85–110	50–70
6	19–24	116–122	16–26	75–115	85–110	50–70
8	23–31	124–134	16–24	70–110	85–110	55–70
10	28–38	130–144	15–22	70–100	95–120	60–75
12	34–48	140–156	12–21	60–90	95–120	65–80

exposed (air conditioning in theatre should be turned off or set at a much higher temperature). Small infants cannot yet produce heat by shivering. Cover the child with blankets and avoid exposure of the body during anaesthesia induction and venous cannulation. A bonnet on the head is very helpful. IV fluids may be warmed before infusion (but not >37 °C). Disposable gloves can be filled with hot water (around 40 °C) and put around the patient, but wrap them to avoid burns caused by direct contact with the skin. Devices such as radiant warmers are also used to keep patients warm. Measure the body temperature at least during all major procedures.

Table 14.1 lists average body weight, height, respiratory rate, heart rate, and blood pressure (not anaesthetised) depending on age. As oxygen consumption per kilogram is higher while tidal volume is the same for all ages (6–8 ml/kg), respiratory rate is inversely related to age and is highest in neonates.

Due to genetic and environmental variations around the globe, some populations would show smaller or bigger average sizes than in the table. Unfortunately, more and more children are getting obese and showing higher BW than in the table.

14.2.1 Respiratory System

Anaesthesia-related respiratory complications are commonest in small infants. The lungs are mature after >36 weeks of gestation, but accessory muscles of respiration are still ineffective, and the diaphragm is more likely to become fatigued due to increased work of breathing. Airway resistance is 20 times higher than in adults while lung compliance (elasticity) is 20 times smaller, causing much more work of breathing for the infant and especially the neonate.

Hypoglycaemia, low body temperature, anaemia, and prolonged hypoxia may depress respiratory drive. Keep newborns warm under all circumstances. Early body contact with the mother is not a tradition in all cultures but the best for both mother and neonate. Allow the newborn also to suck within the first hour after birth.

The lung volumes of small infants during apnoea are smaller per kilogram than in adults. That means, there is little oxygen reserve in the lungs when the patient stops breathing and is not ventilated. Additionally, oxygen consumption is higher in infants, so hypoxia develops more quickly than in larger children or adults, e.g. during anaesthesia induction. Neonates and infants are prone to get bradycardia when their oxygen saturation drops. In that case, immediate ventilation with oxygen is required to prevent cardiac arrest. As soon as saturation normalises, heart rate usually increases promptly to normal values.

The respiratory drive is not mature at birth, and drugs that have respiratory depressant side effects, especially opioids, may be dangerous for small infants.

14.2.2 Circulatory System

See Table 14.1 for normal heart rate and blood pressure at different ages.

The foetal circulation is undergoing marked changes immediately after birth. Inside the uterus, only a small portion of the cardiac output is flowing through the lungs. Blood from the venous side of the circulation is flowing through three different shunts to the arterial part of the circulation. At birth, the lungs are receiving the first breath, and pulmonary blood vessels dilate. Pulmonary blood flow increases until it is the same as the cardiac output. Instead of receiving venous blood from the placenta as relatively oxygen-rich blood (but with lower oxygen saturation than in the arterial blood after birth), the neonate starts breathing so that the lungs let oxygen enter the arterial part of the circulation leading to much higher oxygen saturation than during intrauterine life. Systemic vascular resistance increases, and the shunts between the venous and arterial systems and from the right to the left heart are closed. These changes are not immediately stable. During the first days, hypoxaemia or acidosis may lead to the reopening of the arterio-venous shunts causing a vicious circle with persistent foetal circulation, a life-threatening condition.

The neonatal myocardium cannot easily increase stroke volume. Increases in cardiac output are mainly achieved by and depending on increasing heart rate. There is an imbalance between parasympathetic and sympathetic nervous systems rendering the neonate prone to bradycardia. Atropine (or glycopyrronium which has the same effects and can be used instead of atropine) should always be given to prevent bradycardia during laryngoscopy, insertion of nasogastric tube (NGT), orogastric tube, or suctioning of the airways. Hypoxia may cause bradycardia and finally asystole. The first-line treatment is ventilation with oxygen; if there is no immediate improvement in heart rate, give atropine. If bradycardia or asystole persists or there is no pulse despite sufficient ventilation and atropine injection, the patient needs adrenaline. Give adrenaline 10 μg/kg IV (0.1 ml/kg of adrenaline 1:10,000 = 0.1 ml/kg of a 10 ml dilution of adrenaline [1 mg = 1 ml ampoule diluted with 9 ml to make 10 ml]), perform cardiac compressions and repeat adrenaline every 3 min until stabilization is achieved.

14.2.3 Kidneys and Liver

These organs are not yet mature at birth. At the age of 2 years, kidney function is fully established. In younger infants, the ability to excrete water and sodium and to concentrate urine is limited. Drugs with renal elimination show a longer duration of action in infants. Liver blood flow and enzyme activity for drug metabolism are lower before the age of 1 year. Synthesis of coagulation factors is with lower capacity so that the level of coagulation factors is significantly lower in infants. It is recommended to give vitamin K IM to all neonates to facilitate the synthesis of coagulation factors in the immature liver.

14.3 Preoperative Assessment and Preparation

Preoperative evaluation is very important and should always be performed and recorded (see Chap. 4), at least briefly even in emergencies. Ideally, every child scheduled for surgery should be seen by a paediatrician. However, not all hospitals have a specialist paediatrician which means that correct diagnosis, especially in children with any syndrome, is sometimes lacking and the decision about whether to operate or not to operate is dependent on the knowledge and experience of the surgeon. The AP may experience a difficult situation if a visiting surgeon/paediatric surgeon wants to operate major surgery without considering significant anaesthesia risk, especially if equipment for paediatric anaesthesia is incomplete, and there is no anaesthesiologist. The AP should dare to refuse anaesthetising a child if he/she anticipates a high and not manageable risk for severe complications but aim for constructive dialogue with all involved including the patient's parents.

Age and body weight must always be obtained, plus length if possible. Weighing scales are inexpensive and should never be missing in the preoperative assessment area because airway equipment, IV fluids, and drugs are chosen according to age and weight. If BW is unknown, over- or underdosing is a serious and avoidable complication.

The patient's history is taken with special emphasis on gestational age at birth (prematurity?), weight at birth, growth, physical and mental development, complications in the neonatal period (on oxygen during first days of life?), congenital malformations or disease/syndrome, lung disease, severe infectious disease, sleep-disordered breathing, snoring during sleep (especially children scheduled for ENT operations), and previous surgery/anaesthesia-related complications? Ask about drug allergies, family history of malignant hyperthermia, recent airway infection, diarrhoea, or fever.

Vital signs are measured and recorded. Heart and lung auscultation is important to check for heart murmur, abnormal breathing sounds such as wheezing or crackles. Heart murmur in combination with at least one clinical symptom such as shortness of breath, poor BW for age, SpO_2 below 96%, bluish skin colour, prolonged capillary refill, history of syncope or frequent chest infections, and reduced exercise tolerance are highly suspicious of congenital heart disease with high anaesthesia risk. Only acute life-threatening conditions should be operated on locally in those children and parents must be informed about the risk.

Abnormal breathing sounds: Ask for a history of airway infection or asthma and consider postponing the operation and improving the patient's condition. Upper respiratory tract infections are common in children, especially those for ENT surgery. While a child with a runny nose usually can be operated for adenoidectomy or tonsillectomy, patients should be postponed for several weeks if they are suffering from productive cough, fever, or decreased SpO_2.

Airway assessment: Carefully check for any abnormalities such as micrognathia, cleft lip/palate or other facial malformation, mouth opening, neck movement, and position of the laryngeal cartilage.

Do not accept a child for general anaesthesia if a difficult airway is anticipated and seems not to be manageable with local resources.

Laboratory testing is often not necessary but check all patients for clinical signs of anaemia such as pale tongue, nails, palm of the hands, and conjunctivae. However, if major bleeding is anticipated or the operation of a sick or anaemic child is planned, Hb or full blood count, and depending on the case, other lab tests such as creatinine, glucose, sodium, and potassium should be performed. In regions with endemic malaria or HIV, respective tests may be indicated.

Before surgery with anticipated significant blood loss, have blood cross-matched.

Fasting before anaesthesia is mandatory before elective surgery to minimise the risk of vomiting or regurgitation of gastric contents and pulmonary aspiration. Fasting can be very stressful for children and their parents. Instead of having all patients scheduled for surgery "fasting from 10 PM," it is better to avoid unnecessary fasting by following the 6–4–2 h rule for patients without gastric or bowel problems:

Up to 6 h before starting anaesthesia solid food (in small quantities), porridge, yoghurt, formula or cow milk, or soup is allowed.

Up to 4 h breastfeeding, tea, or similar fluids are allowed;

Up to 2 h before anaesthesia induction, clear fluid like water is allowed.

An exception should be made for infants <3 months, and small-for-age infants or former preterm infants up to 6 months of age without access to breastmilk. They should be allowed to feed with formula or cow milk up to 4 h before induction of anaesthesia because 6 h is too long and increase the risk for hypoglycaemia and dehydration. An experienced anaesthetist should perform induction and intubation in these small infants. Accidental oesophageal intubation would increase the risk of regurgitation and pulmonary aspiration. Alternatively, they may receive a glucose/saline infusion.

Very small quantities of water may even be allowed up to 1 h before anaesthesia as it is common practice in paediatric anaesthesia in Europe, Australia, and New Zealand. Oral premedication may be taken with little water without a time limit. The problem is planning (and surgeons who like to change the order of the list at the last moment). It may prove difficult to know in advance when the operation will really be starting. In order to avoid having patients not ready due to insufficient fasting, many patients are forced to starve longer than necessary. Realistic planning should be aimed together with the surgeon, anaesthesia team, and scrub nurses. The smallest patients should be allowed to breastfeed "at 4 AM" and then be operated on as the first case in the morning as soon as the list is starting. The intake of water should be encouraged for all patients (even adults) when the theatre team knows surgery will not be started within the next 2 h. Good communication between theatre and wards is key.

Premedication is useful for patients with anxiety before surgery. Perioperative stress can be reduced significantly if the patient and parents/caregivers remain calm. Sedatives can be given to patients >1 year while they are together with their parents in the waiting area. Midazolam 0.5 mg/kg (max dose 10–15 mg) can be given as oral suspension with little juice and is effective after approximately 20 min. Diazepam 5 mg or lorazepam 1 mg can be used for children old enough to swallow tablets. The effect will be sufficient after 30 min and last some hours; however, some children do not respond well to sedative drugs. Promethazine 1 mg/kg is sometimes more effective than the before-mentioned agents and can be used for children >2 years, if possible, with oral suspension instead of IM injection, 1 h before anaesthesia induction. Ketamine 5 mg/kg can be injected IM and is highly effective within 5 min, but consider that children do not like syringes and use them only if mask induction with a volatile anaesthetic seems to be impossible or more traumatising than IM injection. Ketamine 7–8 mg/kg can also be given orally, but the effect is less predictable. After injection of ketamine, the anaesthetist must not leave the patient unobserved.

14.4 Airway Management and Ventilation

14.4.1 General Considerations

The head of an infant is large while the neck is short. Therefore, one should use a pillow under the shoulders during induction of anaesthesia to facilitate a free airway (see Fig. 14.1a) and a ring

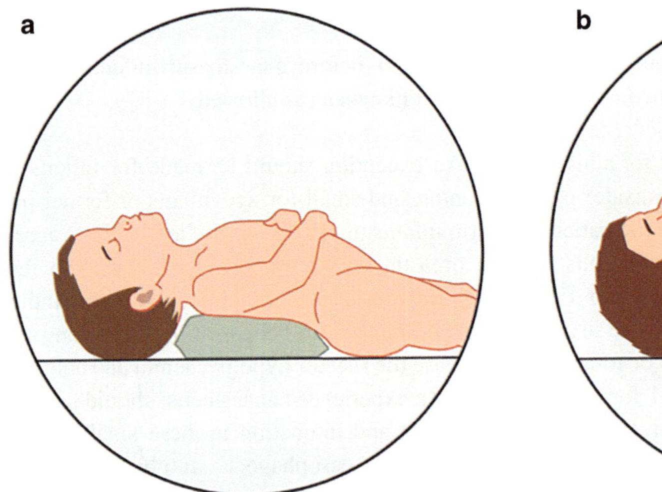

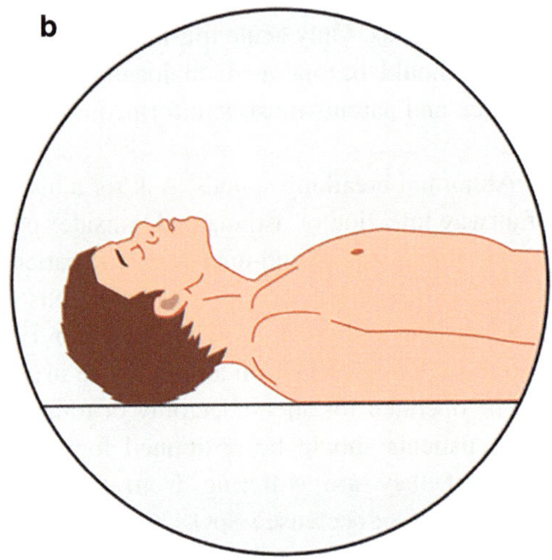

Fig. 14.1 Infant (**a**) and child (**b**), position for airway management. Infants have large heads. For infants and small children, a pillow under the chest facilitates keeping a free airway

(which can be made easily from a piece of cloth formed like a "donut") under the head. Children >1–2 years can often be placed supine without a pillow (see Fig. 14.1b). In relation to body size, the tongue is larger than in adults, making it more difficult to keep a free airway during anaesthesia without using an oropharyngeal airway device (Guedel tube), laryngeal mask, or endotracheal tube. Especially in small infants, the tongue is very prone to fall back to the posterior pharyngeal wall, leading to airway obstruction. The larynx is located more cranially than in adults and the epiglottis is longer making laryngoscopy more difficult. Up to the age of 6 months a Miller blade is better suitable than the curved Macintosh blade, as the straight Miller blade is passed beneath the laryngeal surface until the epiglottis is elevated to facilitate view towards the vocal cords. The Macintosh blade is used for infants after they get the first tooth, and it is advanced into the space between the base of the tongue and the pharyngeal surface of the epiglottis (above the epiglottis), and then the epiglottis is elevated to make the glottic opening visible. Pressing the laryngeal cartilage slightly with the fifth finger of the left hand while doing the laryngoscopy facilitates intubation. The narrowest part of the air passage is at the level of the vocal cords in adults while it may be at the level of the cricoid cartilage in small children.

The trachea is short: newborn 4 cm, at 2 years 5 cm, at 6 years 6 cm (adults: 12 cm). That means, the endotracheal tube may be falsely positioned in one of the main bronchi but can also dislocate easily upwards and out of the trachea, especially during changing position of the patient on the operation table. Auscultation after intubation, after taping the tube, and after each change of positioning of the head or chest is therefore vital.

The lung compliance is reduced, while the airway resistance is increased. The mucous membranes of the respiratory tract are irritable, which means they can swell very easily, e.g. as a consequence of intubation with too large a tube which may cause airway obstruction after anaesthesia. Laryngospasm or bronchospasm is also more common than in adults, and the risk is highest during intubation and after extubation. It can be avoided by intubating in deep anaesthesia with muscle relaxation and by extubating after regaining consciousness. Spontaneous breathing during anaesthesia and after the end of surgery is often insufficient and needs assistance. Always give oxygen!

Anaesthesia in small infants without using a pulse oximeter is dangerous and should be avoided, even for very short procedures in spontaneous ventilation. (Of course, a pulse oximeter should always be used for anaesthesia, not only in small infants!) Additionally, a precordial stethoscope is very useful. In any case of doubt, listen to both lungs. If ECG is available, always use it at least for anaesthesia for major surgery. If disposable electrodes are O/S, use cotton wool made moist with NS to be put on the skin instead and have adhesive tape fixing the ECG cable with its metal bit at its end. If a small BP cuff is available, always use it. If the smallest available BP cuff is too large, it can be used on the leg instead. A too small BP cuff can be used at the wrist. Monitoring end-tidal CO_2 is regarded as mandatory if available.

The functional residual capacity (FRC) of the lungs is small and decreases by anaesthesia while the oxygen consumption per kg BW is threefold higher than for adults. Therefore, apnoea leads very quickly to desaturation.

Preoxygenation with 2–4 l/min oxygen for at least 3–5 min is vital before induction of anaesthesia.

The tidal volume per kg BW is the same for all ages (7 ml/kg), while respiratory frequency is increased. Thereby, the dead space ventilation per minute is also increased, while the dead space of each single breath is 30% of tidal volume as in adults. As the absolute volumes are small, any increase of dead space caused by anaesthetic apparatus, face mask, and so on increases the dead space significantly. Always use the smallest fitting face mask and use the smallest possible connectors between the airway and breathing system/breathing circuit/ventilator tubing.

Infants under the age of 1 year should not breathe spontaneously through an endotracheal tube over longer periods because of the increased resistance. Their respiratory muscles are relatively weak, and the ribs are soft, increasing the risk for respiratory insufficiency during and after anaesthesia. Newborns and young infants show a reduced reaction to hypoxia, especially during hypoglycaemia or hypothermia, which may lead to hypoventilation or apnoea, e.g. after anaesthesia or delivery (especially caesarean section in air-conditioned theatre). The theatre must be warmer than for adults: for newborns at least 28 °C, infants 26 °C, and children >4 years 24 °C unless the patient is lying on a warming blanket and covered with a second warming blanket with adjustable temperature. Always cover the head and body of small infants with cloth, and never have a child naked (uncovered) in the theatre at any moment.

14.4.2 Sizes of Artificial Airways

For the size of airways, length of the ETT at lips, tidal volume, and breaths per minute, see Sect. 6.4, Table 6.1. Oropharyngeal airways and nasopharyngeal airways are easily inserted and may be very helpful to provide a patent airway or to facilitate manual ventilation. They are available in many sizes. Correct size is vital for good effect. The size of the oropharyngeal airway is equivalent to the distance from the corner of the mouth to the earlobe, and the nasopharyngeal airway is placed near the laryngeal entrance. The correct length is approximately equivalent to the distance from the tip of the nose to the earlobe. The correct position is confirmed by exhaled air coming out.

Appropriate size of the endotracheal tube (ETT): From the age of 4 years, the size for uncuffed ETT may be calculated according to this formula: ETT = age/4 + 4 mm internal diameter. For ETT with cuff, age/4 + 3.5 applies.

A rough indicator is the diameter of the child's little finger; however, the correct size correlates better with age (see Table 14.2).

One size larger and one size smaller must be at hand if the planned size is not fitting.

If cuffed tubes are used for children below 8 years, the size may be 0.5 less than stated in the table. Use tubes with cuff only if you can measure the cuff pressure with a cuff pressure manometer, or inflate as little as possible, just to keep it tight at ventilation pressure < 20 mbar. A too high cuff pressure can damage the tracheal wall and lead to severe obstruction after extubation. When uncuffed tubes are used, consider the use of a throat pack (with gauze moistened with water or saline) which can be useful to prevent pulmonary aspiration and dislocation of the tube. After packing, both lungs must be auscultated once more to make sure that the tube is still placed correctly, and bilateral air entry is confirmed. Do never forget to remove the pack before extubation: Leave a bit of the gauze outside the mouth and attach a tape written "pack" on it. From the age of 6–8 years, a cuffed tube is recommended even if no cuff pressure monitor is available. Gently feel the cuff and assess if it is

Table 14.2 Bodyweight and respiratory rate during anaesthesia depending on age; average sizes for endotracheal tubes (ETT) and laryngeal mask airways (LM)

Age (year)	BW (kg)	RR	ETT size	Intubation depth (cm from lips)	LM size
Premature	<2	40–50	2.5	8–9	NA
Neonate	2.5–4	40	3	10	1
1/12–5/12	3.5–7	30–35	3.5	10–12	1–1.5
6/12–1	7–12	30	4	12–13	1.5–2
1–2	9–15	25–30	4–4.5	12–14	2
3–4	14–17	22–25	4.5–5	12.5-14.5	2–2.5
5–6	18–24	20–22	5–5.5	13–15	2.5
7–8	25–30	18–20	5.5–6	14–16	2.5
9–12	>30	14–18	6–6.5	16–18	3

For neonates <2 kg, LM is not applicable (NA). See Sect. 6.4, Table 6.1 for more details. The tidal volume of each single breath is the same for all ages with 7 ml/kg not inflated too much. The trachea of a child < 8 years has a nearly round cross section, while after the age of 8 years, it is more oval. The round trachea does not necessarily require an inflated cuff of the tube, but a gently cuffed tube prevents better from pulmonary aspiration of gastric contents even in small children. The correct depth of intubation that is how many centimetres the tube is inserted (measured from the lips) is also provided in Table 14.1.

Laryngoscopes: Infants below 6 months or before they have teeth are best intubated with a straight Miller blade size 0 for prematures, size 1 for term neonates, and infants up to 6–9 months, Macintosh curved blade size 1 from 6 months up to 2 years and size 2 from 3 years. Children >6 years require size 2 or 3 mac blades.

During mechanical or manual ventilation, the tidal volumes tend to be a little larger; oxygen consumption is decreased by anaesthesia, so the respiratory rate is often somewhat lower than during spontaneous breathing.

14.4.3 Appropriate Size of the Laryngeal Mask Airway (LMA)

LMA is available in sizes for all paediatric patients >2 kg. It is recommended for surgery of the limbs and the genitourinary tract as well as for inguinal hernia repair and as alternative airway in case of failed intubation. It does not protect from pulmonary aspiration as safe as an ETT does.

LMA size 1 can even be used for prolonged neonatal resuscitation in hospitals without a neonatologist and a fully equipped NICU.

For proper sizes, please see Table 14.2. In some patients, the next smaller or bigger size fits better than the one according to the BW.

The cuff should be inflated as little as necessary to avoid damage to tissue and nerves in the throat. Anaesthesia must be deep before insertion of the LMA; otherwise, the patient might start coughing and the device dislocates; even laryngospasm might occur. A muscle relaxant is not necessary to insert LMA but have it at hand in case of severe laryngospasm. With laryngospasm, hand ventilation is often easier with a face mask than with LMA. Do not forget to turn vaporiser on or continue with intravenous anaesthetics to keep anaesthesia sufficiently deep.

14.4.4 Artificial Ventilation in Children

The tidal volume (TV) for controlled ventilation is 6–10 ml/kg BW. Respiratory frequency (approximately): neonates 30–40/min; infants 30–35/min; children 1–2 years 25–30/min; 3–4 years 22–25/min; 5–6 years 20–22/min; and 7–8 years 18–20.

For children <15–20 kg of bodyweight or 6 years of age, use paediatric breathing systems and bellows. During manual ventilation, avoid too high tidal volumes which may cause high intrathoracic pressure that leads to decreased venous return and decreased cardiac output. The higher the risk, the smaller the infant. The smallest ventilation bellows have 0.5 l volume, so squeeze gently to avoid too high tidal volumes. However, in cases of small infants or infants <10 kg, manual ventilation with careful observation of airway pressure, respiratory frequency, and tidal volumes is probably the safest way of ventilation unless well-maintained anaesthesia machines with ventilators suitable for small children are used. A ventilator for children must be able to deliver low tidal volumes at high respiratory frequencies and with a PEEP of 5 cm H_2O to keep alveoli open and prevent atelectasis formation. During intubation anaesthesia with intermittent positive pressure ventilation (IPPV), always use the plateau pressure valve to achieve a constant upper pressure limit of 12–20 mbar to keep the tidal volumes within the physiological range of 6–10 ml/kg BW (not more!). A sudden high tidal volume delivered at high pressure (>30–40 mbar) might cause a pneumothorax. Before extubation, be sure that spontaneous breathing is sufficient even without extra oxygen. Disconnect the tube and wait a few minutes while the patient is breathing air, observing chest movements and pulse oximetry. If the saturation is stable, give again oxygen for a few minutes, suck the oropharynx, inflate the lungs manually, and extubate while squeezing the bellows. The child must then breathe out immediately after extubation, which prevents usually from getting a laryngeal spasm. Leave the oropharyngeal airway device in place until the infant is fully awake. During extubation, always have suction ready and everything including drugs for mask ventilation and reintubation in case of respiratory insufficiency (caused by residual effects of anaesthetics or muscle relaxants, laryngospasm, bronchospam, or aspiration). After extubation, support the jaw (forward displacement) to maintain a clear airway, give oxygen, and wait at least 5 min. If saturation remains stable, wait additionally at least 5 min without extra oxygen. If saturation remains stable (>94%), the patient may be transferred to the recovery area. Do never leave the child unattended until the nurses from the ward have fetched it. It is recommended to have the mother/caretaker at the bedside. Beware child might move and fall from the bed or stretcher. If possible, work always as a team of two professional anaesthesia officers during the induction and emergence of children. In case of a lack of trained anaesthesia staff for assistance, ask other theatre staff or the surgeon to stay with you during these critical phases. Working alone is neither safe nor allowed.

14.4.5 Rapid Sequence Induction

Rapid sequence induction (RSI) is indicated in patients with a full stomach, e.g. the infant for pyloromyotomy due to pyloric stenosis, or laparotomy because of obstructed inguinal hernia, acute appendicitis, or ileus (bowel obstruction), and for acute patients after trauma. After trauma, gastric motility is impaired, so RSI applies even if the patient has not been eating during the past 6 h.

Risks in the RSI situation are higher than for elective intubation. The most experienced, available AP should always be the one to perform intubation after RSI. In patients with distended abdomen, an NGT should be inserted prior to anaesthesia induction and suction performed to empty the stomach.

There are two different approaches for RSI in infants and children: The classical approach is the same procedure as that for adults (see Sect. 6.7) with several minutes of preoxygenation via a tight-fitting face mask, applying cricoid pressure, nearly simultaneous injection of induction agent (propofol, thiopentone, or ketamine) and a rapidly acting muscle relaxant (usually suxamethonium), and intubation without manual ventilation before the ETT is in place and secured.

During recent years, a second approach of securing the airway when RSI is indicated has been established for children below 4–5 years: if no IV line yet, use a precordial stethoscope, pulse oximeter, and inhalational induction with halothane or sevoflurane in pure oxygen, and attach more monitoring (BP, ECG, and capnography if available). As soon as anaesthesia is deep enough, insert an IV cannula, start a drip, and administer IV anaesthetic and MR like suxamethonium, then gently ventilate with a peak pressure <10–15 cm H_2O, and intubate with optimum conditions in deep anaesthesia with sufficient muscle relaxation and a well-oxygenated patient. If the child has already a well-functioning IV line on arrival in the theatre, induction can be intravenous followed by gentle mask ventilation with 100% oxygen until the muscle relaxant is fully effective.

This second way of modified RSI has several advantages: Intubation is performed without cricoid pressure so that the view of the laryngeal entrance is not compromised. Intubation is performed with the full effect of MR. The chance of successful intubation with the first attempt is significantly higher than with the classical approach where the patient is more likely to desaturate because preoxygenation via a poorly fitting face mask in a patient who is uncooperative during induction was ineffective. No mask ventilation is performed with the classical approach, and saturation is already dropping so that the AP would not wait for the effect of suxamethonium and is handicapped by cricoid pressure. The outcome may be a patient who is not successfully intubated but hypoxic. The smaller the patient, the higher the risk. Plan in advance which approach will be best in the given situation.

14.4.6 Laryngospasm, Bronchospasm, and Post-Extubation Stridor

Always call immediately for help if there is a problem with breathing/ventilation/oxygenation of a patient. During anaesthesia induction and immediately or shortly after extubation, there is a risk for airway obstruction, especially in neonates and infants as their airways are small and narrow so that any further narrowing would lead to severe respiratory insufficiency or failure, most often caused by laryngospasm or bronchospasm. Patients with recent airway infections or with a history of asthma are especially at risk. Bronchospasm can also be caused by allergic or anaphylactoid reactions (which can even be caused, e.g. by antibiotics or some anaesthesia drugs and muscle relaxants). Laryngospasm can also occur if anaesthesia is too light. LMA does not prevent from getting laryngospasm, while ETT does. Closure of the glottis may occur within seconds as a reflex that shall prevent the entry of secretion into the trachea. Any irregular breathing or coughing can be an early sign of laryngospasm. Get anaesthesia deeper, ideal with a small dose of propofol. Later symptoms are stridor or chest and diaphragm retractions like paradoxical breathing. Saturation drops a bit later. It is important to immediately diagnose the problem and take action as the condition is potentially life-threatening if untreated. Prevention: Adequate depth of anaesthesia during any kind of surgical or airway stimulation. Suction and clear the throat from secretions prior to extubation. Removing the endotracheal tube or laryngeal mask airway when the patient is fully awake is the best prevention. Treatment: Apply manual ventilation via tightly fitting face mask with positive pressure and pure oxygen. Jaw thrust and a nasopharyngeal airway, sometimes oropharyngeal airway may be helpful. If the situation does not improve within a minute, or saturation drops further/patient looks bluish, consider atropine 0.02 mg/kg plus suxamethonium 0.5–1 mg/kg IV. In the situation of lacking IV access, give suxamethonium as injection sublingually, alternatively IM (IM onset of effect is a few minutes delayed compared with sublingual injection when the onset of effect is nearly as fast as after IV injection). Within a minute after suxamethonium, ventilation should be possible and be continued until the patient is breathing sufficiently himself. As soon as ventilation is possible, avoid too high ventilation pressure but hyperventilate with a high respiratory rate to get rid of the high end-tidal CO_2. In rare cases, reintubation is needed. Before the second attempt of extubation, consider 1 mg/kg lidocaine IV. Hypoxia may lead to cardiac arrest. If that happens, ventilate with 100% oxygen, call for help, start chest compressions at a rate of 100–120/min, and continue ventilation. One person alone gives 30 compressions followed by 2 inflations with 4 cycles per min. Two persons give 15 compressions followed by 2 inflations with 8 cycles/min. If the patient is intubated, compressions are not interrupted by ventilation so that a higher ventilation rate, dependent on the patient's age, can be achieved. Give atropine and repeated doses of adrenaline 0.01 mg/kg (10 μg/kg) every 3–5 min (see Sect. 14.8 for dilution of adrenaline).

Laryngospasm can even occur during ketamine anaesthesia with spontaneous breathing. Airway and respiratory drive are usually unaffected by ketamine, and the patient remains able to swallow and cough, and ketamine has a bronchodilating effect. Airway reflexes, however, are increased so that laryngospasm is possible, especially if procedures are performed in the mouth or oesophagus (e.g. removal of foreign body) when little secretion reaches the larynx entrance. Ketamine is therefore not well suitable for such procedures. Airway equipment, bag ventilation, oxygen, and suxamethonium should be available even if anaesthesia is planned with spontaneous breathing.

Post-extubation croup is a more serious and more seldom complication with initially similar symptoms as laryngospasm. It is caused by oedema of the larynx or trachea as a consequence of intubation, e.g. with too large ETT which was forced into the trachea or after repeated attempts for intubation. The condition is life-threatening if untreated. The patient needs oxygen, if possible, humidified. Sedation is needed with low doses of diazepam, midazolam, or propofol if the child is already awake and obviously stressed. Give adrenaline 1 mg (1 ml 1:1000) through a nebuliser. Repeat treatment, if necessary. Or put 2.5 ml adrenaline 1:1000 into the nebuliser for infants <1 year and 5 ml above 1 year. Up to 400 μg/kg BW adrenaline total dose may be needed. Give hydrocortisone 10 mg/kg or dexamethasone 0.5 mg/kg IV. In cases with severe hypoxia, reintubation with a smaller tube may be indicated and needs to be performed by the most experienced, available anaesthetist. The patient must be intubated for several hours until dexamethasone is fully effective. Gently ventilate manually and monitor oxygen saturation. The patient should be treated in the operation theatre unless a fully equipped PICU is available. Before extubation, have a team of experienced APs and two assistants at the patient's bedside.

If cardiac arrest occurs caused by hypoxia: call for help, start chest compressions, ventilate with 100% oxygen (30:2 compressions: breaths like in adults), atropine 0.02 mg/kg once, and adrenaline 10 μg/kg every 3–5 min. Aim for intubation provided the correct size of ETT and laryngoscope are available. Unfortunately, the prognosis is usually poor once a cardiac arrest has occurred.

14.5 Perioperative IV Fluid Management and Blood Transfusion

14.5.1 Venous Access

Peripheral venous cannulation can be challenging in infants and small children due to size, poor visibility of veins through fat in a chubby infant, vasoconstriction in hypovolaemia, or patients not being cooperative. Ultrasound devices for facilitating cannulation with veins made visible are more and more popular but still expensive. In not anaesthetised children, the use of a special local anaesthetic cream like EMLA® or Ametop® 1 h before intended cannulation is helpful but not available everywhere and may add to the costs for the parents.

Keep the needle out of sight of the child, but tell them something like "it hurts a little" when you proceed with it. Have the child distracted by the caregiver or an assistant and have an assistant holding it and keeping the limb immobile and congested. Rapid securing with good tape is essential before the child is moving. Test the cannula with a flush of NS. Small needles do not always show backflow of blood, so, initially, it may be difficult to know if cannulation was successful.

Sizes of the venous cannula for children are 24–20 gauge, but, for neonates, 26 G is sometimes best fitting. Max flow per min is approximately 12–13 ml/min for 26 G (purple), 15–20 ml/min for 24 G (yellow), 30–36 ml/min for 22 G (blue), and 60 ml/min for 20 G (pink).

Some special sites can be used for cannulation in infants: Scalp veins are often prominent but may require shaving of part of the hair. Remember that blood flow is always directed towards the heart, so from the scalp veins in the direction to the neck not the opposite way.

In anaesthetised infants, the veins on the feet can also be used.

External jugular vein cannulation is used in sick children or children with severe dehydration or anaemia. It is usually well visible. Put a small pillow or roll under the chest and have the neck and head extended with a slightly head-done position and the head turned to the other side. You need to create a horizontal line from the site of needle insertion into the vein. This vein is a central vein but accessible with a standard venous cannula. Aseptic technique is required. The assistant must keep the head and neck immobile. A finger may occlude the vein just above the clavicle to get it congested. The cannula is advanced when the backflow of blood is visible. Often this is not the case, but the vein is transfixed. Then the inner steel is withdrawn partly, and the cannula is slowly drawn back until blood is visible and thereafter advanced into the vein. Correct placement is proven by gentle aspiration of blood with a 2-ml syringe while keeping the vein somewhat extended and flushing with NS. Blood samples can also be obtained from this vein. It is not easy to secure a jugular cannula in a moving child who may be sweating. Use the best tape available. A short venous line extension with a three-way stopcock and optional non-return valve (which needs to be removed before desired blood aspiration for sampling), prefilled with saline, is very useful and should be connected, placed in a half-moon shape, and then secured with tape (steri-strips® or fixomull® stretch are very good); then, infusion or blood transfusion can be connected. If venous access is needed for several days, fixation may be with skin sutures. Often, infusion is only going if the head is turned to the contralateral side. In a freely moving child, the infusion is often not dripping. Therefore, this type of venous access is for emergencies, such as the sick and apathetic child, the child in shock, and perioperatively. It can very easily disconnect, and infusion may then run subcutaneously. Close observation is necessary. Air embolism must carefully be avoided as it may cause arrhythmia, cardiac arrest, or cerebral embolism. All syringes and lines must be filled without air bubbles before connecting to the venous cannula.

Femoral vein cannulation is another method of central venous access, especially in neonates and infants. For children >1 year, venous cannulae are often too short. Special catheters are needed for femoral vein access in larger patients. In some patients, the femoral vein is located behind the artery making cannulation almost impossible. The femoral catheter can be used for several days. Kinking or displacement due to movement of the legs and displacement during changing of diapers and cleaning are possible. Infection risk is high if the patient has diarrhoea. The patient must be immobile during insertion. Unless the patient is apathetic, short GA is required which can be administered with ketamine IM. A small role is placed under the hips plus slight abduction and outwards rotation.

Procedure: A head-up position of 30° enables venous congestion in the legs. An assistant may gently apply pressure between the umbilicus and the inguinal region. Draw a line from the anterior iliac spine to the symphysis pubis (inguinal ligament). Notably, 1–2 cm below the midline of that ligament, the femoral artery is palpated, and the cannula is inserted just medial to the artery with a 45° angle. Have a small syringe attached to the needle and aspirate continuously. Do not advance the needle more than 2.5 cm because of the risk of injury to the intestine or the hip joint. If blood is aspirated and freely flowing out of the cannula when the syringe is removed, the cannula can be advanced further and secured. A short line extension with a three-way stopcock and no-return valve is ideally connected between the cannula and infusion. Instead of or additionally to tape, sutures can be used for fixation. If no blood is aspirated from the syringe and the needle is advanced 2.5 cm, remove the syringe, assume transfixation of the vein, slowly withdraw the needle under continuous gentle aspiration until blood is coming, and then advance the cannula.

Air embolism must carefully be avoided as it may cause arrhythmia, cardiac arrest, or cerebral embolism (same risk as with jugular vein access). Internal jugular or subclavian vein access is only possible with special, sterile sets for central venous catheters for insertion under sterile conditions with surgical drapes. The procedure should be performed ultrasound-guided and is beyond the scope of this book.

Intraosseous cannulation is used to gain venous access when other methods prove unsuccessful, and time is limited due to an emergency. It can only be used short-term, not more than 24 h. Complications: wrong placement not inside the bone marrow but subcutaneously or subperiostally. Infection is possible if sterility is impaired during insertion or used for longer than 24 h. Injury of nearby structures is rare but possible; the most feared is injury of the growth plate which could stop the growth of the bone (tibia). See Fig. 14.2 for landmarks and correct placement.

Specially designed intraosseous needles in different sizes are available. If they are not stocked, for infants, a 19 G butterfly needle, a blood transfusion access needle, or, in children >1 year, a large bore venous cannula can be used instead. The main disadvantages are the length of

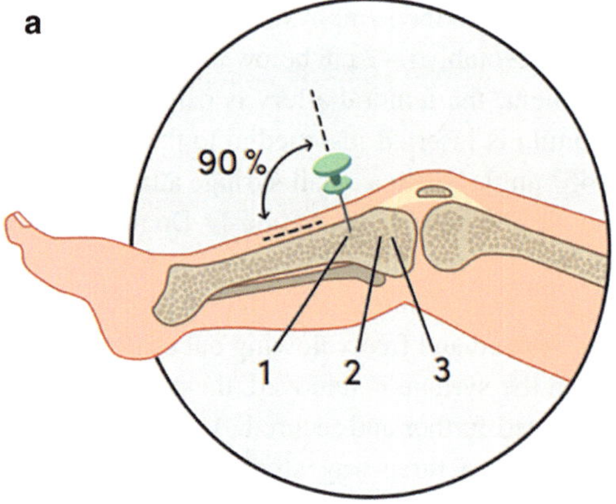

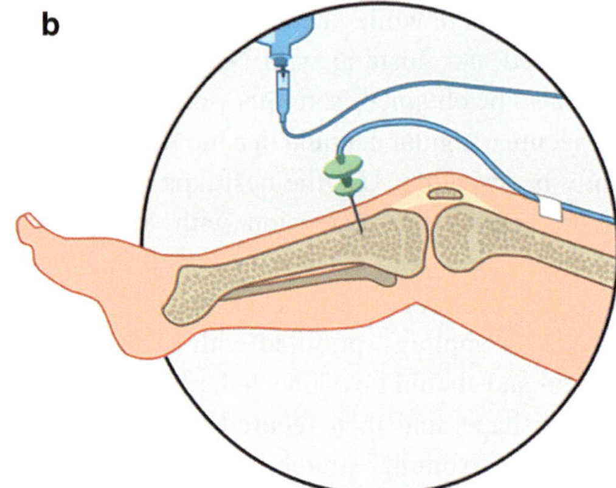

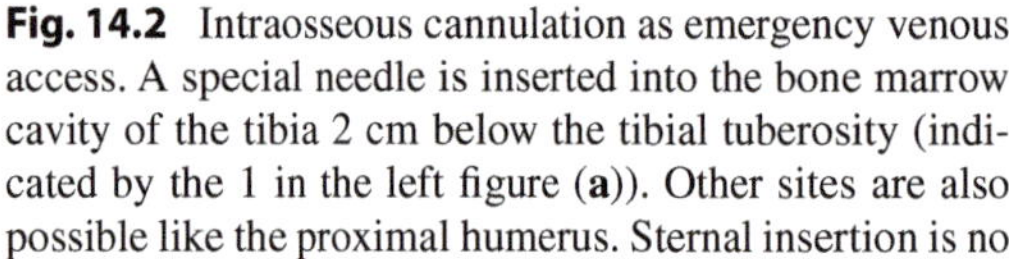

Fig. 14.2 Intraosseous cannulation as emergency venous access. A special needle is inserted into the bone marrow cavity of the tibia 2 cm below the tibial tuberosity (indicated by the 1 in the left figure (**a**)). Other sites are also possible like the proximal humerus. Sternal insertion is no longer recommended. 2 = tibial tuberosity and 3 = tibial growth plate. Right figure (**b**) shows the infusion connected to the cannula with fixation of the infusion line on the thigh by adhesive tape

Table 14.3 Distribution of water in % of body weight (BW)

	ECF (extracellular fluid)	ICF (intracellular fluid)	Plasma volume as % of body weight	Total body water as % of body weight
Neonate	35	40	5	80
Infant	30	40	5	75
Adult	20	40	5	65

the large bore cannulae and difficulty securing without kinking. Intraosseous cannulation is very painful. Either the child is unconscious, or ketamine IM 3 mg/kg should be administered prior to cannulation. Preparation and skin disinfection can be performed immediately after ketamine has been injected.

The needle is placed perpendicular to the bone surface under constant pressure with a rotational, screwing movement. When a sudden loss of resistance if felt, remove the inner steel needle (in case of a venous cannula) or unscrew the cap of the special needle and confirm the correct position by aspirating blood/bone marrow. Sometimes, aspiration is impossible in spite of the correct needle position. Flush with 10 ml saline. If that is easy, and no swelling is visible, use the cannula. The correct position is also indicated by the needle keeping its position 90° to the bone when unsupported. It is easier to secure the infusion line rather than the needle itself with adhesive tape. A short connector with a three-way stopcock is advantageous and must be prefilled with saline or infusion.

14.5.2 Fluid Management and Blood Transfusion

Small infants have more total body water than adults and the turnover of fluid is higher. Dehydration can develop more quickly if intake and losses are not balanced. The higher percentage of total body water is only due to increased extracellular fluid volume, while the intracellular space is almost equal to that in adults per kg BW. Blood volume per kg is also higher in small children (see Tables 14.3 and 14.4). Normal blood volume is 90 ml/kg at birth, 80 ml/kg in infants, and 75 ml/kg until 8 years, thereafter around 70 ml/kg BW.

Baseline Fluid Requirements Different fluid schedules and formulas are used for calculating

Table 14.4 Weight-based fluid and dextrose amounts for baseline infusion perioperatively and blood volumes of children

BW (kg)	Dextrose 5% in NS (ml/h) (DNS)	RL (ml/h)	Total infusion (ml/h)	ml of total blood volume	Max ml allowable blood loss without transfusion	Amount of 20 ml/kg blood transfusion (ml)
1	6	NA	6	100	25	20
1.5	9	NA	9	140	35	30
3	12	NA	12	270	70	60
5	20	NA	20	425	150	100
8	20	12	32	640	240	160
10	20	20	40	800	300	200
15	20	30	50	1200	450	300
20	NA	60	60	1400	550	400
30	NA	70	70	2100	800	600

Maximum allowed blood loss before transfusion is estimated for normal Hb before bleeding. As a rough estimate, 20 ml/kg transfusion of packed red blood cells is adequate; the respective number is given in the table. However, for larger children, not always 20 ml/kg of blood needs to be transfused; half that amount will often do provided that the remaining loss is replaced with crystalloids like NS/RL. *NA* not applicable. Note that a combination of DNS and RL would provide a sufficient but not too large amount of glucose for infusion

perioperative fluid requirements. Larger children do not need glucose infusion routinely during operation. Hyperglycaemia must also be avoided as it causes harm. On the contrary, small infants and especially preterm neonates do need uninterrupted glucose intake as they are prone to hypoglycaemia which may cause damage to the CNS. Table 14.4 gives the needed glucose amount calculated for dextrose 5%. *Infusions need to contain salt as well.* It is potentially dangerous to give dextrose 5% without any electrolytes perioperatively. The example in the table is DNS, containing 5% dextrose in NS. Other combinations of glucose and normal saline, e.g. half normal saline (NS 0.45%) with glucose = 1/2 NS dextrose 5% or with dextrose 2.5%, are also available but not ideal during surgery because of too little sodium. In some countries, Plasmalyte A or Benelyte, a combination of Ringeracetate with a little glucose (around 1%), is used perioperatively for children except neonates who need a higher concentration of glucose. *Glucose requirements for infants <3 kg are 5 mg/kg/min.*

Table 14.4 gives the basal fluid and glucose requirements and as an example the maximum acceptable blood loss if Hb before bleeding is normal, around 12 g/dl (120 g/l), which means Hb 7–8 g/dl (70–80 g/l) after blood loss. Preterm infants have higher Hb (up to 19 g/dl, 190 g/l) and are dependent on higher Hb values. They must not drop Hb below 12–14 g/dl (120–140 g/l). The amounts of blood loss and transfusion in the table are estimated accordingly. Of course, the minimum Hb also depends on the general condition of the child and disease state. Fluid losses during operations need to be added into the calculation and replaced with NS or RL/Plasmalyte® or, in case of blood loss, partly with albumin or FFP. The amounts of Dextrose and RL are suggestions and aim to prevent hypoglycaemia and keep a normal plasma concentration of sodium. From the age of approximately 2 years, intraoperative infusion of glucose is no longer necessary unless the child is fasting very long or is malnourished. Postoperatively, all children should receive glucose- and salt-containing infusions until they are allowed to eat. Maintenance requirements of fluids are approximately 100 ml/kg BW per day <5 years and 60–80 ml/kg/day >6 years.

***Drip rate during anaesthesia*:** Too fast infusion should be avoided in order to prevent fluid overload. During the first hour of anaesthesia, around 5 ml/kg/h is appropriate + replacement of losses. For maintenance, give around 3 ml/kg/h + replacement of losses, e.g. from drainage or from NGT. Table 14.4 shows the exact amounts of fluid based on BW. If available, use paediatric infusion sets or infusion pumps to administer exact volumes. Adult infusion giving sets: 1 ml is equal to 20 drops and paediatric infusion set: 60 drops/ml.

If paediatric infusion sets or infusion pumps are unavailable and adult infusion giving sets must be used, Table 14.5 helps you to administer the correct amount of fluid. It is also useful to mark the volume to be infused per hour on the infusion bottle with a pen. The basal fluid requirements are given in the table and are average approximations. Any losses of fluids or bleeding during or after surgery or increased requirements due to fever or vomiting must be added. It is easier and more exact to inject the required fluid volumes slowly at set intervals in small infants below 5 kg (record the given amounts together with the time on a form at the bedside) than to have an uncontrolled drip running.

Fluid deficits need to be replaced with NS, RL, or similar. Patients with fever, bowel obstruction, or vomiting, after trauma with blood loss or with burns, need to be checked for signs of dehydration: tachycardia, low urine output (nappies/diapers do not need to be changed often), few or no tears when they cry, sunken eyes, sunken fontanelle, CRT > 2 s prolonged, weak pulse, lethargy, and decreased skin turgor. Patients with fluid losses should be weighed daily to calculate fluid balance and changing infusion requirements.

Table 14.5 Drip rate during anaesthesia if adult infusion giving sets are used

Bodyweight (kg)	Initial drip rate (drops/min)/(ml/h)	Maintenance rate (drops/min)/(ml/h)
<5	9 drops/min 25 ml/h	5 drops/min 15 ml/h
5–10	18 drops/min 50 ml/h	10 drops/min 30 ml/h
11–15	30 drops/min 90 ml/h	15 drops/min 45 ml/h
16–20	35 drops/min 100 ml/h	20 drops/min 60 ml/h
21–30	50 drops/min 150 ml/h	27 drops/min 80 ml/h
>30	80 drops/min 250 ml/h	30 drops/min 90 ml/h

14.5.3 Blood Transfusion

Before starting anaesthesia, calculate the appropriate size of units for blood transfusion according to the BW of the patient and let units be prepared with a volume of 10 ml/kg BW. For small patients, adult blood units can be split in the lab to create several units from the same donor which can be transfused on demand. Each such unit of packed RBC would increase Hb by around 2 g/dl (20 g/l). Leukocyte reduction and irradiation of erythrocyte concentrates are recommended for children and infants to reduce the risk for dangerous transfusion reactions related to white blood cells and transmission of the cytomegalovirus.

14.6 The Conduct of General Anaesthesia

14.6.1 Induction of Anaesthesia for Major Surgery

Thiopentone (alternative propofol, see below) is used for IV induction of anaesthesia if insertion of LM or ETT is planned. Doses of 3–5 mg/kg for combination with ketamine, fentanyl, or volatile anaesthestic (mask induction and then insertion of the venous cannula); higher doses of 5–6 mg/kg thiopentone are required as sole induction agent before intubation. Intubation is facilitated with a dose of muscle relaxant, e.g. 1.5–2 mg/kg ***suxamethonium,*** or a non-depolarising NMBA, e.g. 0.1 mg/kg ***vecuronium*** or 0.5 mg/kg ***atracurium***. Many anaesthesiologists worldwide do not like to use suxamethonium because of its potential side effects, but this is controversial, and it is still good clinical practise to use the drug. However, with atropine premedication and considering contraindications (burns, any muscle or neuromuscular disease, and history of MH), suxamethonium is safe, and the great advantages are fast onset and short duration of action; patients are able to breathe spontaneously again within few minutes while, after longer-acting MR, the AP must ventilate the patient for at least 45 min. Additionally, before extubation, long-acting MR needs to be reversed with atropine 0.02 mg/kg and neostigmine 0.05 mg/kg which may cause PONV in patients >2 years. If available, PONV may be prevented by 0.1 mg/kg ondansetrone or other antiemetic agents (more details in Sect. 7.10). Succinylcholine/suxamethonium 2 mg/kg may even be given IM in combination with atropine in case of difficult venous access after mask induction with a volatile anaesthetic. ***Atropine*** 0.015–0.02 mg/kg (max 0.5 mg) is recommended as the first drug to be injected during induction in order to decrease the risk for bradycardia, reflex asystole, and reflex airway obstruction. With a short onset of action within 1 min after IV injection, atropine is also effective within 3 min after IM injection (in case of difficult venous access and inhalational induction).

Propofol is very popular in most countries and sometimes used even in patients where thiopentone or ***ketamine*** would be better. For the AP, propofol is easier to use as it is ready for injection while thiopentone is a powder and needs a few minutes to dissolve. For emergency patients with blood or fluid losses, ketamine is advantageous as it produces vasoconstriction and increases heart rate. The dissolved thiopentone, however, is stable and remains sterile for more than 24 h as an advantage compared with propofol. Often, leftovers in propofol ampoules or vials must be discarded since they must not be used after 12 h because bacteria would multiply quickly in the fatty acid emulsion of propofol. That applies even if propofol is stored in a fridge. If you have only one of the three induction agents propofol, thiopentone, and ketamine, you may use it for almost all patients (for contraindications, see Chap. 7). If you have all these drugs, use propofol for IV induction only for children >2 years and in all patients with risk for PONV. Use a relatively large cannula, placed preferably in a large cubital vein if possible. Propofol may be mixed with 1 ml of lidocaine 10 mg/ml (1%) or 0.5 ml lidocaine 20 mg/ml (2%) per 10 ml propofol to reduce pain on injection. Lidocaine is even useful in preventing laryngeal reflexes. Combination with a strong analgesic, such as fentanyl 1 μg/kg or ketamine 0.5–1 mg/kg, produces better-quality anaesthesia. The induction dose of propofol for children is 3–4 mg/kg. For neonates, the dose is reduced to 2 mg/kg; however, propofol is not well suitable for small infants. Propofol causes vasodilatation and decreased cardiac output and may thereby cause hypotension. Propofol can also be used to facilitate intubation or LMA insertion for children if induction is with inhalation, so they would not feel pain on injection. Especially in small veins, propofol may cause severe pain during injection. A child who remembers that pain is likely to refuse future anaesthetics. Thiopentone, on the contrary, is unlikely to cause pain on injection, and the remaining dose in the vial will not get contaminated and can be used later for other patients. Thiopentone in a smaller dose of 3 mg/kg can safely be used for premature infants <3 kg as it shows milder cardiovascular side effects than propofol. The same is true for *ketamine*; however, the combination of ketamine and halothane may cause severe cardiac depression in neonates and infants with cardiac disease and should be avoided. Ketamine for induction instead of thiopentone or propofol is given at 2 mg/kg IV for children >6 months and 1 mg/kg below 6 months.

Inhalational induction with halothane or sevoflurane is suitable if IV access is not established before induction. Isoflurane is not suitable for mask induction as it has a very unpleasant odour and irritates the airways, and patients may stop breathing during induction without getting adequate depth of anaesthesia. The rapid uptake of inhalational anaesthetics compared with adults is due to increased ventilation, low FRC (functional residual capacity of the lungs), and increased cardiac output.

All inhalational anaesthetics produce different *stages of anaesthesia:*

Stage 1: Amnesia, analgesia, sedation. This earliest stage lasts from a minute after beginning induction until loss of consciousness. At this moment, the parent/caregiver must leave the operation theatre.

Stage 2: excitement; uncontrolled movement, increased breathing rate, widened pupils, eyes looking in divergent directions (breath holding, coughing, laryngospasm, or vomiting are complications during this stage that can be prevented by NOT stimulating the patient with cannulation or inserting oropharyngeal airway). During stage 2, the aim is to deepen anaesthesia quickly and not to stimulate the patient.

Stage 3: surgical anaesthesia with small to normal size pupils and fixed eyes, no eyelid reflex, no movements, decreasing but still sufficient breathing rate, and some muscle relaxation; the patient needs chin lift or jaw thrust/oropharyngeal airway may be needed, and after cannulation and giving atropine, muscle relaxant and analgesic like ketamine 1 mg/kg intubation can be performed.

Stage 4 is called asphyxia and is to be avoided. It means overdose causing respiratory arrest and circulatory collapse.

How to perform inhalational induction of anaesthesia: Start with pure oxygen via a face mask and add halothane/sevoflurane stepwise. Halothane: 0.5% at the vaporiser and then every 3–5 breaths increase by 0.5% until 2.5% is reached. Gently provide a chin lift and keep the airway free. Halothane may take up to 10 min until anaesthesia is deep enough for insertion of an IV cannula, and another 5–10 min until intubation can be performed unless IV anaesthetics are added, which is more common and safer. Sevoflurane: start with 1.5% at the vaporiser and increase every 3 breaths to 3%, 4.5%, and 6%. With sevoflurane, induction is a bit faster than with halothane but would also take several minutes. If manual ventilation is performed during induction, the risk of overdose is higher than with spontaneous breathing. Avoid "bagging" the patient with high concentration at the vaporiser. Cardiac failure and even arrest can occur. Never forget to reduce the concentration at the vaporiser immediately after stage 3 is reached or after intubation/insertion of the laryngeal mask airway and during the prolonged phase of IV cannulation.

The MAC and therefore the required concentration at the vaporiser is increased compared with adults because the immature brain is less sensitive to the anaesthetic effects of these agents. On the contrary, the side effects on the cardiovascular system and respiratory drive are not less than in older patients, so the required concentration of the volatile agent needs to be carefully titrated. Especially halothane in neonates does often depress the heart, and cardiac output would decrease markedly while the anaesthesia may still be not deep enough. Sevoflurane and isoflurane (after IV induction) are safer for small infants than halothane, but the safety margin for all inhalational agents is significantly reduced. All volatile anaesthetics can cause malignant hyperthermia which is a very rare but often deadly complication and must not be used in children with known neuromuscular disease, especially muscular dystrophy, or a family history of malignant hyperthermia. Nitrous oxide is the only inhalational anaesthetic that does not cause MH, but it is not used much nowadays.

Intubation without muscle relaxant is possible for elective patients with no difficult airway anticipated. After induction with halothane or sevoflurane, 2–3 mg/kg propofol is injected, inhalation anaesthetic continued, and 60 s later the trachea is intubated.

Opioids during induction: In combination with ***fentanyl*** 1 µg/kg or ketamine 1 mg/kg as a strong analgesic, the doses of thiopentone and propofol may be reduced by around 25%. ***Morphine*** has a slow onset of action and is therefore not suitable as analgesic for intubation but is effective as an intraoperative analgesic instead of fentanyl or incremental doses of ketamine. A single dose of 0.1–0.2 mg/kg is given after anaesthesia induction and will provide some postoperative analgesia as well due to its long duration of action. Opioids like fentanyl or morphine should be omitted in premature infants up to the age of 6 months after birth for increased risk of postoperative respiratory depression. If opioids are used for children >2 years, when the vomiting centre is mature, an ***antiemetic*** drug should be given as prophylaxis during anaesthesia, e.g. promethazine 1 mg/kg, ondansetrone 0.1 mg/kg, or dexamethasone 0.1 mg/kg. Promethazine may cause a long-lasting sedative effect that has to be considered if it is used instead of other antiemetics.

14.6.2 Maintenance of Anaesthesia

Maintenance can be with inhalational or intravenous agents or both (as balanced anaesthesia) using the same drugs as for adults.

IV Maintenance Ketamine as a sole anaesthetic agent can be used for maintenance during major surgery, approximately 5 mg/kg/h during the first hour and 2.5 mg/kg during the second hour of surgery. For children >30 kg, it can be given as an infusion with 1 mg/ml (500 mg ketamine into a 500 ml infusion) at a drip rate of around 1.5 drops per kg/min (use the timer or stop-watch function of your mobile phone). For smaller children or to avoid overdose if no infusion pump is available, ketamine may be injected in small incremental doses of 0.5 mg/kg every 6 min (use a timer!) during surgery until 30 min before the end of the operation. Combine with diazepam 0.1 mg/kg and promethazine 0.5–1 mg/kg as single doses in the beginning to prevent agitation and nightmares during recovery.

TIVA with Propofol Total intravenous anaesthesia (TIVA) with propofol infusion and a strong analgesic like ketamine 2–4 mg/kg/h or fentanyl 0.001–0.002 mg/kg/h is an alternative to inhalational anaesthesia. Propofol dose for TIVA: Induction with 3–4 mg/kg, followed by 15 mg/kg/h for 10 min, then 10 mg/kg/h for another 10 min, and then 6–8 mg/kg/h for maintenance up to 10 min before the end of surgery. Ketamine can be administered as a continuous infusion with a syringe pump. Fentanyl is given as intermittent bolus doses. Postoperative observation in a recovery unit with oxygen and pulse oximetry available is mandatory. TIVA is indicated for patients with an increased risk for malignant hyperthermia and as a general alternative to inhalation anaesthesia. Special equipment is needed: syringe pumps, special syringes fitting to the pumps and lines, and three-way stopcocks, all of which the AP must be familiar with.

Fentanyl 1–2 μg/kg (=0.001–0.002 mg/kg) is suitable as an intraoperative analgesic for most surgical procedures (as part of balanced or total intravenous anaesthesia) and for induction of anaesthesia in combination with a hypnotic drug. Onset after 2–3 min, duration 30–60 min, risk for accumulation. Fentanyl produces no effects on haemodynamics but profound respiratory depression, especially after repeated doses. A total amount of 2 μg/kg should be regarded maximum if the patient is planned to be nursed in the normal ward soon after surgery. The drug should be used for small infants only by experienced paediatric anaesthetists, and the patient must be ventilated after fentanyl has been administered. Infants must be monitored after extubation because of the risk of prolonged respiratory depression. Premature neonates <44 weeks of gestation must not be extubated if they get any fentanyl but stay intubated in the NICU until fully awake. Fentanyl must not be given to neonates or previous premature infants <6 months of age if a fully equipped NICU is not available.

14.6.3 Inhalational Anaesthesia

The different inhalational agents have different potency, halothane being strongest, followed by isoflurane and then sevoflurane, and nitrous oxide is very weak with a theoretical MAC of 105% which of course is impossible to apply. For safety, at least 30% of oxygen must be administered, leaving a maximum of 70% for N_2O at which this drug causes amnesia, sedation, and analgesia but not anaesthesia for surgery.

Nitrous oxide (N2O) which is delivered in cylinders and administered via calibrated flowmeter at the anaesthesia machine can be used in combination with IV anaesthetics or more potent inhalational agents for induction and maintenance. Not all anaesthesia machines are equipped with a flowmeter for N_2O. Nitrous oxide alone is not strong enough to produce a state of GA for surgery, but it causes amnesia and analgesia, and some sedation, and the doses of other anaesthetics can be reduced by around 50% if nitrous oxide is administered at a concentration of 60–70% in oxygen. Unfortunately, the drug, although used for anaesthesia for more than 150 years, is expensive, and it is not safe to use N_2O without reliable measuring of the inspired oxygen concentration to avoid hypoxic gas mixtures delivered to the patient. It does not irritate the airways and has a sweet smell. Therefore, it is better tolerated for mask induction than sevoflurane or halothane if the child is not premedicated. The combination of nitrous oxide and halothane produces a faster uptake of halothane, and a surgical level of anaesthesia is achieved earlier. Recommendation for inhalational induction if N_2O available: Begin with oxygen and nitrous oxide (around 70%) for at least 1 min, and when loss of eye contact and nystagmus indicates that light anaesthesia is achieved, add halothane or sevoflurane. Before intubation, turn off nitrous oxide and give 100% oxygen for 2 min. After intubation or insertion of a laryngeal mask, N_2O may be continued, or, to save money and in case no oxygen monitor is available, do not continue with N_2O. The only significant side effect of N_2O is increased risk for PONV, which may be another reason not to use it for maintenance of anaesthesia but only for induction. It is contraindicated for operations in the middle ear and for craniotomies because it would increase the volume of air-filled spaces.

Halothane has a pleasant smell and is well suitable for inhalational induction and for maintenance of anaesthesia. It is by far the cheapest inhalational agent (several times cheaper than isoflurane and sevoflurane) as it is not only cheaper to buy but also the consumption per hour of anaesthesia is much less than with the other agents. The negative impact on global warming is many times less than with other inhalational anaesthetics. Contraindications: Raised intracranial pressure (e.g. in head trauma), severe cardiac disease, liver disease, and circulatory shock. About 20% are metabolised in the liver; however, severe halothane-associated liver disease is extremely rare in children even after repeated exposure. *The minimum alveolar, anaesthetic concentration (MAC) is higher than in adults: neonates 1%, infants 1.2%, and children 1% (adults 0.75%).* For maintenance of anaesthesia with inhalational agents, around 1.5 MAC is needed, e.g. 1.5% of halothane. Halothane may lead to cardiac failure and cardiac arrest when given in overdose, especially in neonates. Therefore, a pulse oximeter and precordial stethoscope are mandatory (the volume of heart sounds correlates well with cardiac output; if heart sounds become quiet, switch off halothane or reduce the dose at the vaporiser significantly). It is highly recommended that, whenever possible, the anaesthesia monitor should be equipped with ECG, blood pressure measurement, and measurement of anaesthesic gas concentrations as well as capnography (end-tidal CO_2).

In small infants, using a precordial stethoscope is very important. The heart sounds would die away if the cardiac output was decreasing. Systolic blood pressure is a useful indirect measure for CO in infants. If a small BP cuff is available, take BP every 5 min.

Never forget to reduce halothane concentration at the vaporiser a few minutes after induction and whenever the heart sounds quiet, the SPO_2 reading is poor, or SBP <70 mmHg.

Isoflurane irritates the airway and is not suited for mask induction but for maintenance. During emergence and shortly after extubation, there is risk of breathholding and laryngospasm. Isoflurane produces less cardiac side effects than halothane; therefore, it should be preferred for maintenance anaesthesia in small infants if available. It is more expensive than halothane but much cheaper than sevoflurane. If the anaesthesia machine is equipped with two vaporisers, induction can be with halothane or sevoflurane, and isoflurane can be used for maintenance. *MAC: premature neonates 1.3%, neonates 1.6%, infants 1.9%, children 1.6%, and adults 1.2%.* Isoflurane can also be used for neurosurgery, e.g. insertion of a ventriculoperitoneal shunt in infants with hydrocephalus, or in cases with increased intracranial pressure like subdural haematoma evacuation after head injury with a maximum dose of 1–1.2 MAC (e.g. infant 1–1.2 × 1.9 = 1.9–2.3%).

Sevoflurane is very expensive and therefore often used for musk induction only. Its low blood solubility makes uptake and recovery rapid. Excitation and agitation during recovery occur more frequently than with isoflurane or halothane. It responds well to small doses of propofol

(0.5 mg/kg) or, if the patient is likely to suffer from pain to opioids such as tramadol, pethidine, and morphine. In rare cases of severe agitation, 2 mg/kg thiopentone or 1 mg/kg propofol IV is an effective treatment, but proper size SIB and face mask must be available. Sevoflurane causes less side effects to the circulation than halothane and can be used for neurosurgery including cases with increased intracranial pressure with a maximum dose of 1–1.2 MAC.

For induction, high concentrations of up to 6% are used. They must immediately be reduced to approximately 1.2–1.5 MAC after intubation; otherwise, there is a risk of cardiac failure or cardiac arrest. *1 MAC sevoflurane is equal to: neonates 3.3%, infants 3.2%, children 2.5%, and adults 2%.*

For maintenance, around 1.2–1.5 MAC is sufficient depending on the type of surgery. This dose can be reduced by around one-third if balanced anaesthesia is performed, that is, a combination of inhalation anaesthetic with IV analgesics such as ketamine or fentanyl plus a dose of an antiemetic such as ondansetrone 0.1 mg/kg, dexamethasone 0.1 mg/kg, or promethazine 0.5–1 mg/kg for children >2 years. Ketamine is advantageous as it preserves respiratory drive so that many patients can breathe spontaneously (with assistance and gentle manual ventilation if breathing shallow) for procedures not much longer than 1 h. Doses for fentanyl 1 μg/kg (0.001 mg) every 40 min up to 1 h before the end of surgery (for the duration of surgery <1 h only one dose) (controlled ventilation required) and ketamine 0.5–1 mg/kg every 10–20 min dependent on surgical stimulation. Ketamine may be given up to few minutes before the end of the surgery. Sevoflurane may react with *dry soda lime*. Dry soda lime, e.g. old soda lime, or soda lime after accidentally flushing with fresh gas overnight, must not be used. If sevoflurane reacts with it, soda lime gets hot, and due to a chemical reaction, sevoflurane would lose anaesthetic effect while being an irritant for the airways. Soda lime must be exchanged regularly. It is recommended every week or when the colour is changing to purple, or if capnography shows an inspiratory concentration of CO_2 >0.5%.

Muscle relaxation for surgery is sometimes necessary, depending on the type of operation and the experience of the surgeon. More than one dose of a long-acting MR should be avoided unless the child is admitted to a fully equipped ICU and delayed extubation is planned. It is often safer to increase the depth of anaesthesia, add a strong analgesic, or give a small dose of propofol instead of long-acting MR. Drugs such as diazepam or midazolam or volatile anaesthetics, especially isoflurane, also produce a central muscle relaxant effect. Experienced anaesthetists give repeated doses of suxamethonium 0.5 mg/kg during surgery, but only during special phases such as opening or closing of the peritoneum, or when the patient is pushing the intestine, and because of the risk for marked bradycardia always in combination with atropine 0.02 mg/kg once per hour. If a long-acting MR is to be used, atracurium 0.5 mg/kg, vecuronium 0.1 mg/kg, or pancuronium 0.1 mg/kg should be given once only (the same applies for tubocurarine 0.5 mg/kg). At the end of surgery, reversal with atropine 0.02 mg/kg and neostigmine 0.05 mg/kg IV is mandatory, but the patient can remain weak in spite of reversal agents. Carefully observe if the patient is coughing effectively and keeping eyes open before extubation.

14.6.4 Recovery from Anaesthesia

The speed of recovery or emergence from anaesthesia is dependent on the choice of the anaesthetic drugs used and the duration of surgery. Towards the end of the operation, gradually decrease the concentration at the vaporiser until it is switched off when the skin sutures are made. During emergence from inhalational anaesthesia, after the vaporiser has been switched off, the three phases are passed through in the opposite order from surgical anaesthesia through a phase of excitability with increased risk of laryngospasm and bronchospasm through the phase of amnesia and analgesia until the patient is fully awake. The excitation phase is clinically distinguished by wider pupils, divergent eye movements, and optional, uncoordinated movements.

However, these three phases of anaesthesia are not so clearly distinguishable if other anaesthetic agents are combined with inhalation agents as it is most often the case. After surgery near the patient's airways, e.g. adenectomy or tonsillectomy, it is safest to perform extubation in a lateral position with a pillow under the pelvis, and when fully awake. After most other procedures it is sufficient to wait until the patient is breathing spontaneously and keeping a free airway, meaning the ability to swallow and cough. Avoid extubation during the excitation phase after inhalation anaesthesia because of the very high risk of airway obstruction/laryngospasm. Recovery in a lateral position is advantageous. PONV, agitation, shivering, pain, restlessness, post-extubation stridor, or bronchospasm/laryngospasm may complicate the recovery phase. Patients should wake up in a calm environment and never be left alone, not even for seconds.

14.7 Postanaesthesia Care

14.7.1 Postoperative Observation

After surgery and extubation, the child is brought to the recovery area or, if the condition is critical, to a paediatric intensive care unit if available. Close observation is needed, and vital signs, treatment, infusions, and so on are recorded on an observation chart. A parent or caregiver should be at the bedside to reduce the stress for the child and to prevent the patient from falling from the bed. Pain, nausea, vomiting, postoperative complications of surgery like bleeding, and problems with breathing or circulation must be observed and treated accordingly. At the end of the surgery, prescription for analgesic drugs must be ready so that they can be administered by the AP and, later, by the nurses in the ward without delay. Nausea can be quite agonising and should be prevented if likely (with dexamethasone 0.1 mg/kg at anaesthesia induction) and treated if presenting. Drugs such as promethazine, droperidol, metoclopramide, and ondansetrone can be used IV or, later, orally (Chap. 7 for details). With any obvious or suspected bleeding after the operation, call the surgeon immediately and have saline or RL going IV. For difficulties in breathing, poor oxygen saturation, respiratory depression, weak pulse, and prolonged capillary refill time, immediately call the AP.

14.7.2 Postoperative Analgesia

Analgesia after operations is necessary but not always easy to provide. Even neonates can feel pain, but small infants cannot express their pain directly. Indirect signs such as crying, sweating, not drinking, and restlessness can also be caused by other distress than pain. Analgesic drugs can cause severe side effects that may be dangerous, especially if overdosed.

Wound infiltration with local anaesthetic drugs, analgesics such as paracetamol (acetaminophen), ibuprofen, diclofenac, and others, and opioid drugs such as pethidine (meperidine), tramadol, and morphine are the main pharmacological means. Specialists for paediatric anaesthesia use blocks such as caudal epidural or peripheral nerve blocks; however, these techniques are beyond the scope of this book. Additionally, to calm a child, to comfort and distract is also helpful. The presence of at least one parent or other caretaker with close relation to the child is essential and should be made possible even in recovery areas of operation theatres and in the PICU.

Most children are afraid of getting IM injections. Always use the smallest size of the injection needle and do not let them see the syringe. Skin disinfection of course is mandatory before injection to prevent infection/abscess.

As soon as possible after surgery, analgesics should be given orally or, if available as suppositories, rectally. In the recovery area and PICU, drugs can often be administered by IV instead of IM. However, most analgesics must be injected slowly or in small, titrated doses when given IV to avoid high peak concentrations in the blood causing nausea, respiratory depression, and other side effects such as hypotension or dizziness.

14.7.2.1 Wound Infiltration with Local Anaesthetic

At the end of the surgery, the surgeon may infiltrate the skin around the incision with local anaesthetic. This is highly effective after hernia repair, appendectomy, and some other procedures. Maximum doses of LA must be considered to avoid toxic side effects on the brain and heart (toxicity can lead to convulsions, coma, and cardiac arrest). The doses are given in Table 14.6. The following drugs are commonly used: lidocaine 10 mg/ml or bupivacaine 2.5 mg/ml. Lidocaine may be available as a 20 mg/ml solution only. In that case, it must be diluted for infants to avoid overdose. If possible, adrenaline 5 μg/ml should be added to lidocaine 10 mg/ml 10 mg/ml to extend its effect.

How to add adrenaline to lidocaine: Put 20 ml of lidocaine 2% (containing 20 mg/ml) in a small sterile bowl. Dilute adrenaline 1 ml plus 9 ml NS into a 10-ml syringe to make 0.1 mg/ml, and then add 2 ml of that dilution to the 20 ml of lidocaine. Add 18 ml NS *to make 40 ml of lidocaine 1% with adrenaline 5 μg/ml.* In some countries, lidocaine 1% with adrenaline is available as a mixture in 20 ml vials which must be stored in a fridge. The duration of analgesia is 1–6 h. The recommended maximum dose of lidocaine without adrenaline is 3 mg/kg and 7 mg/kg with adrenaline because adrenaline produces vasoconstriction and thus prolonged action and reduced absorption into blood circulation.

Table 14.6 Safe maximum doses of local anaesthetics in children given as ml dependent on body weight

Local anaesthetic	max ml LA: BW 3–5 kg	max ml LA: 6–10 kg	max ml LA: 11–15 kg	max ml LA: 16–20 kg	max ml LA: 21–30 kg
Lidocaine 10 mg/ml	1–1.5	2–3	3–4.5	5–6	7–9
Lidocaine 10 mg/ml with adrenaline	2.1–3.5	4.2–7	7.7–10.5	11.2–14	15–21
Bupivacaine 2.5 mg/ml	1.8–3	6–10	11–15	16–20	21–30
Bupivacaine 5 mg/ml	0.9–1.5	3–5	5.5–7.5	8–10	10.5–15

Alternatively, *bupivacaine* may be used (or other LA drugs). Bupivacaine has a longer duration of action and does not need adrenaline to be added. The maximum dose is 2.5 mg/kg and in neonates only 1.5 mg/kg. Bupivacaine 0.5% = 5 mg/ml should be diluted 1:1 ml to make 0.25%=2.5 mg/ml.

Pethidine (or *meperidine* as it is called in some countries) in ampoules with 50 mg/ml is a strong and effective analgesic drug which also has a sedative effect. The duration of action is approximately 4 h. 1 mg/kg IM or 0.5 mg/kg IV + 0.5 mg/kg IM at the end of painful major surgery when sufficient spontaneous breathing is regained and postoperative observation in a recovery unit with pulse oximetry and recording of breaths per minutes and pulse/BP are regularly done. For children < 20 kg BW, make a dilution of pethidine with 50 mg = 1 ml into a 5-ml syringe + 4 ml water for injection resulting in a concentration of 10 mg/ml. Then draw the required amount into a 2-ml syringe. Notably, 1 ml of that dilution is equal to 10 mg; 0.5 ml of the dilution is equal to 5 mg; and 0.25 ml of the dilution is equal to 2.5 mg. For doses, see Table 14.7. In an intermediate care unit or ICU, the drug can be repeated when required, e.g. every 2 h 0.5 mg/kg IV. In the peripheral ward, subsequent doses are usually injected IM at set intervals, 6 or 8 h. Respiratory depression can be a dangerous side effect if overdosed. Therefore, observe the infant at least 30 min after the IV injection of pethidine before sending it to the ordinary ward. Count respiratory rate/min. If possible, use a pulse oximeter, and give oxygen if required.

In countries with alternative strong opioids like morphine available, pethidine is no longer recommended as the first choice for children. In rare cases, its active metabolite may cause reversible neurotoxicity with tremor, myoclonus, hallucinations, agitation, or (very rare) seizures. Small infants and children with renal insufficiency are more prone to those side effects, and with higher doses of pethidine, the risk would increase.

Tramadol in ampoules with 50 mg/ml can be used the same way as pethidine and with the same

Table 14.7 Average doses of analgesic drugs

Bodyweight	Pethidine dose	Morphine dose	Diclofenac dose
Neonate-5 kg	2.5 mg (diluted)	0.25 mg (diluted)	Contraindicated
6–10 kg	5–10 mg (diluted)	0.5–1 mg (diluted)	12.5 mg = 0.5 ml
11–15 kg	10–20 mg (diluted)	1–2 mg (diluted)	12.5 mg = 0.5 ml
16–20 kg	15 mg (diluted)	1.5–3 mg (diluted)	25 mg = 1 ml
21–25 kg	25 mg = 0.5 ml	2.5–4 mg	25 mg = 1 ml
26–30 kg	25 mg = 0.5 ml	3 – 5 mg	37.5 mg = 1.5 ml
>30 kg	50 mg = 1 ml	5 – 6 mg	50 mg = 2 ml

Please note that opioids may be administered to infants and small children only if they are under continuous observation by trained staff including pulse oximetry and have oxygen and ventilation equipment available. Diclofenac is a NSAID which is contraindicated below 6 months

doses. It is slightly less effective than pethidine and respiratory depression is unlikely. Avoid fast IV injection as it is likely to cause nausea and vomiting.

Morphine (ampoules with 10 mg/ml) is 10 times stronger than pethidine and has almost the same effects, side effects, and duration of action as pethidine. Morphine and pethidine must not be combined. The best way of using morphine for injection is to make a dilution by drawing 1 ampoule = 10 mg + 9 ml NS into a 10-ml syringe to make 1 mg/ml and give small doses IV thereby titrating the drug to the desired effect. A total dose of around 0.1–0.2 mg/kg is usually sufficient to treat severe pain (see Table 14.7). Observation with a pulse oximeter and counting respiratory rate at regular intervals is highly recommended. If the respiratory rate decreases markedly, stimulate the child. If unresponsive, start bag-mask ventilation and call for help.

Codeine should be used with caution for children <12 years as fast metabolism to morphine may cause respiratory depression in genetically susceptible patients (>10% of the population). The average dose is 1 mg/kg IM. The effect is less predictable than with all other opioid drugs.

Diclofenac is well suited for moderate pain relief for children >6 months. It has a different mechanism of action than opioids and enhances the effect of pethidine or morphine in cases of severe pain without adding to side effects. Severe pain can therefore be treated with a combination of an opioid and diclofenac. The duration of analgesia from diclofenac is approximately 8 h; 1.5 mg/kg IM at the end of the surgery should be administered as a routine to avoid painful awakening from operation except for operations with risk for rebleeding. For doses, see Table 14.7. It is contraindicated in renal insufficiency, known allergy, asthma, and platelet dysfunction. Usually, 1 ml is equal to 25 mg. The average dose is 1–1.5 mg/kg IM for children >6 kg. Some preparations of diclofenac may even be used for IV administration with an infusion or slow injection over several minutes. Read the label of the ampoule to check if that preparation may be used IV or not. Diclofenac is more effective for pain relief and has a longer duration of action than ibuprofen and paracetamol. ***Ibuprofen*** 10 mg/kg may be used orally or rectally from 3 months on.

Paracetamol rectal needs some time for onset of effect. The 24 h dose must not exceed 100 mg/kg; below the age of 3 months, the maximum dose of paracetamol is 60 mg/kg/day. A large loading dose of 40 mg/kg rectally (<3 months 30 mg/kg) is more effective. Every 6 h maintenance doses of 15 mg/kg (<3 months 10 mg/kg) should be given until the patient is pain-free. Paracetamol is also produced in vials for infusion. The dose is 15 mg/kg every 6 h.

14.8 Pharmacological Characteristics and Their Implications for Anaesthesia in Paediatric Patients

14.8.1 General Considerations

Due to higher total body water and extracellular fluid volume in children, many drugs have a higher volume of distribution. That means a higher initial dose per kg is required for some drugs, e.g. atropine and suxamethonium. Due to high cardiac output, the distribution of drugs is faster, leading to faster onset and shorter duration of effect. Initial doses of thiopentone and propofol are therefore higher. Neonates have lower levels of plasma proteins, so the free, unbound concentration of propofol is higher and may cause cardiac depression. Propofol is until now not recommended for use in neonates and would need to be given in smaller doses. Kidneys and liver are immature during the neonatal period and first months of life. Many drugs are eliminated more slowly, e.g. morphine, pancuronium, vecuronium, rocuronium, diazepam, midazolam, and fentanyl. The level of coagulation factors is decreased in neonates, so vitamin K should be given prior to surgery. The blood–brain barrier is more permeable in neonates. That means some drugs cross the barrier easier, e.g. barbiturates and opioids, and may exert a more pronounced effect at lower doses. On the contrary, the immature brain may respond more variable and less predictable to drugs. Because of the generally greater variability of drug response in children than in adults, the required doses need to be titrated carefully to the desired effect.

For detailed pharmacology of the most commonly used drugs, see Chap. 7.

14.8.2 Dilutions and Doses of Drugs Used During Anaesthesia and Resuscitation

Many drugs need to be diluted to facilitate exact dosing for small children. Tables 14.8, 14.9, 14.10, and 14.11 are suggestions for easy and logical dilutions and doses depending on age or body weight for some of the most common drugs during anaesthesia. It is very important that only one way of dilution/drug concentrations/labelling syringes is used throughout a hospital. If different APs are using different concentrations/dilutions of drugs, the risk for wrong dose is high if anaesthetists are changing. Label the syringe with the name of the drug (may be with a common abbreviation), the concentration, the date, the hour, and your initials.

Table 14.8 Dilution and doses for atropine

Bodyweight (kg)	Atropine dose (mg)	ml (0.1 mg/ml)
2.5–4	0.05–0.08	0.5–0.8 ml
5–10	0.075–0.15	0.75–1.5 ml
11–15	0.15–0.2	1.5–2 ml
16–20	0.2–0.3	2–3 ml
21–30	0.3–0.4	3–4 ml
31–40	0.4–0.5	4–5 ml
>40	Undiluted 0.5	Depending on the ampoule size

Diazepam: Injection is painful, but pain on injection can be reduced by mixing 0.5 ml of lidocaine with 10 mg diazepam.

Atropine: Presentation of atropine can be 0.5 mg/ml or 0.6 mg/ml or 1 mg/ml ampoules. Draw 1 ml of the 0.5 mg/ml ampoule with 4 ml of water for injection or NS into a 5-ml syringe, or 1 ml of 0.6 mg/ml atropine with 5 ml NS = 6 ml into a 10-ml syringe or 1 ml of 1 mg/ml atropine with 9 ml NS in a 10-ml syringe, respectively, resulting in a concentration of 0.1 mg/ml. Give a dose of approximately 0.015 mg/kg (neonates 0.02 mg/kg) according to Table 14.8.

Adrenaline (epinephrine) is used for resuscitation and treatment of cardiac failure during anaesthesia. Dilute the drug to make 2 μg/ml (0.002 mg/ml). You need to sacrifice a 500-ml infusion bottle of NS or D5%. Inject 1 ampoule = 1 mg of adrenaline inside, clearly label the bottle, shake it a few times, and draw syringes from it to inject increments of 1 μg/kg = 0.5 ml/kg every 3–5 min for patients with extreme bradycardia, low cardiac output as indicated by > capillary refill over 2 s, quiet heart sounds, or very low BP. In patients with cardiac arrest, 10 μg/kg = 5 ml/kg may be required. For children > 10 kg, a dilution as for adults can be used with 0.1 mg/ml of adrenaline (1 ampoule = 1 mg diluted with 9 ml NS to make 10 ml at 0.1 mg/ml). The dose is 1 ml per 10 kg or 0.1 ml /kg of adrenaline 0.1 mg/ml. Note that dilutions of adrenaline are stable for max 24 h after which they lose effect and must be discarded.

Thiopentone: For infants >3 kg BW, thiopentone may be diluted in the same way as for adults (20 ml in the vial of 0.5 g resulting in a concentration of 25 mg/ml; 1 g vials need to be dissolved with 20 ml first making 50 mg/ml and then diluted once more (10 ml thiopentone 50 mg/ml + 10 ml NS or water for injection to make 25 mg/ml). Draw 2-ml syringes from that dilution to give exact amounts for bodyweights <15 kg and 5 ml syringes for bodyweights >15 kg. For newborns <3 kg dilute the 25 mg/ml thiopentone once more to make 5 mg/ml: 1 ml thiopentone 25 mg/ml + 4 ml NS or water for injection in a 5-ml syringe. The dose for induction is 3 mg/kg for BW <3 kg. For doses, see Table 14.9.

Table 14.9 Average doses of thiopentone for induction of newborns, infants, and children, given as mg and as ml of the respective dilution

Bodyweight	Thiopentone dose	ml (25 mg/ml)	ml (5 mg/ml)
Premature 2 kg	6 mg	NA	1.2
Premature 2.5 kg	7.5 mg	NA	1.5
Newborn 3kg	9 mg	NA	1.8
3–5 kg	12.5–25 mg	0.5–1 ml	2.5–5 ml
6–10 kg	37.5–50 mg	1.5–2 ml	NA
11–15 kg	50–75 mg	2–3 ml	NA
16–20 kg	75–100 mg	3–4 ml	NA
21–25 kg	100–125 mg	4–5 ml	NA
26–30 kg	125–150 mg	5–6 ml	NA
31–35 kg	150–175 mg	6–7 ml	NA

NA not applicable. Syringes must be labelled clearly with the dilution of the drug. Bodyweight must be known exactly as a wrong dose is dangerous

Ketamine: For IM injection, use the undiluted 100 mg/ml solution or 50 mg/ml solution (dependent on the preparation of ketamine) and draw the amount into a 2- or 5-ml syringe together with atropine. Use undiluted atropine for children > 10 kg to avoid too large a volume for injection. For IV injection, the drug is diluted: 1 ml ketamine 100 mg/ml + 9 ml water for injection or NS is drawn into a 10-ml syringe to make 10 mg/ml. If ketamine is available in 50 mg/ml vials, dilute 1 ml ketamine + 4 ml saline to make 10 mg/ml. Alternatively, 10 mg/ml ketamine vials can be used undiluted. Doses are given in Table 14.10.

Suxamethonium (succinylcholine): In order to facilitate exact dosing, the drug should be diluted: 1 ml containing 50 mg + 4 ml saline into a 5-ml syringe to make 10 mg/ml or 2.5 ml containing 20 mg/ml + 2.5 ml NS into a 5-ml syringe to make 10 mg/ml. Neonates can often be intubated without muscle relaxation in spite of reduced induction doses of anaesthetics. Small children need 2 mg/kg while patients older than 10–12 years need 1 mg/kg, same dose as for adults. Doses are given in Table 14.11.

Table 14.10 Average doses (mg) and volumes (ml) for IV or IM injection of ketamine. Ketamine is often available in 50 mg/mL vials but sometimes in 100 mg/mL vials. For IV injection prepare a dilution to 10 mg/mL

Bodyweight	Ketamine mg IV	10 mg/ml IV	Ketamine mg IM	ml IM (50 mg/ml)	ml IM (100 mg/ml)
3–5 kg	2.5–5 mg	0.25–0.5 ml	NA	NA	NA
6–10 kg	10–15 mg	1–1.5 ml	30–50 mg	0.6–1 ml	0.3–0.5 ml
11–15 kg	15–20 mg	1.5–2 ml	50–75 mg	1–1.5 ml	0.5–0.75 ml
16–20 kg	20–30 mg	2–3 ml	80–100 mg	1.6–2 ml	0.8–1 ml
21–25 kg	30–40 mg	3–4 ml	100–125 mg	2–2.5 ml	1–1.25 ml
26–30 kg	40–50 mg	4–5 ml	125–150 mg	2.5–3 ml	1.25–1.5 ml
31–35 kg	50–60 mg	5–6 ml	150–175 mg	3–3.5 ml	1.5–1.75 ml

Ketamine IM for neonates is not recommended (*NA* not applicable)

Table 14.11 Average doses and volumes to be injected for diluted suxamethonium

Bodyweight	Suxamethonium dose	ml (diluted to 10 mg/ml)
Neonate-5 kg	5–10 mg	0.5–1 ml
6–10 kg	10–20 mg	1–2 ml
11–15 kg	20–30 mg	2–3 ml
16–20 kg	30–40 mg	3–4 ml
21–25 kg	40–50 mg	4–5 ml
26–30 kg	50 mg	5 ml
>30 kg	50 mg	5 ml

14.9 Anaesthesia for Some Typical Procedures

14.9.1 Hernia Repair

Inguinal hernia, hydrocele, and umbilical hernia are common reasons for elective surgery in children. Premature infants are especially prone to inguinal hernia. Aim to wait with surgery until the infant is >6 months old to reduce anaesthesia-related risk. In neonates and small infants, inguinal hernia can be strangulated (obstructed). *Strangulated hernia* may lead to incarceration with necrosis of the obstructed bowels. That would mean an *emergency procedure* for which anaesthesia is the same as for the ileus (Sect. 14.4.4; RSI after IV access). Elective hernia repair can be performed with LMA in spontaneous breathing. Inhalation anaesthesia is preferred. Postoperative pain relief can be obtained by local wound infiltration and NSAID. Bupivacaine produces a longer-lasting effect than lidocaine. Bupivacaine should be diluted to make 2.5 mg/ml; otherwise, overdose is possible (Sect. 14.7, Table 14.6).

14.9.2 Appendectomy, Intussusception, Ileus

IV access prior to induction is advantageous, and infusions should already be given in the ward preoperatively to avoid or treat dehydration. Patients may have fever and a distended abdomen. The general condition may be impaired, especially with late presentation. Preoperative restoration of fluid volumes should be performed, and broad-spectrum antibiotics should be given. Vomiting is common. It is not safe to operate on these patients with ketamine anaesthesia under spontaneous breathing. If you do not have equipment (anaesthesia machine/draw over device with oxygen, endotracheal tubes and laryngoscope correct size, suction machine, and suction catheters) or drugs (induction agent, suxamethonium, and inhalational agent), the patient should better be transferred if a higher-level health facility is not too far away. Intubation anaesthesia with RSI is performed, although for infants often gentle ventilation via a face mask may be necessary to avoid hypoxia before intubation. For balanced anaesthesia with IV induction, inhalation anaesthetic plus muscle relaxation plus IV analgesic (ketamine 1 mg/kg boluses or a total maximum of two bolus doses of fentanyl 1 μg/kg before painful surgical stimuli like opening of the peritoneum and pulling at inner organs) is used. For fluid management, see Sect. 14.5. The patients need calculated amounts of fluids IV during the whole perioperative period. During abdominal surgery, spontaneous breathing is impaired, and controlled ventilation, manually or mechanically, is performed. Notably, 20 ml/kg RL or NS is initially needed for fluid replacement, and during surgery, often another 20–40 ml/kg is needed. Blood transfusion is not often necessary but check Hb before operation. The risk for hypothermia is high. Switch the AC off or set it at a higher temperature, cover the patient with blankets and the head with a bonnet, and place warm infusion bottles, wrapped in cloth, around him. Aim to give warm infusions (but not hot, around 37 °C is optimal). Postoperative care depends on the intraoperative findings and the operation performed. Postoperative analgesia is necessary, preferably with opioids such as pethidine, morphine, or tramadol (see Sect. 14.7). After uncomplicated surgery and emergence from anaesthesia, the patient can be sent to the ward, while febrile patients with peritonitis or after bowel resection and anastomosis should receive a second venous line (will be needed for several days) and a urinary catheter and should be monitored closely with a vital signs observation chart and monitoring fluid balance (risk for acute kidney injury with decreased urine production), if possible in a PICU or HDU. They might also need oxygen via nasal prongs for some time.

14.9.3 Colostomy in Neonates with Imperforate Anus

Anorectal malformations are among the most common major congenital malformations presenting for surgery. The missing anus with rectal atresia is often combined with other malformations like fistula between the rectum and urinary bladder or vagina or other malformations, even of other systems in the body. Initial surgical treatment for this life-threatening condition is colostomy, and repair of the underlying malformation can be performed at a later stage. Due to the delayed presentation of many of these patients, intestinal obstruction may have caused complications such as bowel perforation, aspiration pneumonia, and difficulties in breathing due to abdominal distension. Anaesthesia should be intubation anaesthesia with modified RSI, reduced doses of anaesthetic drugs, and inhalational anaesthesia for maintenance. IV induction and controlled infusion of IV fluids (avoid overinfusion), e.g. glucose with normal saline, are mandatory for all patients; for amounts of infusion, see Sect. 14.5. If facilities for safe neonatal anaesthesia are unavailable, especially if the patient is preterm, a colostomy can be performed under local anaesthesia plus oxygen via nasal prongs. The surgical conditions under LA are not very good, but mortality would be significantly less than with GA under suboptimal conditions. Notably, 0.5 mg/kg of diluted ketamine IV may be added to LA and may be repeated after 15 min. Postoperative analgesia with wound infiltration (if surgery was with GA) and paracetamol 15 mg/kg.

14.9.4 Pyloromyotomy

Patients are between 6 weeks and several months old and may present with malnutrition and dehydration due to vomiting after feeding. The condition is caused by congenital hypertrophic pyloric stenosis. Dehydration should be treated before starting surgery which does not need to be performed immediately and never during the night. The patient should get IV access and infusion, NS with dextrose or RL with glucose or similar around 20 ml/kg before the operation should be administered. NGT should facilitate gastric emptying before anaesthesia induction, and of course, the patient must be fasting before surgery. Measure the bodyweight on admission and after treatment of the dehydration. Carefully calculate doses of all drugs and prepare syringes with diluted anaesthetics and atropine (see Sect. 14.8). Anaesthesia is with endotracheal intubation after modified rapid sequence induction (Sect. 14.4). Maintenance with inhalation anaesthesia is best, ketamine is an option if the surgeon is performing the procedure quickly, but surgical conditions and quality of anaesthesia are much better with inhalation anaesthesia. The operation does usually not cause significant bleeding and does not take a long time. The NGT is removed immediately before extubation while suctioning is performed. After recovery, the infant can usually return to the general ward, and oral feeding be started soon afterwards. Postoperative analgesia can be with wound LA infiltration and paracetamol 15 mg/kg. Avoid opioid drugs as these infants are prone to respiratory depression.

14.9.5 Trauma and Fractures

Damage Controlled Resuscitation (DCR) Assess the child with (c)ABC approach (see Chap. 13) and take a short history. What happened when? Which signs of injury are obvious? Which damage is likely after the type of accident? Is there ongoing bleeding? Is the child unconscious? Pale? Pulse normal or fast and weak? If yes, assume bleeding, call for help, and make efforts to stop the bleeding. Give oxygen and keep the airway patent. A short clinical examination is listening to heart and lungs (bilateral equal breathing sounds, normal or silent heart sounds?), checking pulse and SPO_2, and measuring BP. As it is often impossible to put the injured child on weighing scales, estimate BW with the formula (age + 4) × 2 = kg BW. Fill in the most important parameters in a record form, but without losing much time.

If there is major bleeding, surgery must be started as soon as possible. Consider early blood transfusion, preferably fresh warm blood if massive bleeding.

If a patient has no vital signs or develops cardiac arrest caused by trauma, ALS resuscitation, although of course usually practiced, is seldom successful. The team leader needs to decide when to stop.

Venous access is vital but may be difficult to establish. If the veins on hands, forearms, or feet cannot be used for access, in small infants, a scalp vein may be chosen. Alternatively, the external jugular vein is often a good choice, or the femoral vein. If venous access fails within minutes, insert an intraosseous needle (see Sect. 14.5). These procedures may need sedation, e.g. with ketamine IM. A blood sample is taken from the first venous cannula inserted, Hb is measured, and blood is sent for blood grouping and cross-match. After severe trauma, full blood count, potassium, and coagulation parameters are checked as well.

Blunt Abdominal Trauma If ultrasound can be performed, it is ideal to get diagnoses at the bedside quickly. Free fluid in the abdomen is very well visible with ultrasound, and likely diagnoses can be made, e.g. ruptured spleen, liver, or kidney. Emergency laparotomy requires intubation anaesthesia with rapid sequence induction and a sufficiently large bore venous access prior to induction as well as blood available for transfusion. BP should be recorded every 5 min, and fluid management aims for normovolaemia, Hb >7–8 g/dl (70–80 g/l), normal capillary refill time, and normal BP. Consider tranexamic acid (20 mg/kg slowly IV over 10 min) if bleeding is severe and not more than 3 h elapsed since the trauma happened. Urinary catheter insertion is mandatory at least at the end of the operation.

Anaesthesia for ORIF, open reduction, and fixation of fractures: If the child is fasting and the fracture to be operated on is on a limb, anaesthesia can be with laryngeal mask airway and without muscle relaxation. Antibiotic prophylaxis before the start of the surgery, and postoperative analgesia, e.g. with a combination of NSAID and opioid, should be provided at the end of the operation.

Head Trauma In a hospital with CT scan, surgery for evacuation of epidural or subdural haematoma may be performed. Usually, a hospital with CT scan has also an ICU but may be without anaesthesiologist. Anaesthesia for head trauma is preferable with isoflurane or sevoflurane for maintenance. Ketamine is only used in small doses as it can increase intracranial pressure, especially if combined with spontaneous breathing. Patients with severe head injury should be intubated and ventilated with controlled IPPV. In ventilated and intubated patients, a single dose of morphine 0.2 mg/kg or pethidine 2 mg/kg can be given at the beginning of surgery, and the concentration of isoflurane can be reduced to 1 MAC, around 1.5% at the vaporiser. For neurosurgical operations, the anaesthesia working station is placed near the left leg of the patient, as the surgical team is working at the head. The breathing tubes are placed straight towards caudal direction without using an angle piece. Excellent fixation is vital as the AP does not see the airway after sterile drapes are placed. A straight connector between ETT and y-piece can be used. Capnography is highly recommended, and end-tidal CO_2 should be kept between 4 and 5 kPa (30–35 mmHg) in consent with the surgeon. Two venous lines are recommended with an extension and a three-way stopcock to facilitate IV administration of drugs and blood transfusion when access to the forearm is not possible due to sterility issues. IV cannulae must also be perfectly fixed with the best tape available, especially if they are invisible under sterile drapes. An IV cannula on a foot is ideal for the anaesthetist. A urinary catheter is also mandatory, and an orogastric tube instead of NGT is inserted after intubation if injury to the skull base is suspected. Postoperative care in an intensive care unit is needed for several days. Patients who are not fully awake after surgery need to remain intubated and ventilation be assisted with PEEP/CPAP. Feeding via gastric tube is advantageous for patient outcomes compared with IV nutrition. Dehydration as well as overinfusion must be avoided. The "5 H" hypotension, hypoxia, hyperthermia, hypercapnia, hypoglycaemia, and low Hb would cause secondary brain injury and must be avoided.

14.9.6 Burns

Unfortunately, burns are not rare, and all efforts should be made to improve prevention. They often affect small children and patients with epilepsy in areas with cooking over open fire but also in places where cooking is done with electrical plates or with gas. Acid burns are also not uncommon and often very severe. Scalds are mostly happening to toddlers with hot beverages or cooking oil. The body surface area in relation to weight is two to three times larger than for adults making fluid losses and requirements greater. The skin of children <2 years is thinner, so full-thickness burns causing contractures during healing are more likely to occur.

Initial Survey ABCDE approach as for other trauma patients. Check for other injuries than burns. Are there any signs of inhalational trauma especially with burns of face/neck (hoarseness, coughing, wheezing, shortness of breath, runny nose, and chest pain)? How much time has elapsed since the burns, and how much % of the body surface area is affected? Was any treatment already performed at a referring health centre? The area affected by partial or full-thickness burns is estimated. "Rule of nines" functions best for adults but is different for children as their head is larger (up to twice the % of body surface area compared with adults) and limbs are smaller. A burns chart like the Lund and Bowder chart is a useful tool and should be filled in as exactly as possible. If that tool is not available (can be downloaded and printed), a simpler (and less exact) chart is Wallace's rule of nines for children: The head is 18% and each leg is 14% for age 1 year. The head is 1% less for each year thereafter until a minimum of 9%, while 0.5% more per year is added for each leg. Each arm is 9%, and front of the trunk and the back make 18% each.

Fluid Resuscitation During the first 24 h, infusion of RL or similar has to be calculated according to the size of the burned surface area, e.g. with the Parkland formula: 4 ml × BW × % of the burned area as RL over 24 h; the first half of that during the first 8 h and the second half during the next 16 h. Additionally, a maintenance infusion with dextrose in saline or glucose in RL/with electrolytes needs to be administered continuously with approximately 100 ml/kg/24 h up to 10 kg BW plus 50 ml/kg/24 h for each kg >10 and <20 kg, and 25 ml/kg/24 h for each kg >20 kg BW until the child is able to feed orally or via NGT which should be started as soon as possible. In the days thereafter, blood transfusion, FFP, or albumin might be necessary. Check Hb regularly. A urinary catheter is needed, and urine output is recorded. Notably, 1 ml/kg/h urine output is regarded as a target and means fluid therapy is sufficient. If a urine catheter of adequate size is unavailable, feeding tubes may be used instead for small children (not ideal); diapers should be weighed to estimate urine output, and the urine of older children should be collected in a urinal and measured. Carefully record urine output on the patient's observation chart! Urine output of more than 2 ml/kg/h is a sign of overinfusion. Under- and overinfusion are to be avoided.

Consider Referral Referral should be early, that is, after initial stabilising and initial treatment during the first 24 h. Referral to a better-equipped health facility is to be considered for all severe cases, and the option of receiving free treatment at that facility is to be evaluated if health insurance or funds are lacking. Patients with inhalational trauma should be intubated if possible and always be referred to a burn centre/fully equipped ICU if possible. Patients with burns on the face or hands should be referred to a hospital with the availability of plastic surgery. All patients who need skin grafting should be referred early if skin grafting cannot be performed locally. Patients with a huge surface area of burns but a realistic chance of surviving when treated at a burns unit should be referred. Children with >10% of body surface area involved should be referred to a regional hospital/the best-equipped hospital in the area. Patients who cannot be referred should get the best possible care including the best possible pain treatment.

Surgical Procedures and Anaesthesia Unfortunately, full-thickness burns heal slowly and with debilitating contractures if not operated on several times by a physician who is skilled in plastic surgery. Patients need to stay in the hospital often for several months, needing frequent dressing, several operations such as skin grafting, flaps, drugs for pain relief and antibiotics, repeated blood transfusion, and good, protein- and energy-rich nutrition. It is wise after the initial phase to make a realistic plan about which treatment is manageable for the hospital and affordable for the relatives, considering both the medical and the economic impact. It is in severe cases sometimes better not to start expensive, resource-consuming treatment than having a patient suffering for several months, dying despite the effort, and leaving the family desperate and bankrupt.

Several operations may be needed such as wound cleaning, debridement, escharotomy (to prevent compartment syndrome), skin grafting, flaps, and finally surgery for contractures. Depending on the site of surgery and the patient's position on the operation table (supine or prone), endotracheal intubation or laryngeal mask airway is used. Anaesthesia can be balanced with an inhalational agent plus ketamine for analgesia same way as for any other major surgery except using suxamethonium which is strictly contraindicated. Blood loss is often significant. Be prepared for blood transfusion and have Hb checked.

Suxamethonium is absolutely contraindicated up to several months after the burns, in severe cases up to 1 year, because of the risk for severe hyperkalaemia with cardiac arrest and not responding to resuscitation. Other muscle relaxants may be used but are long-acting and need to be reversed.

Burns involving the face can lead to difficult airway access and difficulty with mask ventilation, especially after some time when contractures restrict jaw and neck movement. In such cases, the release of contractures must sometimes be performed with ketamine and LA, and oxygen administered via sterile nasal prongs, if possible.

Venous access can also be challenging.

Analgesia is necessary and may be difficult to provide adequately. Drugs are paracetamol or ibuprofen (>3 months of age) QDS plus opioids like morphine 0.2 mg/kg regularly and on request. Pain level should be assessed and recorded regularly so that analgesic treatment can be adapted to requirements. If available, oral morphine or another opioid orally should be preferred over syringes which children do not like to receive.

Short GA for painful procedures with ketamine is ideal, e.g. dressing and wound cleaning which are very painful. Children who have an IV access should receive ketamine plus diazepam or midazolam IV before the procedure (see Chap. 9, short GA for doses). After several days, when IV access is no longer required or possible, analgosedation can also be provided by ketamine orally. The effect is more variable than for IM or IV ketamine but for children who are responding well, it is a nice method if they are afraid of syringes. For oral ketamine, the dose is 7–8 mg/kg mixed with a little sugar and water or sweet juice. The onset of effect is after 15 min.

Patients with burns need a lot of calories with nutrition and should be omitted from fasting before sedation/short GA with spontaneous breathing if it is not possible to perform the procedure early in the morning before breakfast. An alternative to ketamine for short GA is halothane or sevoflurane via a face mask with spontaneous breathing although it may take around 10 min until anaesthesia is deep enough to perform the procedure (check eyes—when they are looking in the same direction and pupils are normal size, anaesthesia is sufficient). Nitrous oxide (65–70% in oxygen), if available, is advantageous since onset is faster (around 3 min) than with other inhalational anaesthetics. Elderly children for repeated procedures will have preferences that should be followed if possible.

14.9.7 Adenotomy and Tonsillectomy

Patients present with recurrent throat infections or with upper airway obstruction due to hypertrophy of the tonsils, adenoids, or both. These patients may even suffer from obstructive sleep apnoea (OSA) . Although a common and rather short procedure, anaesthesia may be challenging and prone to complications especially if the patients are younger than 3 years and have OSA or any other chronic disease or congenital health problem.

Elective ENT operations must not be performed if sufficient equipment for paediatric anaesthesia is lacking. You need a laryngoscope with blades size 1 and 2, ETT of adequate size, paediatric stylet to facilitate difficult intubation, stethoscope, suction device, anaesthesia machine, reliable oxygen and electricity, pulse oximeter, BP cuff (right size for the child; a too big cuff may be used on the leg to get reliable results), and especially in children with OSA, airway obstruction during the night, ECG is mandatory. Two APs are always needed of which one must be experienced.

While mild respiratory tract infection with a runny nose but without fever and productive cough is no hinder to performing surgery and anaesthesia, a sick child should be postponed to avoid risk for serious postoperative problems such as difficulties in breathing with a tendency to hypoxia and even pneumonia.

The safest type of anaesthesia for these procedures is with endotracheal intubation. Patients may be breathing spontaneously after the effect of the muscle relaxant has worn off or may be ventilated manually or mechanically. Inhalational anaesthesia with halothane or isoflurane (isoflurane after intubation but not for inhalational induction) is suitable. Sevoflurane is also good but expensive. Before intubation, a bolus dose of ketamine 1 mg/kg can be added to the hypnotic drug (halothane or propofol or thiopentone) or ketamine 2 mg/kg IV can be used as the sole induction agent followed by 1.5–2 mg/kg suxamethonium. If fentanyl is available and the anaesthetist is familiar with it, 1 µg/kg (0.025 mg in a 25 kg child) may be used instead of ketamine, but do not use opioids in children with obstructive sleep apnoea syndrome OSA (risk for prolonged respiratory depression after surgery). Patients with OSA should not receive diazepam or midazolam, and they must not be operated on as day case surgery but stay at least 24 h in the hospital after the operation. Close monitoring of breathing during the whole period is essential; if available, additionally with a pulse oximeter.

Special pre-shaped RAE tubes may be used if available or armoured tubes with a metallic spiral. Even ordinary ETTs are suitable, but you need carefully to check that the mouth gag is not kinking or displacing the ETT.

After intubation and careful fixation of the tube in the middle of the lower lip (a small swab on the chin under the ETT can facilitate keeping ETT in the correct position), a small pillow or infusion bag is placed under the back to facilitate head extension. A ring (homemade from a cloth is suitable) under the head keeps it in position. Make sure the ETT is not dislocated during head extension and listen on both lungs after insertion of the gag by the ENT doctor. In doubt, have a look with your laryngoscope to reassure the correct position.

For postoperative pain relief, tramadol 2 mg/kg can be given or diclofenac 2 mg/kg if the surgeon agrees (risk of impaired blood coagulation). Later, paracetamol or ibuprofen orally can be given. Dexamethasone 0.1–0.15 mg/kg at the beginning of the operation is very useful as an antiemetic and anti-inflammatory and adds to the analgesic effect. Ondansetrone 0.1 mg/kg IV is used as an additional antiemetic if available, or clonidine 2 µg/kg IV which has analgesic and antiemetic effects.

At the end of the operation, the patient is placed laterally head down for waking and extubation. Carefully suction the airways and extubate when the child is fully awake. Few hours after the surgery, the child may start to drink and eat if possible. Ice cream is exceptionally good as an anti-pain and is highly appreciated.

14.9.7.1 Bleeding After Tonsillectomy

Severe bleeding is a potentially life-threatening complication after tonsillectomy and rarely after adenectomy. It occurs either within the first 6 h after the operation or after 1 week.

Hypotension is a late sign and means the patient is in severe shock and needs infusion at full speed and blood transfusion as soon as possible. Rapid sequence induction (because the stomach is likely to be full of blood) and intubation can be difficult as the view can be blurred with fresh blood and coagulated blood near the entrance of the larynx. If vascular access is impossible, an intraosseous cannula must be inserted (painful; ketamine IM may relieve the pain). Alternatively, venous access is possible in the femoral vein (assure not to mistake the artery for the vein), external jugular vein, or (rare) with a venotomy operation by the surgeon. Rapid infusion of RL or NS is needed; cross-match and transfusion if necessary. Avoid anaesthesia drugs which are producing vasodilatation. Better give ketamine for induction and maintenance of anaesthesia. If the patient is circulatory stable, inhalational anaesthetic at <1 MAC may be added to increments of ketamine every 5–10 min. Wake the patient when fully awake and in a lateral position with the head down. Perform orogastric suction of the stomach before extubation. No NSAID because of the risk of re-bleeding. Tramadol or paracetamol can be given as an antipain together with a prophylactic antiemetic drug. A throat pack must be removed before extubation.

14.9.8 Removal of Foreign Body from the Oesophagus or Airways

Infants with foreign bodies are typically below 3 years old, more often boys than girls. The most common foreign body is a coin in the upper oesophagus. Small coin-shaped batteries are more dangerous if they get stuck in the oesophagus or bronchus. Lithium-containing button batteries still have a strong current. If the battery gets in contact with saliva, tissue damage will occur quickly as there is a physicochemical reaction occurring which frees poisonous substances such as lithium, cadmium, and others. Without prompt removal in a hospital (if available with an ENT department), the infant is at risk of dying. A foreign body in the airways is the most likely diagnosis in cases of acute respiratory distress in small children. The foreign body is often a peanut or a cashew nut. Bronchoscopy needs to be performed urgently if the patient has severe respiratory distress. In that case, the foreign body is often in the trachea. If the foreign body is suspected to be in a main bronchus (patients with cough but without severe respiratory distress), the patient should be fasting >6 h, and the procedure can be performed during the daytime.

The person who is to perform the foreign body removal needs to be used to do that (e.g. a trained ENT doctor or a trained anaesthetist or paediatrician).

Ventilation and sufficient oxygenation can be very challenging during the procedure.

Anaesthesia for Removal of Foreign Body in the Oesophagus These patients are sometimes dehydrated as they have difficulty swallowing. Give infusion, e.g. DNS. The patient is anaesthetised in the same way as for any other operation, full monitoring is attached, and the trachea is intubated. The ideal is an armoured endotracheal tube that cannot be kinking. Then the oesophagoscope is inserted and the foreign body is removed. Deep anaesthesia is necessary to prevent airway reflexes and reflex bradycardia. During emergence, place the patient in a lateral position and provide thorough suction before extubation of the fully awake child. For muscle relaxation, use a single dose of suxamethonium only for intubation as the procedure is often short-lasting.

14.9.8.1 Procedure for Removal of Foreign Bodies From the Airways With Anaesthesia

A rigid oesophagoscope/bronchoscope of appropriate size with a light source and a side port for ventilation is needed and prepared. Have different sizes at hand if available according to the size of the patient.

Location: In most hospitals, the safest location to perform the procedure is an operation room with equipment for paediatric anaesthesia. Anaesthesia in a unit for endoscopy can only be performed safely if complete anaesthesia equipment including drugs is available at that place. Oxygen, SIB, suction machine, vital signs monitor, and complete airway equipment are mandatory.

Team: ENT doctor and no less than two, better three anaesthesia staff, at least one of them experienced, are mandatory; one theatre nurse.

Anaesthetist: Short assessment and auscultation of heart and lungs. Allergies known? Patient otherwise healthy? Previous anaesthesia/surgery uneventful? Anatomy of the face and neck normal?

Switch on the oxygen source/concentrator. No less than 4 l pure oxygen should be used during the whole procedure. Prepare laryngoscope, suction machine with suction catheters (small and large bore), ETT different sizes (3.5, 4, 4.5, 5), LMA (1.5 and 2), facemask, oropharyngeal (Guedel) airway, infusion (DNS or Ringer), and drugs. Check vital signs, and always use a pulse oximeter and precordial stethoscope. Apply oxygen via a face mask. Have a well-functioning and well-secured venous cannula with a drop established.

Anaesthesia record and preparation: Documentation of vital signs, drugs, and exact time. Give one dose of hydrocortisone 5 mg/kg or dexamethasone 0.1 mg/kg.

During bronchoscopy and removal of foreign body from the airways, deep anaesthesia with muscle relaxation is required. The procedure can take some time. Therefore, after intubation, a longer-acting non-depolarising muscle relaxant such as atracurium, vecuronium, rocuronium, or pancuronium may be administered. Alternatively, increment bolus doses of suxamethonium are given (see Table 14.12). After the procedure, the trachea is intubated, a non-depolarising MR is reversed with atropine and neostigmine, and the patient is kept intubated and ventilation assisted until full emergence is achieved, that is, a child who is fully awake and moving spontaneously. This may require several hours of work for the anaesthesia team. Two persons are mandatory until the child is fully alert and all vitals stable.

Conduct of anaesthesia: IV access functioning → intravenous induction. No IV access is possible preoperatively → inhalational induction

Table 14.12 Drug doses for anaesthesia induction and maintenance for foreign body removal from oesophagus or airways

Bodyweight	10 kg	12.5 kg	15 kg
Drug doses for induction of anaesthesia			
Atropine 0.1 mg/ml	0.2 mg = 2 ml	0.25 mg = 2.5 ml	0.3 mg = 3 ml
Diazepam 1 mg/ml	2 mg = 2 ml	2.5 mg = 2.5 ml	3 mg = 3 ml
Thiopentone 25 mg/ml (thiopentone *or* propofol)	50 mg = 2 ml	62.5 mg = 2.5 ml	75 mg = 3 ml
Propofol 10 mg/ml	40 mg = 4 ml	50 mg = 5 ml	60 mg = 6 ml
Ketamine 10 mg/ml	20 mg = 2 ml	25 mg = 2.5 ml	30 mg = 3 ml
Suxamethonium 10 mg/ml	20 mg = 2 ml	25 mg = 2.5 ml	30 mg = 3 ml
Drug doses for maintenance every 5 min or with signs of light anaesthesia			
Thiopentone 25 mg/ml (thiopentone *or* propofol)	25 mg = 1 ml	30 mg = 1.2 ml	37.5 mg = 1.5 ml
Propofol 10 mg/ml	20 mg = 2 ml	25 mg = 2.5 ml	30 mg = 3 ml
Ketamine 10 mg/ml	10 mg = 1 ml	15 mg = 1.5 ml	20 mg = 2 ml
Suxamethonium 10mg/ml	10 mg = 1 ml	12 mg = 1.2 ml	15 mg = 1.5 ml

Patients are usually 1–3 years old (10–15 kg BW)

if the patient still is breathing sufficiently and $SPO_2 > 90$, IV cannulation as soon as anaesthesia is deep enough.

Maintenance of anaesthesia should be IV/TIVA as it may be difficult to obtain a sufficient alveolar concentration of halothane, and light anaesthesia would cause coughing and bronchospasm/laryngospasm. For drugs and doses, see Table 14.12. The airway is shared between the anaesthetist and the surgeon! Good communication is essential.

Start IV infusion. Give oxygen via face mask 4 l /min. Give one dose of hydrocortisone 5 mg/kg or dexamethasone 0.1 mg/kg and atropine 0.02 mg/kg, diazepam 2.5 mg or midazolam 2 mg.

Anaesthesia induction is with ketamine 2 mg/kg and thiopentone 5 mg/kg, or propofol 4 mg/kg. Propofol provides better quality of anaesthesia and less irritation of the airway than thiopentone or halothane.

Muscle relaxation is necessary to avoid laryngospasm or bronchospasm which are likely to occur without MR. The initial dose of MR is suxamethonium 2 mg/kg or atracurium 0.5 mg/kg. Ventilate the patient via a face mask. After 1 min, the ENT specialist inserts the bronchoscope. Anaesthetist connects the ventilation tube (T-piece circuit) from the anaesthesia machine to the side port of the bronchoscope and manually ventilates the patient. For TIVA, you need either syringe pumps for continuous administration, or you can use the stopwatch on your mobile phone. Record the time of drug injection carefully. Every 5 min (earlier if the patient is moving or coughing) half-dose IV anaesthetics for maintenance:

ketamine 1 mg/kg plus thiopentone 2.5 mg/kg (or propofol 2 mg/kg) and suxamethonium 1 mg/kg) no suxa if MR is with atracurium which does not need to be repeated).

Repeated doses of suxamethonium may cause bradycardia and even asystolia. In that case, give one additional dose of atropine. As the effect of atropine IV lasts around 30 min, repeat it always if the procedure takes a longer time. Have ephedrine ready, double dilution (1:10, again 1:10 to make 0.3–0.5 mg/ml depending on 30 or 50 mg/ml presentation of the drug); give 0.5–1 ml of that dilution if bradycardia develops in spite of atropine).

After the removal of the foreign body and removal of the bronchoscope, intubate the patient with an ETT or a laryngeal mask. Ventilate the patient until fully awake, then extubation in a lateral position after thorough suctioning. Apply oxygen with nasal prongs, and after emergence, send the patient to the ICU/high-dependency area for 24-h observation.

Prepare Diluted Drugs for Induction Propofol 10 mg/ml or thiopentone 25 mg/ml, atropine 0.1 mg/ml, diazepam or midazolam 1 mg/ml, ketamine 10 mg/ml, and suxamethonium 10 mg/ml or atracurium 10 mg/ml. For estimated doses, see Table 14.12. See Sect. 14.8 for how to dilute the drugs.

Sufficient quality of anaesthesia can be achieved with TIVA with propofol plus ketamine plus suxamethonium with doses as in Table 14.12. Close observation after the procedure is necessary in the recovery unit or, better, in an intermediate or intensive care unit depending on the condition of the child. After esophagoscopy, recovery usually is good and rapid; however, after bronchoscopy, the airways may be swelling, and obstruction is possible. Observation for 24 h in an HDU is recommended.

Further Reading

Broadis E, Chokotho T, Borgstein E (2017) Paediatric burn and scald management in a low resource setting: a reference guide and review. Afr J Emerg Med 7:S27–S31

Gottlieb EA, Andropoulos DB (2023) Pediatrics. In: Pardo MC (ed) Miller's basics of anesthesia, 8th edn. Elsevier, Philadelphia, pp 612–641

Jöhr M (2018) Managing complications in paediatric anaesthesia, 1st edn. Cambridge University Press, Cambridge

Kumar PA (2016) Fundamentals of paediatric anaesthesia, 3rd edn. Jaypee Brothers Medical Publishers, New Delhi

Roberts S (ed) (2019) Paediatric anaesthesia. Oxford specialist handbooks in anaesthesia, 2nd edn. Oxford University Press, Oxford

15 Emergencies and Critical Incidents

Abstract

For successful management of emergencies and critical incidents good communication and teamwork are essential and should be trained regularly. A debriefing after the incident is also helpful to learn "what could have been done better".

Initial assessment consists of receiving a short report and performing a structured approach with A—airway, B—breathing, C—circulation, D—disability/drugs, E—exposure. Interventions are needed if the airway is not free, breathing is insufficient/oxygen saturation is low, pulse/BP are inadequate, the patient is unconscious, needs emergency drugs like adrenaline, and shows a condition requiring urgent treatment.

Circulatory shock, most often presenting as haemorrhagic shock, is caused by life-threatening bleeding. Clinical signs: pallor, fast and weak pulse, low BP (late sign), prolonged capillary refill time. Initially, compensatory mechanisms like vasoconstriction and tachycardia help survive. Severe shock must be treated aggressively (elevating the legs, IV fluids, oxygen, ephedrine, adrenaline infusion, blood transfusion), and the bleeding must be stopped as fast as possible.

Circulatory arrest requires immediate recognition, call for help, early starting chest compressions with a depth of 5–6 cm and giving two breaths every 30 compressions, early defibrillation, securing the airway, giving pure oxygen, drugs like adrenaline 1 mg IV every 3 min, and good post-resuscitation care.

Laryngospasm is a common complication during anaesthesia, notably in children. Early recognition of paradoxical chest movement even before desaturation is vital, and giving oxygen, positive pressure ventilation, drugs like propofol, and in severe cases muscle relaxation are essential interventions.

Keywords

ABCDE approach for emergencies · ABCDE approach for critical incidents · Adverse effects of neuromuscular blocking agents in resource-limited settings · Anaesthesia management of circulatory shock · Anaesthesia-related bronchospasm and laryngospasm · ATLS classification of haemorrhagic shock · Basic and advanced life support · Resuscitation in the operation room

Emergencies and critical incidents are happening in all health facilities around the globe and may imply a very stressful burden for the involved personnel. It is highly recommended to create a local hospital critical incident reporting system. For improving quality, audits are useful. The hospital should organise meetings of all involved staff for morbidity–mortality sessions, where all unex-

D. Kietzmann, *Anaesthesia in Remote Hospitals*, Sustainable Development Goals Series,
https://doi.org/10.1007/978-3-031-46610-6_15

pected deaths, cardiac arrests, and unexpected ICU admissions or referrals to larger/regional hospitals are discussed in a friendly, open, and not-condemning atmosphere. Nobody must be blamed during these sessions. A debriefing where every person is heard, and where at the end the moderator (e.g. doctor in charge) would summarise the incident and conclude if the event and outcome were avoidable or unavoidable with the available resources, can create a learning process where prevention and management of critical incidents will improve over time. Always ask "what could have been done better? Communication skills, practical skills, and knowledge are the most crucial resources needed for a favourable outcome. These resources can be supported at every health facility without extra costs.

15.1 Assessment, ABCDE Approach

All patients at risk for deterioration of vital functions should be placed in a way that close observation is possible (e.g. near the nurses' office). A simple observation chart at the bedside for pulse rate (PR = pulse rate or HR = heart rate), blood pressure (BP), respiratory rate (RR), oxygen saturation (SpO_2), body temperature, urine output, remarks (e.g. deteriorated consciousness), and interventions (e.g. giving oxygen) is extremely helpful and should be carefully recorded at least once per hour. The hospital needs to have a clear policy about response to any deterioration in the patient's clinical condition. All staff should be trained in the early recognition and management of patients in critical condition. They should also be encouraged to call for help and to know whom to call in which situation. A structured way of communication is useful and should also be trained, e.g. with the Situation-Background-Assessment-Recommendation (SBAR) or Reason-Story-Vital Signs-Plan (RSVP) approach.

For successful management of emergencies and critical incidents, good communication and teamwork are vital. The team leader should remain calm and communicate clearly although time to solve the problem is usually very limited so that diagnostic and treatment procedures may be required at the same time or with overlap.

When called to an emergency situation, ask for a brief report. Simultaneously perform an initial assessment of the patient according to the A-B-C-D-E approach (see below). Do not hesitate to *call for help* if you are not sure to be able to solve the problem with the persons who are present at the site. In difficult-to-treat life-threatening emergencies, even a person who is not on duty may be called from home to help save the life. During all efforts, regularly re-assess the patient. Use an observation chart with timely documentation of events, vital signs at regular intervals, medications, and interventions during treatment. Use a clock. If no visible clock is in the room, use the timer function of the vital signs monitor (if available), or put your mobile phone on the observation list and start its timer or stopwatch function.

Exception from ABCDE Approach for Trauma Patients with Severe Bleeding The approach used for trauma is *(c)ABC,* which means that catastrophic bleeding needs to be treated first, before assessing airway and breathing with an approach to control the bleeding, e.g. by mechanical compression, tourniquet, or by immediately rushing to operation theatre while one team member calls the OP team to prepare for damage control surgery. If the patient is unresponsive, apply jaw thrust, and use an OPA which does not cost any time. Put IV access when in theatre so that the surgical team can already begin with preparation and sterile draping. If peripheral IV access cannot be established within 2 min, consider cannulation of the external jugular vein or inserting an intraosseous cannula. If IV access is achieved, just give ketamine and oxygen initially, apply a fast-running drip with NS/RL, and focus on stabilising haemodynamics and obtaining blood for transfusion. Consider tranexamic acid 1 g if no more than 3 h have elapsed since injury.

The aim of the initial treatment is to keep the patient alive and achieve some clinical improvement. This will buy time for further treatment and making a diagnosis. Remember that it can take a few minutes for treatments to work, so wait a short while before reassessing the patient after an intervention.

15.1.1 Working Systematically by ABCDE Approach

Recommended video for training: https://www.resus.org.uk/library/abcde-approach www.youtube.com/watch?v=KNqoXboSVUI&t=42s by Resuscitation Council UK.

In the absence of uncontrolled critical bleeding which is addressed before airway and breathing, the primary approach to all deteriorating or critically ill patients is the same.

A—*Airway*—is the patient breathing through a patent airway, or is the airway obstructed? Perform jaw thrust if the patient is unconscious and place the head in a neutral position. Use an oropharyngeal airway if the patient is unconscious and consider endotracheal intubation after having checked B and C.

B—*Breathing*—can you feel breaths with your hand over the patient's mouth and nose? Do you see bilateral breast excursions or the diaphragm moving? If the patient is not breathing use a face mask and SIB to ventilate manually and consider intubation after having checked C. Is the breathing irregular, normal, or fast (>20/min adults)? Wheezing, chest tightness, or other signs of respiratory distress? No breathing on one side of the chest—consider pneumothorax. What is skin colour—nails—tongue—eyelids? Is the patient pink, pale, or cyanotic? If available, use a pulse oximeter to check oxygen saturation.

C—*Circulation*—feel the pulse: Is it strong or weak or absent; slow, adequate, or fast; regular or irregular, arrhythmic? Is capillary refill time (CRT) <2 s? No palpable radial pulse? Check carotid pulse or femoral pulse. If no pulse is detected, start chest compressions, and call for help. Check BP: Is BP detectable or not, systolic pressure > 100 but < 200?

D—Disability—within the ABCDE approach, disability means impaired consciousness. Check consciousness, pupils, and blood glucose. Rule out very low blood pressure or hypoxia as a cause for unconsciousness. Assess according to AVPU or Glasgow Coma Scale (GCS) (see below).

D—Drugs—some of the most important emergency drugs are adrenaline, amiodarone, atropine, dexamethasone, dextrose, ephedrine, furosemide, hydrocortisone, ketamine, lidocaine, and morphine.

E—Exposure—examine to find an explanation for the patient's condition. E applies particularly to injured or burned patients and means to examine the whole patient for injury including front and back. Log-roll the patient if a spine injury is suspected. Be careful not to lose venous access when turning the patient, and do not have the patient lying completely uncovered. Even check the temperature—high fever or low body temperature?

15.1.2 The AVPU Method to Assess Level of Consciousness

While the internationally used GCS is a bit complicated, using the AVPU method is effective and simple. Rapidly estimate the patient to be *alert (A), voice responsive (V), pain responsive (P), or unresponsive (U)*. Record your findings on the observation chart.

Unconscious patients need to get their airway protected, either by turning the patient into a stable lateral position (not applicable for patients with trauma of the spine) or by a device like an endotracheal tube, oropharyngeal, or nasopharyngeal airway. Even a laryngeal mask may be inserted; however, that device can only be used a few hours, not several days. Suction of the airway must be performed if there are any secretions in the throat. NGT should be inserted soon.

15.1.3 The Glasgow Coma Scale (GCS)

GCS is a score to describe the degree of impaired consciousness independent of the cause. It is used for medical and trauma patients. In traumatic brain injury (TBI), the score is a measure

Table 15.1 The Glasgow coma scale. Maximum score = 15 and minimum score = 3

Eyes	Points	Verbal response	Points	Motor response	Points
–		–		Obeys command	6
–		Oriented talk	5	Localises to pain	5
Open	4	Confused	4	Withdraws to pain	4
Open to voice	3	Inappropriate words	3	Abnormal flexion to pain	3
Open to pain	2	Incomprehensible sounds	2	Abnormal extension to pain	2
None	1	None	1	None	1

of severity—mild = 13–15, moderate = 9–12, and severe = 3–8. Table 15.1 shows the details.

15.2 Circulatory Shock

15.2.1 Definition, Pathophysiology, and Compensation Mechanisms

Shock is one of the most important causes of death among surgical patients. Death may occur as a consequence of the profound, irreversible state of shock with resulting circulatory collapse, or be delayed resulting from the consequences and complications of organ ischaemia, e.g. acute renal failure, adult respiratory distress syndrome (ARDS), or severe coagulation disorders (loss of coagulation factors and thrombocytes or disseminated intravascular coagulation).

Shock is an acute life-threatening situation of generalised hypoxia (oxygen deficiency) and acidosis of the cells of all tissues and organs in the body. It is caused by an acute, severe imbalance between the oxygen demand and the oxygen supply of the body or by impaired tissue perfusion.

The underlying cause of a circulatory shock is most often acute blood loss (***haemorrhagic shock***), thereby loss of erythrocytes as oxygen carriers + decrease of cardiac output or any other cause of severe hypovolaemia (***hypovolaemic shock***) leading to cardiac failure due to diminished venous return. If the heart fails to pump enough blood, then the oxygen supply to the organs is insufficient even with normal Hb.

Sepsis can also cause shock *(**septic shock**)* by shunts between arterioles and venules with hypoperfusion of the capillaries leading to hypoxia of the tissues. The generalised hypoxia and acidotic metabolites in the cells then lead to secondary cardiac failure. Those patients need oxygen and vasopressor infusion plus antibiotics and would often require ventilatory support in an HDU or ICU.

Anaphylaxis/severe allergic reaction may cause shock *(**anaphylactic shock**)* by sudden vasodilatation leading to a marked decrease of venous return and thereby to cardiac failure.

The same can happen after a traumatic lesion of the spinal cord or with accidentally total spinal anaesthesia, the so-called *spinal or **neurogenic shock***, where massive vasodilatation is combined with a lack of compensatory tachycardia. Give vasopressor drugs and IV infusions, and ventilate the patients.

Cardiac failure, e.g. caused by lung embolism, tension pneumothorax, or myocardial infarction can lead to a primary ***cardiogenic shock*** and may quickly progress to cardiac arrest. The underlying cause needs to be treated. A pneu requires needle decompression followed by chest drain. If available, the patient should be treated in ICU or HDU after initial resuscitation.

Independent of the underlying cause, the pathophysiology and the reactions of the body to all forms of shock are almost the same.

Shock most commonly occurs as a result of an imbalance between the blood volume and the capacity of circulation and thereby impaired tissue perfusion. Fluid losses reduce the venous return to the right heart and decrease cardiac output. Within not more than 1 min, the body reacts as a response to stimulation of baroreceptors in the carotid arteries with an immediate increase in the activity of the sympathetic nervous system. That results in the release of adrenaline by the adrenal glands, leading to increased heart rate and peripheral vasoconstriction. Cardiac output is redistributed away from skin, muscle, kidney, and bowels, while the blood flow to the vital organs, mainly the heart, lungs, and brain, is maintained as long as possible. The kidneys suffer from hypoperfusion that may result in acute renal failure after survival of shock and, without intermittent haemodialysis, lead to death several days after survival of the initial phase of the shock and reinstitution of normal circulation and oxygenation.

The respiratory system reacts by increasing the respiratory rate and the alveolar ventilation to establish a respiratory alkalosis to compensate for the metabolic acidosis. That means by exhalation of more CO_2, the concentration of carbonic acid in the blood decreases, and thereby the acidosis becomes less. The metabolic acidosis during shock is caused by acidic products that accumulate in the tissues due to their poor oxygenation (anaerobic metabolism is ineffective and produces a lot of lactic acid).

Normal BP does not exclude severe bleeding! Give IV fluids if bleeding is likely. *A decrease in arterial blood pressure is a late symptom of shock* as it is maintained normal until approximately 20% of blood volume is lost and cardiac output has already diminished by 30% if patients are not anaesthetised. Under general or spinal anaesthesia or under antihypertensive drugs, these compensatory mechanisms are disturbed, so volume loss is less well tolerated.

If the blood loss is stopped at a critical level, where survival is possible, for further compensation, the pituitary gland produces increased ADH (antidiuretic hormone) and the adrenal gland produces aldosterone in order to decrease urinary output and to retain water and sodium. Fluid shifts from the intracellular fluid space (ICF) to the extracellular fluid compartment (ECF) resulting in the normalisation of the blood volume within 24 h.

If the cause of the shock is too severe or the blood loss too much, the compensatory mechanisms will fail. In the end stage, hypoxia and acidosis of heart muscle and blood vessel myocytes lead to vasodilatation and bradycardia with a further decrease in cardiac output. This phase has been termed "***irreversible shock***" and means that patients are unlikely to survive when this stage is reached even if maximum resuscitation therapy is performed.

15.2.2 Hypovolaemic Shock

Hypovolaemic shock is most often presenting as haemorrhagic shock caused by life-threatening bleeding. Patients are pale; the pulse is fast and weak, and the blood pressure is low. The pulse rate divided by systolic blood pressure is >1 (so-called "shock index"), which means pulse >100/min and systolic arterial pressure <100 mmHg. The sympathetic stimulation leads to sweating, the skin is cool, and patients are often anxious or restless. Respiratory frequency is increased, and urinary output is decreased. In order to measure urinary output and prevent renal failure, a bladder catheter should be inserted early. Urinary output of at least 0.5 ml/kg BW/h indicates sufficient therapy; therefore, a careful monitoring of urine production is mandatory.

A very good and fast-to-obtain-indicator is the *capillary refill time (CRT)*, assessed at a fingernail: If it takes more than 2 s (that is longer than to say the words "capillary refill"), perfusion of peripheral tissues may be markedly decreased, and if it is normal, severe shock is unlikely. A useful measure to assess the severity of shock is given in Table 15.2.

15.2.3 Management

Elevating the legs will often improve venous return and cardiac output in the hypovolaemic patient.

Replacement of blood volume by aggressive, fast, and uninterrupted infusion therapy with more than one large-bore venous line is essential (exception: cardiogenic shock, which requires specific treatment according to the underlying cause). Ringer's solution and plasma expanders

Table 15.2 ATLS classification of haemorrhagic shock (ATLS means advanced trauma life support foundation, see Chap. 13)

Class	I	II	III	IV
% Blood loss of TBV	<15	15–25	25–40	>40
Heart rate	<100	>100	>120	>140
Blood pressure	>100	Ca. 100	<100	Very low
Urine output ml/kg/h	>0.5	0.25–0.5	Little	None
Mental status	Slightly anxious	Anxious	Confused	Lethargic

are best suited, normal saline (which contains too much chloride to be the first choice) is an alternative when Ringer's solution is not available, while glucose-containing infusions are not suitable. (During shock, patients cannot metabolise glucose adequately. Instead, lactate production increases further and the acidosis is getting more severe due to the anaerobic metabolism.)

The patients are often sweating, so the large-bore IV cannula needs to be taped very well and may be secured even with a gauze bandage if the skin is moist! To lose an intravenous cannula in a patient with severe shock may lead to the death of that patient because it may be impossible to establish a new IV line.

Rapid infusion needs to be continued until the bleeding/fluid losses have stopped and until the whole estimated amount of acute blood loss/fluid loss has been replaced. If the amount of loss is not known, a good measure for sufficient fluid intake is a urinary output of more than 0.5 ml/kg BW/h in combination with systolic blood pressure >100 mmHg and a pulse rate of <100/min (however, tachycardia may also continue longer because of stress and pain). If crystalloid infusions are administered (i.e. NS or RL), they will be distributed in the whole ECR (extracellular space), that is, the threefold volume than the blood volume. Therefore, the threefold amount is needed to compensate for blood loss. For example, if blood loss is 1000 ml, 3000 ml (3 l) of NS or RL is needed to fully compensate for the volume. If bleeding is severe, early blood transfusion is recommended and is better than giving high volumes of crystalloids. Warm blood is advantageous as it contains platelets and coagulation factors. If more than four units of blood are transfused, the patient should receive 1 g calcium gluconate IV which is necessary to keep coagulation sufficient.

In the initial phase, patients may compensate for even very low Hb values if the circulating blood volume is kept normal, and a sufficient cardiac output can be established by compensatory vasoconstriction and tachycardia. Patients die not from low Hb itself but from hypoxia, which is a result of both the lack of oxygen in the blood and low cardiac output. Give the patient oxygen via a face mask (5 l/min) whenever possible. Thereby, the amount of available (physically dissolved) oxygen in the blood may be increased effectively and help the patient to survive.

A blood sample should be taken for Hb as soon as possible and a cross match performed if a blood transfusion is needed. Avoid taking the sample from an arm while infusions are running, because the measurement will then be unreliable. The puncture of the radial or femoral artery or femoral vein to get a blood sample may be an alternative if infusions are running at both arms. Arterial blood gas analysis can be performed if available and gives information of acid–base status and oxygen and CO_2 in the body.

The oxygen consumption of the body may be decreased by sedation with diazepam (if the patient is restless but not suffering from pain) or by pain relief with pethidine (meperidine)/morphine/tramadol/pentazocine. Remember that pethidine and morphine may decrease blood pressure. A combination of diazepam and opioids should be avoided as that combination could lead to severe respiratory depression. Severe pain is not only unpleasant but worsens a shock and should therefore always be treated with analgesics. If all the above-mentioned analgesics are unavailable or unsuitable (e.g. if BP is low), give small increments of ketamine (25–50 mg IV in adults) plus a small dose of diazepam (2.5–5 mg). Blood pressure and pulse rate or heart rate must be taken as often as possible, at least every 3 min. If available, vital signs monitoring with pulse oximetry, ECG, and automatic blood pressure measurement should be performed and all vital signs be recorded on anaesthesia record or observation chart.

Vasoactive drugs = sympathomimetic or vasopressor drugs such as ephedrine, adrenaline (in some countries called epinephrine), phenylephrine, noradrenaline (=norepinephrine), or dopamine are useful if arterial blood pressure remains low in spite of sufficient fluid administration. A systolic blood pressure of >70–90 is regarded sufficient and should not be treated with vasopressors unless the patient is a known hypertensive case, old, or has traumatic brain injury when SBP should be kept >100 mmHg. While ephedrine is administered as an IV or IM bolus, the other sympathomimetic drugs are better administered with continuous infusion because of their very short duration of effect (half-life of around 3 min). Adrenaline is the strongest of these drugs. If you do not have a syringe pump, just put one ampoule into a 500 ml infusion and let it drip with a speed that lets BP stabilise around 80–100 mmHg of systolic pressure; start with 30 drops/min that is one drop every 2 s. Otherwise, one ampoule into 50 ml in a syringe pump, start with 10 ml/h and adjust according to the target effect.

An ***observation record*** should be filled in as exactly as possible. All drugs, infusions, and vital signs should be recorded together with the exact time. Blood pressure and pulse rate/heart rate need to be measured every few minutes until the patient is circulatory stable. If a peripheral pulse is not detectable and BP is not measurable, the heart rate must be measured with the help of a stethoscope if no ECG monitor is available. Use an ECG monitor in all patients if available. If disposable electrodes are O/S, just use a little cotton wool, moist with NS, put it on the skin, put the ECG cable above it, and use adhesive tape to keep it in place; it works very well. The urinary output must be measured and carefully recorded as acute kidney failure is a common and serious complication of shock. After treatment of the underlying cause, the patient needs close observation for at least 24 h, if possible, in an ICU, HDU, or intermediate care unit (even improvised as a place in the ward near the nurse's office).

Treatment of the underlying cause must be done as soon as possible which means, in case of haemorrhage, the source of bleeding must be stopped as quickly as possible (by immediate operation if required).

15.2.4 Anaphylactic Shock

This type of shock is caused by a severe, life-threatening anaphylactoid reaction, often due to severe allergy and exposure to the antigen that causes the allergy. During anaesthesia, it is generally rare, but if it occurs, it is most often caused by muscle relaxants or by antibiotics or atropine. Blood transfusions and contrast for X-rays as well as latex may also cause severe anaphylactic reactions. However, latex is more and more being replaced by plastic or silicone which is safe. Assume anaphylactic shock if you cannot measure BP or observe severe arrhythmia with or without flushing of the skin or bronchospasm very short after administration of a drug which is known to cause allergic reactions in susceptible persons. Severe anaphylactic reactions may lead to cardiac arrest very quickly.

First-line treatment of ***anaphylactic shock*** is IM injection of adrenaline 0.5 mg = 0.5 ml for adults >50 kg BW; infants <10 kg 0.1 mg = 0.1 ml; children 10–25 kg BW 0.15 mg = 0.15 ml; and patients 25–50 kg BW get 0.3 mg = 0.3 ml into the mid-outer thigh. IM adrenaline is the first choice even in patients with IV access. For small doses, you may dilute 1 ml of adrenaline with 1 ml of NS or water for injection or whatever fluid is available and inject twice the volume as stated above. Then, 500–1000 ml of normal saline or Ringer's solution (children 20 ml/kg) is infused at high speed through a large-bore venous cannula. Check pulse and BP.

If no BP is measurable and the pulse is weak or absent, perform chest compressions and give IV injection of adrenaline 0.5–1.0 mg, repeated every 3 min until systolic blood pressure is stable >90 mmHg. Adrenaline IV must be diluted to facilitate exact dosing as it can cause severe arrhythmias. Notably, 1.0 mg is the recommended dose for cardiac arrest, while smaller doses are given in severe hypotension, starting with 0.05 mg or 0.1 mg (i.e. 0.5–1 ml of a dilution of 1 ampoule in 10 ml sodium chloride). The effect of adrenaline is very strong but short-lasting. Therefore, it should be repeated every 3 min until the patient has become stable. After each injection of adrenaline, the blood pressure must be measured to assess the effect and adjust the dose. Alternatively, an adrenaline infusion can be started.

Additional treatment is cortisone as a single shot of 4–8 mg dexamethasone or 100–200 mg of hydrocortisone.

15.3 Circulatory Arrest and Advanced Life Support (ALS)

Cardiac arrest is an emergency among in-patients, approximately around 5 per 1000 patients. The outcome is extremely poor if cardiopulmonary resuscitation (CPR) with chest compressions is not started immediately since the brain would remain with permanent damage already within 3 min of circulatory arrest. However, there is inter-individual variability which means some patients suffer from brain damage although resuscitation was started instantaneously, while others survive in good condition even after 10 min without resuscitation. The latter is yet unusual. Even with well performed timely CPR, less than 20% of patients would survive until discharged from hospital.

If a patient with cardiac arrest shall have a chance, a "chain of survival" is necessary. That means:

- Early recognition and call for help
- Early starting CPR with chest compressions and ventilation
- Early defibrillation
- Good post-resuscitation care, if possible, in an HDU or ICU

Prevention of in-hospital cardiac arrest can be possible in some cases as cardiac arrest is the end of a deteriorating disease state with hypoxia and hypotension that goes often unrecognised if patients are not closely observed and monitored in the wards.

15.3.1 Basic and Advanced Life Support

The diagnosis cardiac arrest is made if a patient is unconscious and unresponsive with no or severely abnormal breathing. It is not mandatory to provide proof for the absence of pulse. Assume cardiac arrest, call for help, and start CPR. High-quality chest compressions are vital and mean compressions with a depth of 5–6 cm and a rate of 100–120/min which are interrupted only very shortly during ventilation with 2 breaths after each 30 compressions and when persons are changing every 2 min as well as for defibrillation if indicated. The hands are in the middle of the lower half of the sternum placing the thenar (heel of the hand) on the sternum and avoiding the fingers to compress the ribs (rib fractures and other injuries may be caused). Between compressions, the chest must be allowed to recoil completely; otherwise, the chambers of the heart would not fill sufficiently.

Recommended video on adult advanced life support: https://www.youtube.com/watch?v=jQYHQr3ebLo.

Initially, in most cases, ventilation will be with a bag and face mask, if possible, additionally with Guedel airway. If a SIB and mask are not at hand, mouth-to-mouth ventilation must be performed until devices have been fetched. Notably, 30 compressions and 2 breaths are alternately provided without longer than a minimum interruption of compressions. A laryngeal mask airway (LMA) or other type of supraglottic airway can be inserted and would facilitate CPR. Patients with LMA or ETT are ventilated 10 times per minute, while chest compressions are continuously provided without interruption. The patient should receive pure oxygen. Tracheal intubation is only beneficial if provided by a skilled and experienced person who can perform it within 10 s (according to the guidelines). Otherwise, facemasks or LMAs are superior for the outcome.

When cardiac arrest is confirmed and help including a defibrillator arrives, chest compressions and ventilation are continued while applying self-adhesive defibrillator electrodes or preparing the paddles.

The rhythm is identified—is it shockable or non-shockable?

If the rhythm is shockable *(ventricular tachycardia or fibrillation)*, the defibrillator is charged with >150 J (3–5 J/kg). During a pause of compressions for no more than 5 s, the shock is applied (make sure that nobody is in touch with the patient or the bed). After shock, immediately continue with compressions and ventilation. Continue CPR for 2 min. Then check the heart rhythm again, continue CPR, and repeat defibrillation (200 J or more) if still shockable rhythm. Continue CPR for another 2 min. This is repeated a third time in the same situation. An IV or intraosseous access is established under continuing CPR. *After the third defibrillation (250–360 J),* give 1 mg of adrenaline which should be diluted to 10 ml and followed by infusion of NS or RL. Give amiodarone 300 mg, if available, or lidocaine 1 mg/kg (50–100 mg), slowly IV as an antiarrhythmic drug. Continue adrenaline 1 mg every 3–5 min as long as CPR is performed. Even a fourth or fifth defibrillation may be indicated and a second dose of amiodarone (then 150 mg) or lidocaine 1 mg/kg.

In cardiac arrest with no shockable rhythm, perform CPR, establish venous access, and give adrenaline 1 mg (diluted to 10 ml to make 0.1 mg/ml) every 3–5 min (children 10 μg/kg = 0.01 mg/kg) with a running infusion to enable the adrenaline to be distributed in the whole blood volume. A flush of at least 20 ml fluid is needed to get a drug delivered from the peripheral vein to the central circulation during cardiac arrest, which is best achieved by also elevating that limb above the heart.

Sodium bicarbonate is no longer recommended for CPR as it does not add any benefit in most cases. The best treatment for acidosis during cardiac arrest is performing chest compressions and ventilation with oxygen.

Give oxygen as soon as possible. Treat reversible causes, e.g. hypovolaemia, hypothermia, and tension pneumothorax (with large bore venous cannula in the second intercostal space midclavicular line or fifth intercostal space anterior axillary line followed by intercostal chest drain as soon as possible).

The team leader/the physician who is responsible for the patient decides how long to perform CPR if no return of spontaneous circulation is obtained. If circulation recovers, start post-resuscitation care at the highest level of care unit in your hospital. Treat underlying disease if possible.

15.3.2 Resuscitating in the Operation Room

Causes for cardiac arrest in the OR:

- Relative overdose of induction agent. Thiopentone and propofol are available in different concentrations which facilitate wrong labelling of syringes and overdose. Wrong dose if body weight is not known may be a second cause, especially in children.
- Hypoxic cardiac arrest. Cannot ventilate—cannot intubate situation or lost airway (dislocated ETT), unrecognised oesophageal intubation. Perform CPR and apply the algorithm for difficult airway (Chap. 6). Pure oxygen and ventilation are vital.
- Hypovolaemia (bleeding), e.g. during caesarean section. Before the infant is delivered, consider aortocaval compression syndrome (see Chap. 11). If bleeding is massive and cannot be stopped quickly by the surgeon, shock

may be severe and lead to circulatory collapse. Perform CPR (unlikely to need a defibrillator) and give infusions and blood at full speed. Give adrenaline infusion. At least two venous cannulae are needed.
- Lung embolism (arrhythmia, low end-tidal CO_2, low BP, and low SPO_2 may precede cardiac arrest). ALS according to the algorithm above.
- Anaphylactic reaction after drugs or blood transfusion. Adrenaline IM plus adrenaline IV and simultaneous CPR according to the ALS algorithm.
- Tension pneumothorax, e.g. during laparoscopic operations. CPR if no pulse/no BP is recordable; cannula inserted in the second intercostal space midline or fifth ICS in the anterior axillary line.

Guidelines for ALS in theatre are the same as elsewhere. In theatre, infrastructure is better, and patients usually have IV access, often plus airway access. Ventilate with pure oxygen and stop anaesthetic agents. Start cardiac compressions at a rate of 100–120/min. Get a defibrillator and use the same algorithm as stated above for patients in other locations in the hospital. Simultaneously, the underlying cause for cardiac arrest in theatre must be treated if possible.

15.4 Laryngospasm, Bronchospasm, and Pneumothorax

15.4.1 Laryngospasm

Presentation is a sudden incident showing inspiratory stridor or absence of breathing sounds and paradoxical respiratory movements with incomplete, then complete airway obstruction caused by spastic contraction of the vocal cords. It occurs most frequently during anaesthesia induction or awakening. Children are more prone to this complication than adults. Chest movements may be excessive, but there is no movement of the reservoir bag and no capnography reading. Desaturation is the most common manifestation. Other symptoms are bradycardia and finally even asystole.

Laryngospasm is impossible with an endotracheal tube inserted, while bronchospasm is still possible.

Management: Give pure oxygen with high continuous pressure via a tight-fitting mask. Make sure you have a skilled assistant or call for help.

During induction: Increase the depth of anaesthesia by an extra dose of propofol or other IV anaesthetic. If there is no improvement and saturation decreases or the patient gets bluish, give suxamethonium 25–50 mg IV (twice that dose IM if no IV access). Add atropine to avoid bradycardia. Intubate the patient instead of using a laryngeal mask. Suction if any secretions are visible with the laryngoscope.

During the wakening of the patient: In many cases, applying high-pressure oxygen via a tight-fitting mask is sufficient. Add a small dose of propofol or thiopentone or ketamine or suxamethonium half intubation dose if saturation decreases without improvement of ventilation/breathing. Add atropine. Use a laryngoscope and remove secretions if there are any but do this quickly and keep an eye on saturation. Reintubation is often not necessary; instead, use gentle manual ventilation as soon as the spasm resolves until the patient is sufficiently breathing spontaneously. Monitor the patient carefully until fully recovered.

Prevention: In patients at risk (e.g. patients with known asthma), give lidocaine 1 mg/KG IV before suxamethonium and intubation. Propofol is superior to thiopentone and ketamine as an induction agent to prevent laryngospasm. Remove all secretions or blood until the larynx is completely cleared before extubation. Wait until the patient is awake and avoid extubation during the excitation phase after inhalational anaesthesia (that means do not irritate the patient when pupils are wide). Children can be put in a left lateral position with an elevated pelvis before wakening, especially if secretions in the airway are expected, e.g. after tonsillectomy or adenectomy.

15.4.2 Bronchospasm

Causes Causes include asthma, airway infections, especially in patients with a history of asthma or COPD; patients during surgery, if GA is performed in spite of respiratory tract infection; children and young adults during wakening from inhalational anaesthesia; and allergic/anaphylactic reaction.

Symptoms Symptoms include difficulty breathing/ventilation in anaesthetised patients with increased airway pressure/high ventilation peak pressure; on auscultation wheezing, prolonged expiration; decreasing oxygen saturation; and capnography without reaching a plateau, looking like a shark fin.

Management Give oxygen, and in severe cases, call for help. Drugs for nebulising need a volume of at least 4 ml, and the patient's dose should be diluted to 4–5 ml. Ventoline® = salbutamol 2.5 mg/ml—dilute 5 mg of it with 2–3 ml NS; or 0.5 mg adrenaline diluted to 5 ml with NS in the nebuliser. The dose may be repeated if necessary. Hydrocortisone 1–2 mg/kg. Aminophylline 1 amp = 240 mg for adults slowly IV or 5 mg/kg over 20 min (fast injection leads to tachyarrhythmia). Bricanyl = salbutamol 0.5 mg /ml = 1 amp SC. Magnesium 1–2 g slowly IV. Ketamine 0.5 mg/kg, followed by ketamine infusion 1 mg/kg/h. Inhalational anaesthetics are strong bronchodilators; however, bronchospasm may occur when they are stopped. In extreme cases, adrenaline 0.1 mg may be injected slowly IV followed by infusion. Side effects are tachycardia and hypertension. Start with one of these drugs, add a second if there is no effect, add a third if there is still no improvement, and add a fourth if it is still not good.

15.4.3 Pneumothorax

Simple pneumothorax means there is air in the pleural space compressing the lung. Tension pneumothorax is the same under pressure. A tension pneumothorax can be caused when a patient with pneumothorax is ventilated with IPPV. A pneumothorax can develop spontaneously in patients who are prone to it, but most often, it is caused by chest trauma. During surgery, pneumothorax is a rare but dangerous complication caused by injury of the lung, the diaphragm, or too high ventilation pressure which would cause rupture of alveoli. Symptoms include high airway/ventilation pressure, hypoxia, uneven chest excursions, and differences between breathing sounds in both lungs. Exclude accidental endobronchial intubation! Patients with pneumothorax must never get nitrous oxide.

A tension pneumothorax would additionally cause hypotension and circulatory collapse. Sometimes, distended jugular veins become visible.

A stable patient may undergo chest X-ray or ultrasound imaging for diagnosis. An unstable patient with suspected tension pneumothorax needs immediate action. Give oxygen. Insert a large-bore cannula in the second intercostal space in the midclavicular line and confirm position in the pleura space by hearing the sound of escaping air. In big patients, the cannula may be too short to reach the pleura, try to use a longer cannula if available. Check pulse and BP and give adrenaline if BP/pulse is low. Perform CPR if pulseless and no BP. Then, as soon as possible, an intercostal drain with an underwater seal should be inserted in the midaxillary line. After stabilising the patient, a chest X-ray may be taken to confirm the correct position of the drain.

15.5 Pulmonary Aspiration of Gastric Contents

Definition Gastric contents enter the airways.

This critical incident can happen during anaesthesia induction, during surgery, or in the early recovery period.

Rule Out Endobronchial intubation, bronchospasm of different causes, pulmonary oedema, or foreign body in the airway.

Complications Bronchospasm, respiratory insufficiency, hypoxia, and pneumonia.

Aspiration During Anaesthesia Induction with Intubation During laryngoscopy, gastric contents regurgitate visibly and enter the trachea. Aim to intubate as fast as possible and inflate the cuff. Then perform suction through the ETT before starting ventilation, even if SpO_2 is decreasing. Of course, suction must not take much time. Then ventilate with oxygen and auscultate both lungs. Gastric contents usually reach the right bronchus and the right lung rather than the left side. The difference in breathing sounds in this case may be caused by aspiration instead of endobronchial intubation. If available, apply capnography. Fix the tube with adhesive tape, insert a nasogastric or orogastric tube, and empty the stomach. If possible, ventilate with positive end-expiratory pressure (PEEP). Persisting bronchospasm is treated as stated under Sect. 15.4.2. Prophylactic antibiotics are not recommended. If ventilation is possible and saturation is adequate, the surgery may be performed as planned. After the operation, a decision needs to be made if the patient should be extubated early or delayed. This depends on the severity of aspiration. If oxygenation and ventilation are quite good, and the patient is able to breathe sufficiently at the end of the operation, extubation may be performed; if not, the tube should be maintained. However, a tube is helping much only provided the patient can be kept on PEEP/CPAP/IPPV ventilation postoperatively.

If there is no ICU with a ventilator, sometimes keeping the patient on an anaesthesia machine can be a good option; alternatively, use an Ambu bag (SIB) for manually assisted and spontaneous ventilation, and give oxygen to keep $SpO_2 > 93\%$. In hospitals without a mechanical ventilator, a PEEP valve to be attached to the SIB is highly recommended. It is cheap and easy to use. Ambu PEEP valves can be obtained single-use or reusable. The positive end-expiratory pressure (PEEP) keeps the lung alveoli open and helps in the prevention and treatment of atelectasis. Patients with severe pneumonia are more likely to survive and recover with PEEP. Then, the AP needs to look after the patient even during the next 24 h or longer together with the staff in the respective ward.

Aspiration During Surgery in Patients on LMA or Face Mask Pregnant women and patients with full stomach are at risk for regurgitation of gastric contents. It depends on the depth of anaesthesia and the general condition of the patient if he/she is able to vomit and clear the throat, or inhales and aspirates the gastric contents. A supraglottic airway device like the LMA must be taken out if there is suspicion of vomiting and regurgitation. Perform suction of the throat and stomach and intubate under sufficient anaesthesia and muscle relaxation if skills and equipment render it possible. Otherwise, the same treatment as above would apply.

Aspiration postoperatively, in a spontaneously breathing, not intubated patient, e.g. in the recovery area: Turn the patient in a left-lateral, head-down position (put a pillow or a folded blanket under the pelvis to get the head at the lowest position). Apply suction and give oxygen via face mask. Treat bronchospasm as stated above. Severe cases require intubation and treatment with PEEP/CPAP/artificial ventilation if available.

15.6 Transfusion Reactions

Blood transfusions need to be blood group compatible and cross-matched with a sample of the patient's blood to prevent antigen–antibody transfusion reactions. The most severe adverse reactions are haemolytic transfusion reactions caused by incompatibility, often by giving blood with the wrong blood group.

Symptoms The symptoms include chills, fever, flashing or urticarial rash, restlessness, anxiety, bronchospasm with difficulty breathing, pain in the chest, or back, haematuria (brown colour of urine) coagulopathy, and circulatory shock.

Antibodies of the recipient destroy the red blood cells of the transfusion if the blood groups are not compatible. The destroyed erythrocytes cause haemolysis, the urine is getting brownish colour, and acute kidney injury may be the consequence of haemoglobin, platelets, and other particles of the damaged red blood cells clogging and obstructing the small capillaries in the glomeruli, thus hindering the kidneys from producing primary urine.

Minor transfusion reactions can be allergic without haemolysis, as there are several antigens and antibodies on blood cells and in plasma besides the antigens/antibodies of the blood groups A, B, 0, and AB.

Management Stop the transfusion; give oxygen, check ABC, give infusion NS or RL full speed, and call for help. Treat low blood pressure or bronchospasm with adrenaline for anaphylactic shock. Monitor and record all vital signs. If transfusion of incompatible blood is confirmed and there is an urgent need for transfusion, try to obtain cross-matched blood for the patient and give it.

Send the patient to the ICU or HDU or improvised higher-level care place. Consider referral to a larger hospital if multiple organ failure seems likely to occur.

Return the blood bag and a blood sample of the patient to the laboratory and inform about the incident. Record the event in the patient's file and inform him/her and the relatives. In many countries, transfusion reactions must be reported according to an incident management and investigation system.

15.7 Malignant Hyperthermia

Malignant hyperthermia (MH) is a very rare but often deadly complication during inhalation anaesthesia. Most AP will never experience a case during their lifetime since the incidence is about 1 in 50,000 anaesthetics where one of the trigger medications is used. The condition for MH is genetic, so family history is important. Some groups of patients show higher susceptibility for MH, most of them having neurological diseases such as muscular dystrophy. In these patients, MH may occur as anaesthesia complication already before they have developed any symptoms of the muscular disease. Therefore, young children are more frequently getting MH compared with adults.

MH is a hypermetabolic condition that is triggered by inhalational anaesthetics such as halothane/isoflurane/sevoflurane and by the muscle relaxant suxamethonium, but not by any other muscle relaxants such as pancuronium or atracurium. Intravenous anaesthetics such as ketamine, propofol, and thiopental or opioid drugs such as pethidine, morphine, and fentanyl do not trigger MH and can safely be used in patients with a positive history.

MH can start immediately after anaesthesia induction or begin delayed, but seldom more than 40 min after the beginning of anaesthesia.

Symptoms Symptoms include increased heart rate, arrhythmias, increased respiratory rate with hyperventilation in spontaneously breathing patients; a steep and marked rise in end-tidal CO_2 (if capnography is used), hypoxia (decreased oxygen saturation as seen with the pulse oximeter), stiff muscles of the jaws (even spasm with difficulty to open the mouth), the thorax, and the limbs; and as a late sign, markedly increased body temperature, sweating, and brownish urine (due to rhabdomyolysis with muscle cell break down and increased excretion of myoglobin). Lab results: acidosis, hyperkalaemia, and coagulation disorders (DIC = disseminated intravascular coagulation).

Differential Diagnosis Inadequate/light anaesthesia, sepsis, anaphylaxis (allergic reaction), and thyroid storm (especially patients with goitres).

Management Call for help if you suspect MH. Inform the surgeon and ask to stop or end the procedure. Stop the trigger agents, that is, switch off the vaporiser. If possible, remove the vaporiser from the anaesthesia machine. Increase fresh gas flow to at least 8 l oxygen/min and increase ventilation by three times. Increase tidal volume until the peak pressure is 20 cm water. If the patient is breathing spontaneously and you do not have an automatic ventilator, ask a theatre nurse to hand-ventilate the patient with one breath every 2 s. If the patient is not intubated, try to intubate or insert an LMA but do not lose too much time with such efforts, maximum two attempts by one person, intermittently manual ventilation.

If the theatre has AC, turn it on to the minimum temperature and expose the patient to reduce body temperature. Give cold infusions quickly, around 3 l RL. Let someone fetch ice from the fridge and mix it with water then instil it into the urinary bladder and the stomach (NGT required) to cool the patient. Stop cooling when the body temperature has decreased to 38.5°C. If the patient needs sedation or anaesthesia, give ketamine and diazepam, fentanyl, or very small doses of propofol or thiopentone. Check BP every 2 min and use vasopressor drugs if required. Use the best vital signs monitor you have. If possible, use a thermometer, ECG, and capnography. Arterial blood gas analysis is also useful if available, but, in severe cases, you can always give 2 mmol/kg sodium bicarbonate. Take blood samples to the lab and ask for blood gas analysis, Hb, potassium, glucose, myoglobin, and DIC parameters, if available. Insert a urine catheter and aim for forced diuresis with around 200–300 ml urine per hour due to rhabdomyolysis (the muscle cells are degenerated to myoglobin which can cause acute kidney failure). Dialysis may be needed if available. FFP and platelets may be needed in severe DIC. Arrhythmias may need treatment with amiodarone (150–300 mg slowly IV), calcium, and magnesium injections/infusions. Severe hyperkalaemia: Dialysis is best; otherwise, insulin/glucose drip with 10 IU insulin per 500 ml glucose 5%.

If dantrolene is available (not likely), give 2.5 up to 10 mg/kg with short infusions.

With that management, a minority of patients (around 25%) may survive. If the patient is surviving, inform him; otherwise, inform the relatives thoroughly and report the incident locally and to the national society of anaesthesiology irrespective of the outcome.

15.8 Local Anaesthetic Toxicity

Local anaesthetic drugs are absorbed from the site of injection. At high blood levels, toxic effects may occur such as seizures, respiratory depression, loss of consciousness, and finally cardiac arrest. Careful administration below the maximum doses is safe. However, if LA is accidentally injected intravenously, blood concentrations can peak above the threshold for toxicity. Lidocaine is the least, but bupivacaine is most likely to cause severe toxicity when overdosed.

Combination with adrenaline leads to prolonged absorption and lower peak concentrations in the blood, allowing higher maximum doses.

15.8.1 Maximum Doses of LA

- Lidocaine without adrenaline 3 mg /kg, with adrenaline 7 mg/kg
- Bupivacaine 2 mg/kg without and 3 mg/kg with adrenaline

Especially small infants are prone to LA toxicity as small amounts can already exceed the maximum dose. Bupivacaine should be diluted to make 2.5 mg/ml for infants.

15.8.2 Early Signs and Management of LA Toxicity

Blurred vision, tinnitus, agitation → give diazepam IV. Call for help. Monitor SpO_2 and ECG if available and measure BP frequently. Give oxygen and observe the patient. Have everything ready for resuscitation. If the patient becomes unconscious, intubate or insert LM and ventilate with oxygen. Mild hyperventilation is advantageous (adults with a frequency of around 16/min). Seizures are treated with diazepam, midazolam, propofol, or thiopentone IV (half the doses for anaesthesia induction). Check pulse. If pulseless, start CPR. If cardiac arrest is caused by bupivacaine, CPR may be needed for more than 60 min. High-quality resuscitation is vital (see Sect. 15.2). If available, a lipid emulsion IV at a rapid infusion rate of up to 300–500 ml total volume (used for parenteral nutrition in the ICU) can be helpful as it can reverse part of the toxic effects of local anaesthetics.

15.9 Prolonged and Severe Adverse Effects of Muscle Relaxants

All muscle relaxants (MR) or neuromuscular blocking agents (NMBAs) cause severe anaphylactic reactions more often than any other drugs used during anaesthesia although still seldom. See Sect. 15.2 anaphylactic shock for symptoms and treatment. Immediately after securing the airway, BP must be measured. If BP is very low, anaphylaxis is possible, and adrenaline should be given immediately.

The effects of NMBAs must have worn off completely before the patient wakes up and is extubated. However, in some patients, the effects of MR are lasting longer than expected. In fact, residual paralysis is quite common when NMBAs are administered, occurring in up to two-thirds of patients. Better keep the endotracheal tube until the patient has completely recovered. After prolonged abdominal surgery in patients with impaired general condition, it may be required to keep the ETT until the next morning to guarantee a patent airway. Pancuronium produces sufficient relaxation for surgery for approximately 45–60 min, but it takes more than 90 min for the patient to regain sufficient muscle strength for swallowing and coughing. Patients with decreased urine output need even longer than 90 min to recover after pancuronium. Atracurium and rocuronium are more reliably and faster eliminated than pancuronium and independent from kidney function.

Serious complications arise if these effects are underestimated. Upper airway integrity is impaired by minimal levels of neuromuscular blockade due to the susceptibility of the upper airway muscles to the effects of NMBAs. Weakness of the airway muscles results in pharyngeal dysfunction with difficulty swallowing. This puts patients at increased risk of pulmonary aspiration.

It is the responsibility of the anaesthesia provider to make sure that the patient is able to breathe, keep a patent airway, keep the eyes open, and swallow and cough to clear the airway from secretions when any artificial airway (ETT or LM) is removed. No patient must die because of the prolonged effect of muscle relaxants, and the anaesthetist is to be blamed if that happens as it is an avoidable anaesthesia complication.

Therefore, the use of muscle relaxants requires a high level of responsibility and practical skills; otherwise, these drugs must not be used! That applies especially for long-lasting MR as pancuronium. It is the responsibility of the anaesthetist to be able to ventilate and oxygenate a patient who cannot breathe because the AP has given him a muscle relaxant drug. If you are not able to ventilate a patient over at least a few hours, you must not use these agents.

Succinylcholine or Suxamethonium is usually short-lasting with onset after 30 s and a duration of effect of 5 min; however, in some individuals, it is up to 20 min. During surgery, smaller doses than for intubation are sufficient, e.g. 25 mg increments for adults. As long as a cumulative dose of 200–300 mg per adult is not exceeded, the duration of effect usually is still short. Higher doses may cause a long-lasting neuromuscular block because an active metabolite of suxamethonium accumulates when high doses are given. For most laparotomies, however, you never need excessive doses. If anaesthesia is sufficiently deep, the patient will not need high doses of any muscle relaxant. *Remember that even propofol boluses and diazepam have some relaxant effect which can safely be used to avoid too high doses of MR.*

Suxamethonium is metabolised rapidly by the enzyme cholinesterase in the plasma (blood). Some patients have a genetic disorder leading to atypical cholinesterase (cholinesterase deficiency). In these individuals, the effect of suxamethonium can be prolonged to 30 min, seldom even to 2 h, and longer. Very rare, but not impossible, the effect can last for 24 h. The condition is not dangerous if recognised. The patient must not be extubated and must be ventilated until the muscle strength has fully recovered. In a hospital where no mechanical ventilator is available (not even within the anaesthesia machine), the patient must be ventilated manually, e.g. with self-inflating bellows. Often, room air is sufficient, or a small amount of oxygen (1–2 l/min) may be added to keep SpO_2 >94%. The patient should be sedated, e.g. with diazepam, and given analgesics if he is likely to suffer from pain. Talk to the patient and assure him/her to recover and not to be afraid.

Suxamethonium is in many respects the best suitable MR in resource-limited settings, but contraindications must be considered, and the AP should be prepared to handle sudden, life-threatening adverse effects although they are very rare (not more than one in a lifetime).

The first one is anaphylactic shock which can happen to any patient. Bronchospasm is not always obvious after anaesthesia induction, and the only symptom of anaphylaxis may be a non-recordable blood pressure, in severe cases followed by cardiac arrest. CPR and immediate injection of adrenaline are often successful. The AP must take non-recordable BP very seriously and should never assume that it is just a technical problem of the BP cuff. Instead, feel the pulse: if it is strong and regular, it is really a technical problem. If no or weak pulse, give adrenaline, ventilate with 100% oxygen, and assume anaphylaxis.

The second one is the excessive release of potassium from muscle cells causing cardiac arrest which is usually not reversible by CPR. Patients > 24 h after burns or massive trauma involving muscle tissue or spinal cord injury are susceptible to that effect, and suxamethonium is strictly contraindicated for these patients for several months after the initial injury. Patients with any neuromuscular disease, with paralysis, or who are bedridden for more than a few days are also at risk and must not receive suxamethonium.

The third one is sudden masseter muscle rigor (increase in the tension of the jaw muscle) when complete mouth opening and laryngoscopy remain impossible and are not responding to pancuronium (give propofol and try LM insertion instead). Masseter muscle rigidity can be an early sign of MH, but it may also occur independently of MH. Inhalational anaesthetics should be avoided if masseter muscle rigidity occurs as differential diagnosis cannot be made to exclude MH. Differential diagnosis is even dysfunction of the temporomandibular joint which could have been obvious at the time of preoperative assessment.

The fourth potentially deadly complication that may be caused by suxamethonium is malignant hyperthermia (see Sect. 15.7).

After successful resuscitation, the patient must get oral and written information and explanation about what happened to avoid such adverse reactions during future anaesthetics.

Pancuronium is the longest-lasting muscle relaxant drug. The effect of a single dose of 0.05 mg/kg or one ampoule that is 4 mg in average adults is lasting around 60 min. However, the effect can be prolonged unpredictably by high age and by decreased renal function or low urine output. During major surgery and postoperatively, decreased renal function is quite common, although often not clinically identified and only temporary. In patients with ileus or other causes of acute abdominal problems leading to emergency operation, the likelihood of acute renal injury is high. Therefore, the use of pancuronium should be restricted to the situation with good postoperative observation of the patients and the possibility of ventilating (delayed extubation) after surgery. Patients who need to be transferred to the surgical ward with no availability of high dependency or intensive care should rather be given only suxamethonium. Atracurium is a safer long-lasting MR because it is eliminated from the body independent of renal and liver function. Rocuronium is also slightly safer than pancuronium but not available in all countries. A small residual effect of long-acting MR but NOT of suxamethonium can be reversed with a combination of atropine 0.5 mg and neostigmine 2.5 mg IV. Even after successful reversal with neostigmine, muscle paralysis may recur after 30–60 min. Patients who received pancuronium should be continuously monitored and observed with a skilled person present at the bedside for more than 1 h in the recovery unit or another suitable place. Patients who are weak after major surgery, especially after abdominal surgery, are prone to hypoxia, developing atelectasis, silent aspiration of secretions, and developing pneumonia.

15.10 Tetanus

Prevention Immunisation of pregnant women prevents neonatal tetanus. Vaccination every 10 years would prevent almost all cases. After five total doses, even a booster every 30 years would prevent severe tetanus infections. Give Tetanol® vaccine to all patients with no confirmed vaccination state and after a trauma with a wound contaminated by soil. Patients with burns or wounds with devitalized tissue also need vaccination. In patients with previous immunisation a couple of years ago, the infection would cause only mild or no symptoms.

Symptoms After an incubation period of 7–10 days post-trauma (sometimes a very small injury that the patient would not even remember), the onset of symptoms is usually mild. Within 1–7 days post-onset of some muscle rigidity, e.g. difficulty opening mouth and chewing, patients develop painful spasms, localised, or generalised. The severity of the disease can vary between four grades from mild to life-threatening and may last several weeks.

Complications Complications include the inability to feed, laryngospasm, spasms of chest muscles with respiratory insufficiency, hypoxia, pneumonia, fractures caused by severe spasms, severe attacks of hypertension and hypotension, and tachycardia, arrhythmia, and cardiac arrest. Severe cases have high mortality.

Management Wound debridement. If available, a single human tetanus immunoglobulin dose is given. Immunisation with tetanus vaccine "tetanus toxoid" or "TT" is given before discharge. Treatment depends on the severity of tetanus. Nurse the patient in a high dependency unit if available but in a quiet place, preferably in a single room with door to protect the patient from noise and any disturbance. Observe vital signs every hour. Nursing care: the patient may need regular gentle suction of the throat, turning the patient to either side to avoid bedsores and pressure ulcers. Nutrition with high-calorie intake is advised, in patients with difficulty swallowing via NGT. Venous access and infusion with, e.g. diazepam 10–20 mg and tramadol 200 mg every 8 h; mild cases can take the medicine orally instead of infusion. Promethazine 25 mg TDS may prevent nausea and add to sedation. For severe cases, additionally magnesium infusion intermittently with 1–2 g. Laryngospasm can be treated, e.g. with IV injection of 50 mg chlorpromazine. Magnesium infusion is also helpful and decreases muscle tone and spasms. The loading dose is 40 mg/kg over 30 min followed by maintenance infusion of 1.5 g/h for patients <45 kg, 2 g/h for 45–60 kg, and 3 g/h for patients >60 kg BW until control over spasms is achieved. Mg may be repeated during the course of the disease. Very severe cases need intubation or tracheostomy, sedation, and muscle relaxation with regular doses of pancuronium 2–4 mg/h. Metronidazole 500 mg TDS is given as first-line antibiotic therapy.

Further Reading

Barley M (2019) Management of critical incidents. In: Thompson J, Moppett I, Wiles M (eds) Smith and Aitkenhead's textbook of anaesthesia, 7th edn. Elsevier, London, pp 572–600

Mai NTH, Warrell M, Newton C, Lockwood D (2021) Neurology. In: Davidson R, Brent A, Seale A,

Blumberg L (eds) Oxford handbook of tropical medicine, 5th edn. Oxford University Press, Oxford, pp 383–443
Meistelman C, McLoughlin C (1993) Suxamethonium—current controversies. Curr Anaesth Crit Care 4:53–58
Monsieurs KG et al (2015) European resuscitation council guidelines for resuscitation 2015 section 1. Exec Summary Resusc 95:1–80
Moos DD. Basic guide to anesthesia for developing countries. Volume 1 of 2. Copyright free anesthesia manual. Free download via http://medbox.org
Nolan J (2019) Resuscitation. In: Thompson J, Moppett I, Wiles M (eds) Smith and Aitkenhead's textbook of anaesthesia, 7th edn. Elsevier, London, pp 601–616
Onyeka TCU (2010) Masseter muscle rigidity: atypical malignant hyperthermia presentation or isolated event? Saudi J Anaesth 4(3):205–206
Singer M, Webb AR (2009) Oxford handbook of critical care. Oxford University Press, Oxford
Soar J et al (2015) European resuscitation council guidelines for resuscitation 2015 section 3. Adult advanced life support. Resuscitation 95:100–147
Thim T, Vinther Krarup NH, Grove LE, Rohde CW, Lofgren B (2012) Initial assessment and treatment with the airway, breathing, circulation, disability, exposure (ABCDE) approach. Int J Gen Med 5:117–121

16 Case Scenarios

Abstract

To make anaesthesia safer, regular group discussions and practical training with simulated cases are highly recommended. Anaesthesia providers should meet from time to time with their colleagues from neighbouring hospitals exchanging ideas and sharing experiences with challenging patient cases. Case scenarios with potentially hazardous situations or deterioration of patient's vital signs are a good measure for discussing causes, treatment, and prevention of anaesthesia complications. This chapter provides 16 short, typical scenarios from anaesthesia everyday life, points of discussion, and suggestions on how to manage the presented problems.

Keyword

Case scenarios for anaesthesia training in limited resource settings

16.1 Case Scenarios for Discussion in Groups

16.1.1 Case 1

A 12-year-old child is scheduled for elective anaesthesia for foot surgery. The patient is ASA 1. Anaesthesia is induced with thiopentone followed by halothane in oxygen and nitrous oxide via a face mask. During the induction, the patient starts to cough and gets laryngospasm. The SpO2, which started at 98%, falls to 88% during coughing and then to 74% when laryngospasm occurs. Discuss why the saturation has fallen and what would be the most appropriate actions.

16.1.2 Case 2

A 56-year-old obese patient is undergoing emergency laparotomy for bowel obstruction.

Preoperatively he is reasonably fit and his SpO2 is 95%. After rapid sequence induction and intubation, the patient is ventilated and anaesthesia is maintained using isoflurane with 30% oxygen. Over the next 10 min, the patient's SpO2 falls to 85%. What are the most likely causes and what action would you take?

16.1.3 Case 3

During a Caesarean section under spinal anaesthesia, a fit 23-year-old primigravida complains of tingling in the fingers and difficulty breathing. The SpO2 falls from 97% to 88%. What are the most likely causes and what action would you take?

Adopted from material with courtesy of the global non-profit Lifebox foundation

D. Kietzmann, *Anaesthesia in Remote Hospitals*, Sustainable Development Goals Series,
https://doi.org/10.1007/978-3-031-46610-6_16

16.1.4 Case 4

A 7-year-old boy is undergoing an open reduction of a fractured radius and ulna.

Anaesthesia is induced with propofol, fentanyl, and suxamethonium. After intubation, you are unable to ventilate the patient. His saturation starts to fall. What is your management?

16.1.5 Case 5

Your colleague asks you to take over an anaesthetic for him as he has to get away to a family event. The patient is a 19-year-old man who suffered major burns 2 weeks ago in a house fire. The patient is breathing spontaneously via a laryngeal mask airway (LMA). The mixture is oxygen and sevoflurane. The surgery—debridement and skin transplantation—has been going on for over an hour. There is an IV of NS in the right arm which also has a BP cuff and a pulse oximeter in place. The left arm, both legs, and part of the left abdomen are involved in the burn debridement. Things continue for another hour, and you notice the pulse rate going up to 110/min and the BP dropping to 80–90 systolic. The pulse oximeter seems to only work intermittently. When it does read, the saturation seems to be steadily decreasing. Your colleague documented the SpO_2 at the start as 97%. It is now reading 92%. What issues are you thinking about as this case proceeds?

16.1.6 Case 6

In the Recovery Room, following a laparotomy under relaxant anaesthesia, a 43-year-old patient is reported to have a SpO2 of 77% and is making twitching, jerky movements. What are the most likely causes and what action would you take?

16.1.7 Case 7

A 2-year-old child is booked for general anaesthesia for an emergency laparotomy. She has been unwell for 5 days and required large amounts of fluid for resuscitation. Just before induction, her pulse rate is 130 and SpO2 is 95% on high-flow oxygen. Anaesthesia is induced with thiopentone and suxamethonium. Just after intubation, her saturation drops to 80%. What is your management?

16.1.8 Case 8

You are giving an anaesthetic for abdominal hysterectomy in a 45-year-old woman. The surgeon asks you to perform general anaesthesia, not spinal due to expected difficulties and duration of surgery.

Preoperatively you notice that she has prominent upper incisors. You induce anaesthesia with fentanyl, propofol, and suxamethonium and then oxygenate the patient via a face mask. When relaxed, you proceed to intubate the patient. With laryngoscopy, all you can see is the tip of the epiglottis. You try to intubate but are unable to. You can hear the pitch of the pulse oximeter getting lower. You look and it is reading 90%. You ventilate the patient via a face mask and get the saturation up to 96%. You try to intubate again using a different blade and with a stylet in the tube. You are unsuccessful. You call a colleague who tries a blind nasal intubation and causes a nosebleed. By now, the oxygen saturation is 80%. It is becoming increasingly difficult to ventilate the patient. What is your management?

16.2 Points for Discussion and Results of the Case Scenarios

16.2.1 Case 1

A 12-year-old child is scheduled for elective anaesthesia for foot surgery. The patient is ASA 1. Anaesthesia is induced with thiopentone followed by halothane in air and oxygen via a face mask. During the induction, the patient starts to cough and gets laryngospasm. The SpO2, which started at 98%, falls to 88% during coughing and then to 74% when laryngospasm occurs. Discuss why the saturation has fallen and what would be the most appropriate actions.

16.2.1.1 Expected Discussion Points

Give 100% oxygen, and assess ABCDE:

A—Is there airway obstruction due to laryngospasm? Apply positive pressure to the reservoir bag, and deepen anaesthesia. If the situation does not resolve, a small dose of suxamethonium (0.5 mg/kg) should be given.

B—The breathing improves after the resolution of laryngospasm.

C—Assess pulse rate—bradycardia may occur due to hypoxia or secondary to suxamethonium. Consider atropine after treating hypoxia.

D—Check the halothane has not run out. Light anaesthesia can cause laryngospasm.

E—Check that the anaesthesia equipment is functioning and connected appropriately.

After treating the laryngospasm, the patient improves and the SpO2 returns to normal. Surgery can be performed as planned.

16.2.2 Case 2

A 56-year-old obese patient is undergoing emergency laparotomy for bowel obstruction. Preoperatively he is reasonably fit and his SpO2 is 95%. After rapid sequence induction and intubation, the patient is ventilated and anaesthesia is maintained using isoflurane with 30% oxygen. Over the next 10 min, the patient's SpO2 falls to 85%. What are the most likely causes and what action would you take?

16.2.2.1 Expected Discussion Points

Give 100% oxygen, and check ABCDE:

A—Check the airway and position of the tracheal tube. Check there is equal air entry to both sides of the chest and that the tube is not kinked. Check that there is no vomit in the mouth to suggest that the patient may have aspirated.

B—Check that there are no added breath sounds to suggest aspiration, lung collapse, or bronchospasm. Give large tidal volumes by hand and listen to the chest. Is ventilation easy?

C—Assess whether the circulation is normal.

D—Assess whether the patient is fully relaxed. Check that there are no signs to suggest drug reaction (particularly wheeze + hypotension + rash, which are signs of anaphylaxis).

E—Check that the anaesthesia equipment is functioning and connected appropriately.

After ventilating the patient with some large tidal volumes and increasing the inspired oxygen, the patient improved. The problem was lung collapse (atelectasis) due to obesity, supine position, and laparotomy pushing the diaphragm upwards.

16.2.3 Case 3

During a Caesarean section under spinal anaesthesia, a fit 23-year-old primigravida complains of tingling in the fingers and difficulty breathing. The SpO2 falls from 97% to 88%. What are the most likely causes and what action would you take?

16.2.3.1 Expected Discussion Points

Give 100% oxygen. Check ABCDE:

A—Check that the airway is clear

B—Assess breathing. A high spinal may paralyse the muscles of respiration. If breathing is inadequate, ventilate the patient, induce anaesthesia, and intubate after rapid sequence induction with ketamine/suxamethonium. Ventilate until the block wears off.

C—Check the blood pressure—hypotension is likely. Check pulse rate—bradycardia is likely. Treat with left lateral tilt, IV fluids, atropine, and vasopressors (ephedrine, phenylephrine, and adrenaline).

D—Check the height of the block. Look for signs of a very high block—difficulty breathing, whispering rather than talking, weak arms, and numbness on the shoulders. All indicate that the nerves to the diaphragm are becoming blocked. This will make it impossible for the patient to breathe. If the block is not this high, the patient can talk in a normal voice and move their arms normally, but breathing may feel difficult due to the paralysis of the intercostal muscles.

E—Always ensure that equipment is ready in case this complication occurs.

After giving oxygen, the anaesthetist determined that the block was not too high and the patient settled with reassurance, left lateral tilt, and IV fluids. The SpO2 improved with oxygen. Any hypoxia in a pregnant patient is dangerous for the baby.

16.2.4 Case 4

A 7-year-old boy is undergoing an open reduction of a fractured radius and ulna. Anaesthesia is induced with propofol, fentanyl, and suxamethonium. After intubation, you are unable to ventilate the patient. His saturation starts to fall. What is your management?

16.2.4.1 Expected Discussion Points

High-flow oxygen is given.

You are unable to ventilate the patient—this could be a patient problem or an equipment problem.

Replace the patient breathing circuit with a self-inflating bag to exclude possible equipment problems. Do not forget to replace the angle piece as this may be where the obstruction is.

Investigate possible patient problems, including a problem with the tracheal tube—Check the correct tube position with a laryngoscope, and check end-tidal CO_2 if available.

This case emphasises the importance of excluding an obvious equipment problem before assessing the patient using ABCDE.

16.2.5 Case 5

Your colleague asks you to take over an anaesthetic for him as he has to get away to a family event. The patient is a 19-year-old man who suffered major burns 2 weeks ago in a house fire. The patient is breathing spontaneously via an LMA. The mixture is air, oxygen, and sevoflurane. The surgery has been going on for over an hour. There is an IV of NS in the right arm which also has a BP cuff and a pulse oximeter in place. The left arm, both legs, and part of the left abdomen are involved in the burn debridement. Things continue for another hour, and you notice the pulse rate going up to 110/min and the BP dropping to 80–90 systolic. The pulse oximeter seems to only work intermittently. When it does read, the saturation seems to be steadily decreasing. Your colleague documented the SpO_2 at the start as 97%. It is now reading 92%. What issues are you thinking about as this case proceeds?

16.2.5.1 Expected Discussion Points

A—The airway is clear.

B—Respiratory depression from sevoflurane; atelectasis from the long procedure; preexisting lung damage from fire. LMA is not safe for extended surgery → consider intubation and mechanical ventilation.

C—Volume loss due to burns; blood loss due to debridement → check Hb, give more IV fluids, and consider blood transfusion. Body temperature prior to surgery? Infection, sepsis → antibiotics?

D—Consider hypoventilation secondary to opioids. Check end-tidal CO_2 if available. Is soda lime still working? When was it exchanged last time?

E—Use of oximeter on the same limb as BP cuff; hypothermia from wide exposure and debridement and inadequate signal due to shivering. → Try to get the patient warm again (warm infusions, air conditioning off, and blankets).

16.2.6 Case 6

In the Recovery Room, following a laparotomy under relaxant anaesthesia, a 43-year-old patient is reported to have a SpO2 of 77% and is making twitching, jerky movements. What are the most likely causes and what action would you take?

16.2.6.1 Expected Discussion Points

A—Open the airway and give 100% oxygen.

B—If chest expansion is inadequate, assist ventilation with a bag and mask.

C—Check pulse and ensure intravenous access.

D—Give anticholinesterase (neostigmine 2.5 mg plus atropine 0.5–1 mg) as relaxant reversal.

E—Check the position of the pulse oximetry probe.

Inadequate reversal is a common cause of breathing problems and hypoxia in recovery if long-acting muscle relaxants were given.

16.2.7 Case 7

A 2-year-old child is booked for general anaesthesia for an emergency laparotomy. She has been unwell for 5 days and required large amounts of fluid for resuscitation. Just before induction, her pulse rate is 130 and SpO2 is 95% on high-flow oxygen. Anaesthesia is induced with thiopentone and suxamethonium. Just after intubation, her saturation drops to 80%. What is your management?

16.2.7.1 Expected Discussion Points

A—The tracheal tube (TT) is a new size 4.0. It does not seem to be blocked. While preparing to listen to the chest, saturation has fallen to 60%. Capnometry is not available.

B—Her abdomen is swollen and chest expansion is difficult to assess. You are unable to hear breath sounds. Saturation is now 45% and heart rate is 60.

It is not certain that the TT is in the trachea. Participants should be prompted to return to A to check the position of the TT.

A—Repeat laryngoscopy shows the TT is not in the larynx. The SpO2 falls to 30% before the patient is reintubated.

B—Chest expansion is now obvious and the saturation quickly returns to 96%.

This scenario highlights the importance of correcting a problem before moving to the next step of the algorithm.

16.2.8 Case 8

You are giving an anaesthetic for abdominal hysterectomy in a 45-year-old woman. The surgeon asks you to perform general anaesthesia, not spinal due to expected difficulties and duration of surgery. Preoperatively you notice that she has prominent upper incisors. You induce anaesthesia with fentanyl, propofol, and suxamethonium and then oxygenate the patient via a face mask. When relaxed, you proceed to intubate the patient. With laryngoscopy, all you can see is the tip of the epiglottis. You try to intubate but are unable to. You can hear the pitch of the pulse oximeter getting lower. You look and it is reading 90%. You ventilate the patient via a face mask and get the saturation up to 96%. You try intubating again using a different blade and with a stylet in the tube. You are unsuccessful. You call a colleague who tries a blind nasal intubation and causes a nosebleed. By now, the oxygen saturation is 80%. It is becoming increasingly difficult to ventilate the patient. What is your management?

16.2.8.1 Expected Discussion Points

A—Management of unanticipated difficult intubation. Discuss management of a "can't intubate, can't ventilate" situation.

B—Aspiration? → suction, gastric tube.

C—Severe bradycardia secondary to hypoxia. Treating A + B should treat the bradycardia. Commence CPR if there is a cardiac arrest. However, without successful ventilation, CPR will not help.

D—Should anaesthesia drugs be continued or stopped?

E—What is your backup plan for an unexpected difficult airway? What equipment would you have nearby? Blind nasal intubation is not recommended in that scenario. Instead, an LMA would have been the airway of choice after two to three unsuccessful attempts to intubate. If ventilation via LMA is not possible, consider emergency coniotomy/tracheotomy → call the surgeon for help.

Appendices

1.1 Pre Anaesthesia Visit Form

(Adopted from St. Benedict Ndanda Referral Hospital, Tanzania, with kind permission)

D. Kietzmann, *Anaesthesia in Remote Hospitals*, Sustainable Development Goals Series,
https://doi.org/10.1007/978-3-031-46610-6

Pre Anaesthesia Visit Form

(adopted from St. Benedict Ndanda Referral Hospital, Tanzania, with kind permission)

______________________________________ name of the hospital **Date**_____________

Patient name__________________ **Gender**____ **Hospital registration No.**_______ **Ward**_____

Pre-op diagnosis____________________________ **Planned procedure**____________________

Present history diseases ______________________________
symptoms ______________________________
medication ______________________________

Past history diseases ______________________________
operations / complications ______________________________
anaesthesia / complications ______________________________
drug allergies ______________________________

Family history congenital disorders ______________________________
history of malignant hyperthermia ______________________________

Social history ______________________________
Consumption of alcohol ____________________ **smoking** ____________________

Physical examination body weight ____ height _____ BP _______ pulse rate _______ temp _____
heart __________________ lungs ______________________
abdomen _____________ peripheral oedema _____________
sites for venous access ______________________________
eyes _____________ Mallampati class ___ thyromental distance _________

Dental status upper R 7654321 / 1234567 L 0 missing x mobile
lower R 7654321 / 1234567 L

Laboratory Hb _______ blood group __________ X-matching ______________
b-glucose ______ other lab findings ______________________________

Nutritional status normal ______ slim _______ weight loss _________ obese ______________

pre-op fasting from ________hr food _______ hr water / tea

ASA class _______ premedication ______________________________
Pre-anaesthesia orders ______________________________

Planned anaesthesia technique spinal ___ GA ___ intubation ETT size _____ LM size ______

Patient's consent for anaesthesia ______________________________ date _______

Patient __________________________ signature **Anaesthetist**____________________ signature

1.2 Anaesthesia Record

(Adopted from St. Benedict's Referral Hospital Ndanda, Tanzania, with kind permission)

Anaesthesia Record

(Adopted from St. Benedict Ndanda Referral Hospital, Tanzania, with kind permission)

Date	Patient
Diagnosis	Hospital reg. no.
Operation	Ward
Surgeon	Age / date of birth
Scrubb nurse	BW height
Anaesthesia team	Hb/Hk
	Blood group x-match
	BP pulse
	Temp preop fasting from

Time [hr]			15	30	45		15	30	45		15	30	45	
Oxygen l/min														Pre-op conditions
														- good / fair / poor
Halo / iso / sevo %														- emergency
Diazepam / midazolam														- ASA class
Ketamine / fentanyl														
Thio / propofol														Start of operation
Suxamethonium														
Panc / atracurium														End of operation
Morphine														
Tramadol / pethidine														Mask
Diclofenac / ketorolac														LM
														ETT RSI yes / no
Atropine														-size
Ephedrine														Oral
Adrenaline														Nasal
SpO_2														Ventilation
$ETCO_2$														- Spontaneous / manual
Syst BP v	220													- controlled
Dias BP ∧	210													- TV / frequency
Mean BP -	200													
Pulse •	190													Draw-over
	180													Rebreathing
	170													Non-rebreathing system
	160													
	150													Spinal
	140													- injection time
	130													- needle size
	120													- site of injection
	110													- drug
	100													- amount
	90													- effect A - B – C
	80													
	70													Patient position
	60													- supine
	50													- prone
	40													- lateral / right / left
	30													- lithotomy
Infusions / transfusion urine output temperature														

1.3 Observation Chart for Critical Care Patients

Observation chart for critical care patients

Name of Hospital___________________________

Name______________________Age_____Gender___Hospital registration no.________Date__________chart no.___

Time hours	BP mmHg	Pulse rate /min	SpO_2 %	Resp rate /min	Temp °C	Infusion NS/RL/ other/ml	Oral fluid intake ml	Urine ml	NGT ml	Drainage ml	Oxygen l/min	CPAP cmH_2O	Observations	Comments
6 AM														
7														
8														
9														
10														
11														
12														
1 PM														
2														
3														
4														
5														
6														
7														
8														
9														
10														
11														
12														
1 AM														
2														
3														
4														
5														
Total input / output per 24 h														

Epilogue

1.1 About the Author

After attending the medical school of Cologne, Germany, and completing a doctoral thesis in neuropathology, **Daniela Kietzmann** specialised in anaesthesiology and intensive care medicine at the University Hospital of Göttingen, Germany, until 1991. She conducted research in clinical pharmacology/pharmacokinetics-pharmacodynamics until she qualified as a PhD and became a senior university lecturer in anaesthesiology at the University of Göttingen. She has been an active member of the examination board for the European Diploma in Anaesthesiology and Intensive Care (EDAIC) since 1996. Currently, she holds the position of consultant anaesthesiologist at the Department of Anaesthesia and Intensive Care, Uppsala University Hospital, Uppsala, Sweden.

Since 2001, the author has been visiting hospitals in East Africa, where she has spent several years in total. She works as a regular visiting anaesthesiologist together with local nurse anaesthetists at two referral hospitals in Tanzania for approximately two months every year. Additionally, she visits other remote hospitals in resource-limited locations, mainly in Africa, providing on-job training and support for local anaesthesia providers.

The idea for this handbook emerged when there was a need to develop teaching material that grew over the years. Now, the material has been completed and updated to create an easy-to understand, concise yet comprehensive handbook for non-specialist anaesthesia providers in places with limited equipment and without specialist anaesthesiologists.

D. Kietzmann, *Anaesthesia in Remote Hospitals*, Sustainable Development Goals Series,
https://doi.org/10.1007/978-3-031-46610-6

Index

A
ABCDE approach, 52
  for critical incidents and emergencies, 192
  for trauma patients, 146
Abdominal hysterectomy, 210, 213
Acute abdomen, 140
Acute kidney failure (AKF), 14
Acute kidney injury (AKI), 149
Adrenaline
  epinephrine, 89
  resuscitation children, 179
  shock, 197
Advanced life support (ALS), 198
Advanced trauma life support (ATLS®), 146
Airway management, obese patients, 68
Airway obstruction, infants, 165
Alfentanil, 78
Alveolar ventilation, 4
Aminocaproic Acid, 97–98
Aminophylline, 97
Amoxicillin, 94
Ampicillin, 94
Anaesthesia
  for patients with burns, 153
  abdominal trauma, 148
  for craniotomy, 151
  for emergency laparotomy, 141
  for ORIF, children, 183
  machine, 24, 44
  record form, 46
  respiratory complications, infants, 157
  risk, children, 155
  safety checklist, 50
Analgesia
  balanced anaesthesia, 107
  for children with burns, 185
Anaphylactic shock, 194
  treatment, 197
Anorectal malformations, infants, 181
Antibiotic prophylaxis, 47, 93
Antiemetic drugs, 92–93
Antihypertensive drugs, 91–92
Aortocaval compression, 124
ASA score, 42
Atelectasis, lung, 6
Atracurium, 86
Atropine, 89

B
Baby bubble CPAP, 133
Balanced anaesthesia, 106
Basic life support, 198
Blood transfusion, children, 170
Blunt abdominal trauma, children, 183
Body temperature, 15
  during abdominal surgery, 137
  monitoring, 34
Body weight, height, children, 157
Bowel obstruction, 209, 211
Bronchodilatation, 96
Bronchospasm, 201
Bupivacaine, 88–89
Buprenorphine, 81
Burns, 210, 212
  children, 184
  management of, 152

C
Capillary refill time, CRT, 10
Capnography, 33
  for patients with craniotomy, 152
Carbon dioxide transport in the blood, 9
Cardiac arrest in the OR
  resuscitation, 199
Cardiac output (CO), 10
Cardiogenic shock, 194
Ceftriaxone, 95
Cefuroxime, 95
Chin lift
  manoeuvre, 58
Chlorpromazine, 84
Circulation, systemic, 11
Clindamycin, 94
Clonidine, 84

D. Kietzmann, *Anaesthesia in Remote Hospitals*, Sustainable Development Goals Series,
https://doi.org/10.1007/978-3-031-46610-6

Cloxacillin, 94
CO_2 absorption, 28
Codeine, 80
Complications
during laparoscopy, 64, 143
LMA, 66
Compressed gas anaesthetic machines, 27
Continuous medical education (CME), 1
Contraindications
LMA, 66
spinal anaesthesia, 116
COPD, 43–44
Cormack and Lehane grades, 60
Coronary artery disease, 9
CPAP, 56
Criteria for transfer, patients with burns, 154
Critical incident reporting system, 191

D
Damage control resuscitation (DCR), 147
Dead space, anatomical, 4
Defibrillator, 39
Delayed extubation
after abdominal surgery, 142
criteria, 56
Desflurane, 105
Dexamethasone, 96
Diabetes mellitus, 43–44
Diazepam, 83
Diclofenac, 81
children, 178
Difficult airway algorithm, 68, 69
Difficult intubation, 67
Difficulty breathing, 209, 211, 212
Dilution/drug concentrations/labelling syringes, 179
Discharge criteria, postanaesthesia care, recovery area, 54
Diuretics, 91–92
Dopamine, 90
Doses of LA for spinal anaesthesia, 119
Draw- over vaporiser, 26–27
Draw-over anaesthesia system, 25
Drip rate during anaesthesia, children, 169
Droperidol, 93
Drugs for short GA, 110–112

E
Electricity, 18
Electrocardiogram (ECG), 32–33
Emergence agitation, 54
Emergence from anaesthesia, children, 175
Endotracheal intubation, 62
Endotracheal tubes, 36
ENT operations, anaesthesia management in children, 186
Ephedrine, 90, 130
Epidural haematoma, spinal anaesthesia, 122
Epinephrine, adrenaline, 89
Essential drugs, for anaesthesia management, 45–46
Essential equipment, operating room, 44–45
Ether, 105
Etomidate, 78
Evacuation of epidural or subdural haematoma, paediatric anaesthesia, 183
External jugular vein cannulation, children, 166
Extracellular and the intracellular fluid compartment (ECF and ICF), 13

F
Face masks, 59
Fasting before anaesthesia
children, 159
fasting, 43
Femoral vein cannulation, 167
Fentanyl, 79
paediatric anaesthesia, 173
Flucloxacillin, 94
Foetal circulation, 158
Foot surgery, 209–211
Fresh frozen plasma (FFP), 98
Front of neck access (FONA), surgical airway, 69
Functional residual capacity FRC, 5
Furosemide, 91

G
General anaesthesia, 210
during pregnancy, 125
Gentamicine, 94
Glasgow Coma Scale (GCS), 193–194
Glyceryl trinitrate, 91
Goal-directed IV fluid therapy, 136
Gum elastic bougie (Eschmann stylet), 68

H
Haematoma, spinal, 122
Haemorrhagic shock, 195
Halothane, 102
paediatric anaesthesia, 174
Hand hygiene, 47
Head tilt manoeuvre, 58
Heart, physiology, 9
HELLP syndrome, 127
Hernia repair, paediatric anaesthesia, 181
High spinal, spinal anaesthesia, 121
High-dependency care, 55
Hospital pharmacy, 75
Hydralazine, 91, 128
Hydrocortisone, 95
Hypertension, 43–44
Hypovolaemic shock, 194

I

Ibuprofen, 82
  children, 178
Indications
  LMA, 66
  anaesthesia IV in children, 170
Infection, spinal anaesthesia, 122
Infrastructure, for hospitals, 17
Inhalational induction, 171
Initial survey, ABCDE, children with burns, 184
Insulin, 96
intermittent positive pressure (IPPV), 5
Intraoperative analgesia, 140
Intraosseous cannulation, 167
Intubation
  complications of, 64
  endotracheal, 60
  without muscle relaxant, children, 172
  without neuromuscular blocking agent, 138
Intussusception, paediatric acute abdomen, 181
Isobaric, local anaesthetics for spinal, 118
Isoflurane, 103
  paediatric anaesthesia, 174

K

Ketamine, 76
  anaesthesia, for caesarean section, 126
  doses paediatric anaesthesia, 180
  for maintenance in children, 106, 173
  for short GA, 110
  TIVA, 106
Ketorolac, 82
Kidney failure, 14

L

Labetalol, 92
Laparoscopy, 142
Laparotomy, 210, 212, 213
Laryngeal mask airway (LMA), 36, 65
  size for children, 66, 163
Laryngoscopy, 36
  children, 163
  infants, 161
Laryngospasm, 200, 210, 211
  children, 165
Lidocaine, 88
Local anaesthetics, hyperbaric, for spinal, 118
Lorazepam, 83
Low- and middle-income countries (LMIC), 1

M

Magnesium sulphate, 128
Maintenance of anaesthesia, general anaesthesia, 101
Malignant hyperthermia (MH), 203
Mallampati classification, 60
Mannitol, 92
Manual ventilation, 6
Mapleson F breathing system, 30
Mechanical ventilator, 24
Meperidine, 79
  pethidine, 177
Metamizole, 82
Metoclopramide, 93
Metronidazole, 95
Midazolam, 83
Miller blade, intubation of infants, 161
Minimal alveolar concentration (MAC), 101
Minimal equipment for safe anaesthesia, 39–40
Minimally invasive surgery (MIS), 142
Minor surgery, 110
Minute ventilation (MV), 6
Morphine, 78
  children, 178
Multi-modal analgesia, 54
Muscle relaxants
  children, 175
  neuromuscular blocking agents, 84, 107

N

Naloxone, 80
Nasopharyngeal airway, 59
Neonatal resuscitation, 131–133
Neostigmine, 87
Neuromuscular blocking agents (NMBAs)
  anaphylactic reactions, 205
  muscle relaxants, 84
NIBP monitor (non-invasive blood pressure monitor), 32
Nifedipine, 92
Nitroglycerin, 91
Nitrous oxide (N_2O), 104
  paediatric anaesthesia, 173
Noradrenaline, 90

O

Observation list, vital signs, 52
Obstructive sleep apnoea (OSA), children for adenotomy, 186
Ondansetrone, 93
Open reduction and internal fixation (ORIF), 149
Opioid analgesics, 78
Oropharyngeal airway, 58
Oxygen analysers, 23, 34
Oxygen concentrators, 19, 22
Oxygen cylinders, 21
Oxygen supply, types of, 19
Oxygen transport in the blood, 7–9
Oxygen-haemoglobin dissociation curve, 7
Oxytocin, 96, 126

P
Pancuronium, 86, 107, 206
Paracetamol, 82
  children, 178
Pathophysiology, compensation mechanisms, 194
PEEP, 56
Pentazocine, 81
Pethidine, 79
  children, 177
  spinal anaesthesia, 119–120
Phenylephrine, 90
Piped gas supply, 21
Plenum vaporisers
  vaporiser, 29
Pneumothorax, 201
Post Dural Puncture Headache, 120–121
Post-anaesthesia care unit (PACU), 51
Post-dural-puncture headache, 127
Post-extubation croup, children, 165
Postoperative analgesia, 54
  children, 176
Postoperative care, acute abdominal trauma patients, 148
Postpartum bleeding, 129
Preeclampsia, 127
Premature infants, anaesthesia risk, 156
Premedication, children, 160
Preoperative evaluation, 41
  children, 158
Preoperative examination, 136
Preoxygenation, 61
Primary brain injury, 149
Primary survey, trauma management, 146
Promethazine, 84, 93
Propofol, 77
Pulmonary and systemic blood circulation, 10
Pulmonary aspiration, during anaesthesia, 201–202
Pulse oximeter, 31
  paediatric anaesthesia, 161
Pyloric stenosis, infants, 182
Pyridostigmine, 87

R
Radius and ulna fracture, 210, 212
Ramped position, airway management, 68
Rapid sequence induction (RSI), 70
  children, 164
Rebreathing circuit, 28
Remifentanil, 78
Residual paralysis, after muscle relaxants (NMBA), 205
Respiratory insufficiency, post-operatively, 56
Respiratory problems, after abdominal surgery, 139
Respiratory rate, heart rate, and blood pressure, children, 157
Rocuronium, 86

S
Saddle block, spinal anaesthesia, 118
Salbutamol, 96–97
Secondary brain injury, prevention of, 150
Septic shock, 194
Sevoflurane, 104
  paediatric anaesthesia, 174
Shock, pathophysiology, compensation, 194
Short GA
  children with burns, 185
  doses for, 112
  ketamine, 110
  patients with diabetes, 112
  patients with hypertension, 112
  patients with kidney disease, 112
  patients with respiratory disease, 112
  without available anaesthesia staff, 111
Skin transplantation, 210, 212
Soda lime, 28–29, 38
  CO_2 absorption, 38
Spinal anaesthesia, 115
  caesarian section, 124
  for abdominal surgery, 137
  indications, 116
Spine injury, 149
Spontaneous breathing during anaesthesia, children, 161
Storage of drugs, 74
Succinylcholine, 205
Suction machine, 38
Sufentanil, 78
Sugammadex, 87
Supine hypotension syndrome, 124
Supraglottic airway device, 65
Surgical airway, 69
Surgical checklist, 50
Suxamethonium, 85, 205
Suxamethonium (succinylcholine), doses paediatric anaesthesia, 180
Systemic vascular resistance, 11

T
Temperature control, during anaesthesia, 15
Temperature regulation, 34
Tetanus, 207
Thiopentone, 76
  paediatric anaesthesia, 179
Thyromental distance, 60
Titrating a drug to effect, 75
TIVA, 106
TOF monitors, nerve stimulator, 37
Tonsillectomy, 186–187
Total intravenous anaesthesia (TIVA), 1, 106
  children, 173
Total spinal anaesthesia, 121

T-piece system for children, 30
Tramadol, 80
  children, 177
Tranexamic acid (TXA), 97, 129
Transfusion reactions management, 202

V
Vaporisers draw-over, 26
Variability in drug response, 107
Vasopressor drugs, 197
Vecuronium, 86
Venous cannulation, children, 166
Venous return, 12
Ventilation in children, anaesthesia, 163
Volatile anaesthetics, 100

W
World Federation of Societies of Anaesthesiologists (WFSA), 1, 2
Wound infection, prevention, 47–48
Wound infiltration with local anaesthetic, 177–178

GPSR Compliance

The European Union's (EU) General Product Safety Regulation (GPSR) is a set of rules that requires consumer products to be safe and our obligations to ensure this.

If you have any concerns about our products, you can contact us on ProductSafety@springernature.com

In case Publisher is established outside the EU, the EU authorized representative is:

Springer Nature Customer Service Center GmbH
Europaplatz 3
69115 Heidelberg, Germany

Batch number: 10371059

Printed by Printforce, the Netherlands